ATLAS OF
Clinical Gynecology

ATLAS OF

Clinical Gynecology

SERIES EDITOR

Morton A. Stenchever, MD

Professor, Chairman Emeritus
Department of Obstetrics and Gynecology
University of Washington Medical Center
Seattle, Washington

Volume II

Gynecologic Pathology

VOLUME EDITOR

Barbara Goff, MD

Associate Professor
Department of Obstetrics and Gynecology
University of Washington School of Medicine
Seattle, Washington

With 20 contributors

APPLETON & LANGE

Developed by Current Medicine, Inc.
Philadelphia

Current Medicine, Inc.
400 Market Street
Suite 700
Philadelphia, PA 19106

Director, Product Development	*Lori J. Bainbridge*
Development Editor	*Susan L. Hunsberger*
Editorial Assistant	*Charlene A. French*
Art Director	*Paul Fennessy*
Design and Layout	*Robert LeBrun*
Illustration Director	*Ann Saydlowski*
Illustrators	*Elizabeth Carrozza, Beth Starkey, Ann Saydlowski*
Production Manager	*Lori Holland*
Production Associate	*Amy Watts*
Index	*Alexandra Nickerson*

Library of Congress Cataloging-in-Publication Data
ISBN 0-8385-0317-9

Gynecologic pathology / Barbara Goff and Morton Stenchever, volume editors.
p. cm.—(Atlas of clinical gynecology ; v. 2)
Includes bibliographical references and index.
ISBN 0-8385-0317-9 (alk. paper)
1. Gynecologic pathology—Atlases. I. Goff, Barbara.
II. Stenchever, Morton A. III. Series.
[DNLM: 1. Genital Diseases, Female—pathology—atlases. WP 17
A8806 1997 v. 2]
RG79.A88 1997 vol. 2
[RG77]
618.1'0022'2 s—dc21
[618, 1'07]
DNLM/DLC
for Library of Congress 97-42377
CIP

Although every effort has been made to ensure that drug doses and other information are presented accurately in this publication, the ultimate responsibility rests with the prescribing physician. Neither the publishers nor the authors can be held responsible for errors or for any consequences arising from the use of information contained herein. Products mentioned in this publication should be used in accordance with the prescribing information prepared by the manufacturers. No claims or endorsements are made for any drug or compound at present under clinical investigation.

Printed in Singapore by Imago Productions (FE) Pte Ltd.

10 9 8 7 6 5 4 3 2 1

Series Preface

The *Atlas of Clinical Gynecology* is an ambitious 5-volume series covering the field of gynecology. Volume topics include pediatric and adolescent gynecology, oncology, pathology, reproductive endocrinology, urogynecology, and reparative surgery. Each volume contains more than 500 images. The images in this collection include not only traditional photographs, but also charts, tables, algorithms, and diagrams, making this collection much more than an atlas in the conventional sense.

The atlas series serves as an excellent teaching tool and resource. In the past few decades, individual learning styles have changed dramatically. In the past, the printed work in book and journal was the primary way in which information was transferred and learning accomplished. In recent decades, however, education has been greatly enhanced by the addition of audio and visual technology. More recently, the advent of personal computers has further enriched the types of learning modalities available.

The *Atlas of Clinical Gynecology* series is designed to use the printed word and visual modalities. The information can be used by individual students and by those who teach physicians, medical students, and other health care professionals. The atlas may also serve as a valuable patient education tool.

The series is comprehensive and includes topics that may be neglected in the literature or absent from some training programs. Often practitioners do not see enough patients with a given condition to develop expertise in diagnosis and management. The series is designed to expose the clinician to the unfamiliar as well as to update information on more common gynecologic problems.

I wish to thank the volume editors for their expertise and dedication—Alvin Goldfarb, Barbara Goff, Daniel Mishell, Benjamin Greer, and J. Thomas Benson. We hope that physicians, health care professionals, and the educators who train them find the quality and format of this series useful in the diagnosis and treatment of women of all ages. They deserve the best care available.

Morton A. Stenchever, MD

Volume Preface

Understanding gynecologic pathology is essential for all practicing obstetricians and gynecologists. Although there have been many advances in the fields of obstetrics and gynecology, histopathology remains the diagnostic gold standard. Without an accurate pathologic diagnosis, clinicians would have significant difficulty managing many gynecologic conditions. Understanding the histopathology is also a prerequisite for effectively counseling patients about their diseases.

Communication between the gynecologist and the pathologist is extremely important, yet often overlooked. Clinicians must provide accurate and detailed clinical information about the patient to assist pathologists in making a correct diagnosis. In addition, it is important for pathologists to discuss their findings with clinicians. Pathologic diagnoses are not always "black and white;" clinicians should frequently review their cases with pathologists. Sometimes the correct clinical management can be determined only after the clinician sits down with the pathologist to look at the histology slides.

This atlas is written for general obstetrician-gynecologists, subspecialists, pathologists, and for residents training in these fields. This is a multi-author book with contributions from both clinicians and pathologists; each of the contributors is an expert in the field that he or she describes. The authors have provided excellent examples of both the common and rare pathologic conditions of the reproductive tract, with a good balance of gross and microscopic photographs.

I would like to thank the contributors to this volume for creating an atlas which can be used by both pathologists and clinicians. I would also like to thank the series editor, Morton A. Stenchever, MD, for his help with this volume, and the staff of Current Medicine, Susan Hunsberger, and Charlene French for their support.

Barbara Goff, MD

Contributors

Jo Ann Benda, MD
Professor
Department of Pathology and Obstetrics and Gynecology
University of Iowa
University of Iowa Hospitals and Clinics
Iowa City, Iowa

Dale Brown, Jr, MD
Clinical Professor
Department of Obstetrics and Gynecology
Baylor College of Medicine
Houston, Texas

Rochelle L. Garcia, MD
Acting Instructor
Department of Pathology
University of Washington
Seattle Veteran's Administration Hospital
Seattle, Washington

Barbara Goff, MD
Associate Professor
Department of Obstetrics and Gynecology
University of Washington School of Medicine
Seattle, Washington

Melissa D. Gordon, MD
Assistant Professor
Department of Pathology
Oregon Health Sciences University
Portland, Oregon

Allen M. Gown, MD
Director
PhenoPath Laboratories
Seattle, Washington

Douglas A. Hansen, MD
Fellow
Department of Pathology
University of Washington
Seattle, Washington

Michael R. Hendrickson, MD
Professor
Department of Pathology
Stanford University Medical School
Stanford Medical Center
Palo Alto, California

Karen Ireland, MD
Professor
Departments of Pathology and Gynecology
and Obstetrics
Oregon Health Sciences University
Portland, Oregon

Raymond H. Kaufman, MD
Professor
Department of Obstetrics and Gynecology
Baylor College of Medicine
Houston, Texas

Nancy B. Kiviat, MD
Professor
Department of Pathology and Medicine
Director of Cytology
University of Washington
Seattle, Washington

Teri A. Longacre, MD
Professor
Department of Surgical Pathology
Stanford University Medical School
Stanford Medical Center
Palo Alto, California

Melinda Mann, MD
Assistant Attending
Department of Obstetrics and Gynecology
Maimonides Medical Center
New York City, New York

Howard G. Muntz, MD
Clinical Assistant Professor
Department of Obstetrics and Gynecology
University of Washington;
Gynecologic Oncology
Virginia Mason Medical Center
Seattle, Washington

Richard Reid, MD
Consultant Gynaecologist
Department of Obstetrics and Gynaecology
Liverpool Hospital
University of New South Wales
Sydney, Australia

Mark Spitzer, MD
Associate Professor
Department of Obstetrics, Gynecology, and Reproductive Science
Mount Sinai School of Medicine
New York City, New York;
Director of Obstetrics and Gynecology
Queens Hospital Center
Jamaica, New York

Hisham K. Tamimi, MD
Professor
Department of Obstetrics and Gynecology
University of Washington School of Medicine
Seattle, Washington

Cornelia Liu Trimble, MD
Assistant Professor
Department of Obstetrics and Gynecology
Johns Hopkins University School of Medicine
Baltimore, Maryland

Nan Ping Wang, MD, PhD
Washington Pathology Consultants, Inc., P.S.
Seattle, Washington

Richard J. Zaino, MD
Professor
Department of Pathology
Penn State University College of Medicine
Chief, Anatomic Pathology
Milton S. Hershey Medical Center
Penn State Geisinger Health System
Hershey, Pennsylvania

Contents

CHAPTER 5

Endometrium

Richard J. Zaino

CHAPTER 6

Mesenchymal Tumors

Teri A. Longacre and Michael R. Hendrickson

CHAPTER 7

Fallopian Tube

Howard G. Muntz

CHAPTER 8

Epithelial Tumors of the Ovary

Melissa D. Gordon and Karen Ireland

CHAPTER 9

Germ Cell Tumors of the Ovary

Cornelia Liu Trimble and Barbara Goff

CHAPTER 10

Placental Tumors

Hisham K. Tamimi

CHAPTER 11

Cytology

Rochelle L. Garcia and Nancy B. Kiviat

CHAPTER 12

Immunocytochemistry

Allen M. Gown, Nan Ping Wang, and Douglas A. Hansen

Human Papillomavirus–Associated Diseases

CHAPTER 1

Richard Reid

Papillomaviruses are small (55-nm) DNA tumor viruses, comprising an 8-kb genome encapsulated by an outer shell of capsid protein. Many subdivisions have been defined within the *Papillomavirus* genus, with different mammalian species serving as hosts for a specific subgroup. There are more than 70 types of human papillomavirus (HPV), which can be grouped clinically according to site, proclivity, and host immunologic status. Subdivisions include *cutaneotropic in healthy hosts* (common and plantar warts), *cutaneotropic in immunosuppressed hosts* (*eg*, flat warts in epidermodysplasia verruciformis), and *mucosotropic in healths hosts* (*eg*, condyloma acuminatum and anogenital neoplasia).

All members of the genus induce benign papillomas; some members ("high-risk" group) also encode oncoproteins that disturb cell cycle control, thereby leading to genetic instability in persistently infected cells. This enhances the risk of mutations within the cellular genome, and may thus trigger or promote tumor formation. More than 95% of cervical carcinoma specimens contain HPV genetic fragments. Furthermore, HPV DNA causes neoplastic transformation in cell cultures, altering growth properties in ways that resemble carcinoma cells.

Three international consensus conferences have evaluated the relationship of HPV to cervical cancer. The World Health Organization organized coneferences in 1991 and 1995, through the International Agency for Research on Cancer (IARC). In 1996, a third conference was sponsored by the U.S. National Institutes of Health. The key conclusion from these three meetings was that epidemiologic and molecular virologic evidence has established the causal relationship between high-risk HPV types and anogenital carcinoma. As a result, there have been many calls to examine the utility of screening for HPV, and to develop prophylactic or therapeutic vaccines to help reduce the massive toll of HPV infection: over 500,000 lower tract cancers per year worldwide and billions of dollars in medical expenses.

BASIC BIOLOGY OF HUMAN PAPILLOMAVIRUS

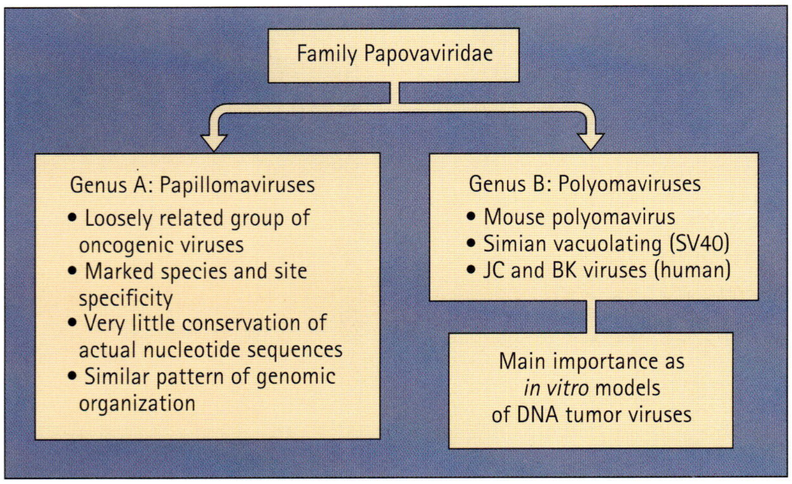

FIGURE 1-1.
Taxonomy of the family Papovaviridae. Papilloma viruses are small, double-stranded DNA viruses, classified in the same family as polyomaviruses because of superficial similarities in electron microscopic appearance and biologic properties. However, molecular hybridization studies have shown that the two groups are evolutionarily different. The polyomaviruses served as important laboratory models of a DNA tumor virus but have little role in human disease. Conversely, papillomaviruses cause important diseases in many species, especially humans. All of these viruses alter cell growth and tissue maturation. Although the overall pattern of genomic organization is similar throughout the genus, there is little conservation in actual nucleotide sequence from one virus to another; hence, papillomavirus infections show profound species and site selectivity.

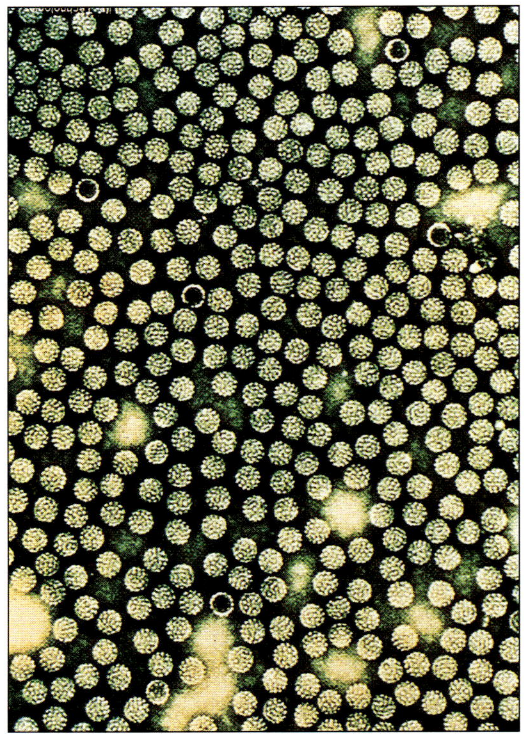

FIGURE 1-2.
Electron micrograph of papillomavirus virions. Each virion is a 55-nm, icosahedral (20-sided) particle composed of a circular, double-stranded, covalently closed DNA molecule, surrounded by a protein capsid. The absence of an outer membrane, such as is found in other viruses, may account for the low antigenicity of papillomavirus infections.

CLINICAL EXPRESSION OF HUMAN PAPILLOMAVIRUS INFECTION

CLINICAL GROUPINGS OF HPV-ASSOCIATED DISEASES

Cutaneotropic—healthy host
- Verrucae (common wart) on nongenital skin
- Plantar warts on nongenital skin

Cutaneotropic—immunodeficient host
- Epidermodysplasia verruciformis
- Skin cancers in transplant recipients

Mucosotropic group
- Anogenital warts, dysplasias, and cancers
- Aerodigestive papillomas and neoplasias

FIGURE 1-3.
Clinical groupings of disease associated with the 70 known types of human papillomaviruses (HPVs). The various HPV types can be divided into three main clinical groupings. First, HPVs 1, 2, 3, 4, and 7 and variously associated with plantar or common warts on nongenital skin of healthy individuals. Viruses in this group produce benign warts that are never carcinogenic. Second, about 30 of the known HPV types were isolated from the skin of immunosuppressed individuals. A quarter to one third of these individuals develop skin cancers, usually in sunlight-exposed areas. The two main types associated with oncogenicity are HPVs 5 and 8. Finally, about 35 known HPV types are mucosotropic, affecting either anogenital skin or mucous membranes.

DISEASE ASSOCIATIONS OF DIFFERENT HPV TYPES

	HPV types	
Disease	**Frequent association**	**Less-frequent association**
Plantar warts	1, 2	4, 63
Common warts	2, 1	4, 26, 27, 29, 41, 57, 65
Common warts of meat, poultry, and fish handlers	7, 2	1, 3, 4, 10, 28
Flat warts	3, 10	27, 38, 41, 49
Intermediate warts	10	26, 28
Epidermodysplasia verruciformis	2, 3, 10, 5, 8, 9, 12, 14, 15, 17	19, 20, 21, 22, 23, 24, 25, 36, 37, 38, 47, 50
Condylomata acuminata	6, 11	30, 42, 43, 44, 45, 51, 54, 55, 70
Intraepithelial neoplasia		
Unspecified		30, 34, 39, 40, 53, 57, 59, 61, 62, 64, 66, 67, 68, 69
Low-grade	6, 11	16, 18, 31, 33, 35, 42, 43, 44, 45, 51, 52
High-grade	16, 18	6, 11, 31, 33, 35, 39, 42, 44, 45, 51, 52, 56, 58, 66
Bowen's disease	16	31, 34
Bowenoid papulosis	16	34, 39, 42, 45
Cervical carcinoma	16, 18	31, 33, 35, 39, 45, 51, 52, 56, 58, 66
Recurrent respiratory papillomatosis	6, 11	
Focal epithelial neoplasia of Heck	13, 32	
Conjunctival papillomas and carcinomas	6, 11, 16	
Others		6, 11, 16, 30, 33, 36, 37, 38, 41, 48, 60

FIGURE 1-4.
Disease associations of different HPV types. More than 70 different HPV types have been characterized, and many others are recognized. Because the viruses cannot be cultured, typing is based on DNA homology. Each type is site-specific and largely associated with a distinct histopathologic process. (*From* Bonnez and Reichman [1]; with permission.)

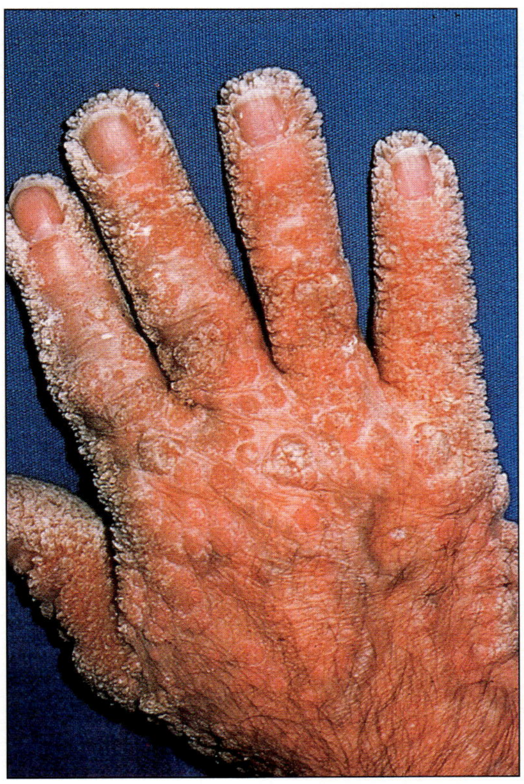

FIGURE 1-5.
Extensive verrucae vulgaris of the right hand. Common warts represent up to 71% of all cutaneous warts and are most prevalent among school-age children. They are believed to be transmitted by close personal contact. (*Courtesy of* R. Ostrow, MD.)

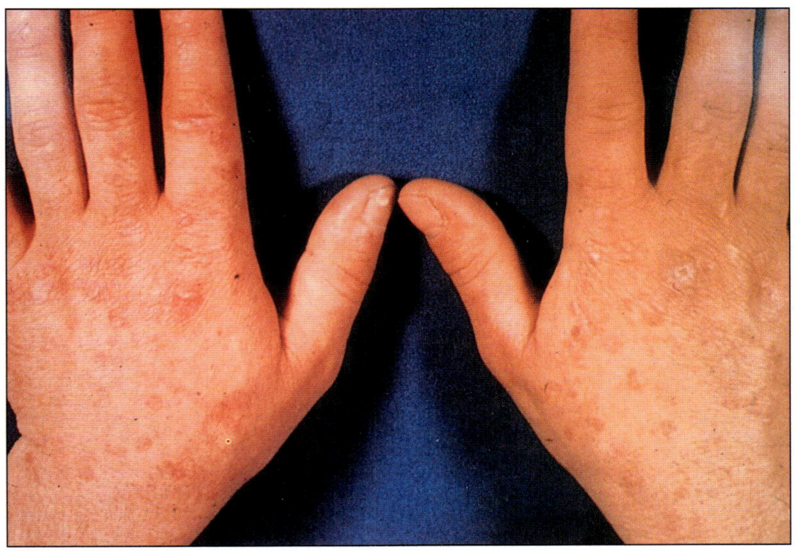

FIGURE 1-6.
Epidermodysplasia verruciformis of the hand. The dorsum of the hand shows multiple flat warts that will persist for life in this congenitally immunosuppressed individual. A large invasive squamous cancer (not shown) also has developed in the sunlight-exposed area of the right forehead. Epidermodysplasia verruciformis is a rare, probably autosomal dominant condition that is characterized by disseminated cutaneous warts and malignant transformation. It usually appears early in life in persons with depressed cellular immunity. (*From* Pfister [2]; with permission.)

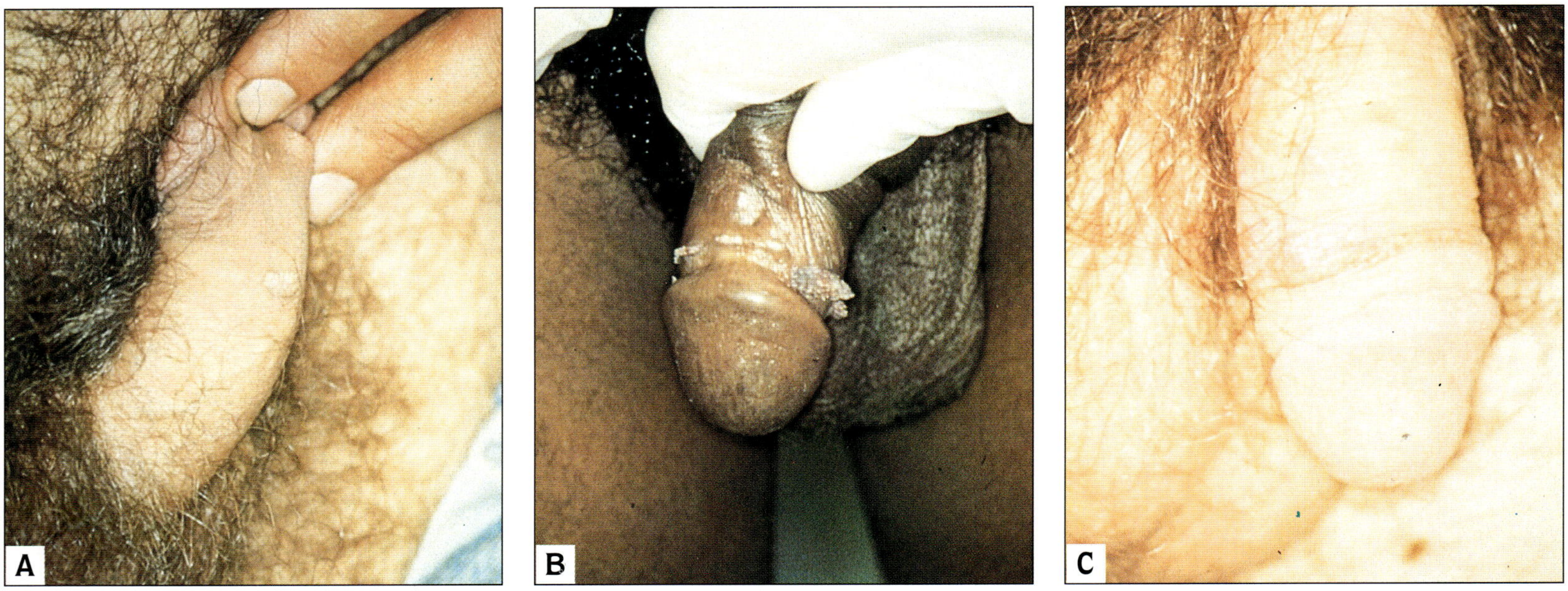

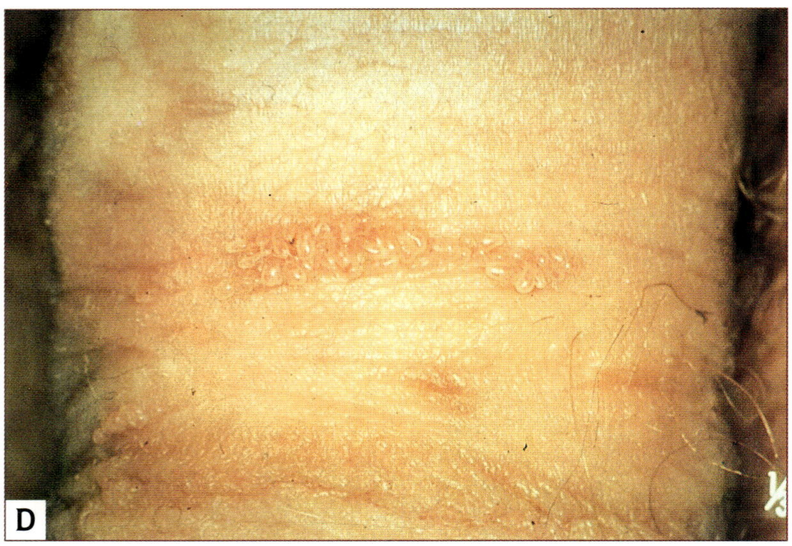

FIGURE 1-7.
Penile warts. **A**, Typical papilliferous wart of the penis in a healthy man. These exophytic lesions are initially soft and fleshy. They occur most frequently on the shaft and coronal sulcus and are commonly found under the prepuce. When lesions have the typical verrucous appearance seen here, a clinical diagnosis is made easily. The lesions may spread linearly or circumferentially. A smaller lesion is seen distally, just beneath the patient's fingers. **B**, Papilliferous warts of the penis involving the coronal sulcus. The coronal sulcus is a common site for condylomata acuminata in men, perhaps because of the susceptibility of this site to subclinical trauma during intercourse. Here, the warts have spread circumferentially, with the inital lesions to the patient's left. These older lesions have become hyperpigmented. **C**, Flatter, more chronic warts on the penis. These lesions were an incidental finding on a man who presented as an asymptomatic contact to a woman with chlamydial cervicitis. Chronic warts are likely to become keratinized. **D**, Recurrent warts on the penile shaft. This patient had been treated 3 months previously, with complete resolution of visible lesions but returned with recurrent, tiny lesions. A blush may be seen at the base of some of the individual lesions, which are highly vascular. The appearance of a tiny blood vessel running along the side of a lesion may assist in identifying it as a wart (as opposed to molluscum contagiosum). (*From* Oriel [3]; with permission; *courtesy of* M. F. Rein, MD.)

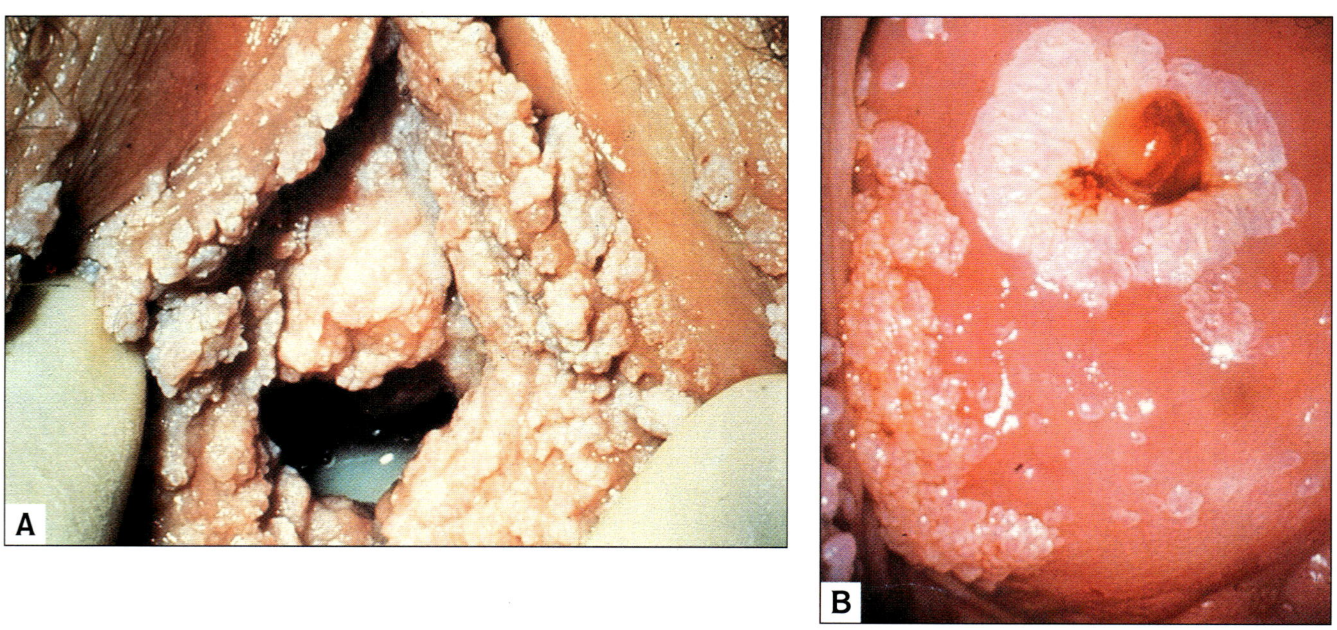

FIGURE 1-8.
Condylomata acuminata. **A** and **B**, Typical papilliferous warts (condylomata acuminata) affecting the vulva and vagina (*A*) and cervix (*B*) of an immunologically healthy young woman. (*Courtesy of* E. Pixley, MD.)

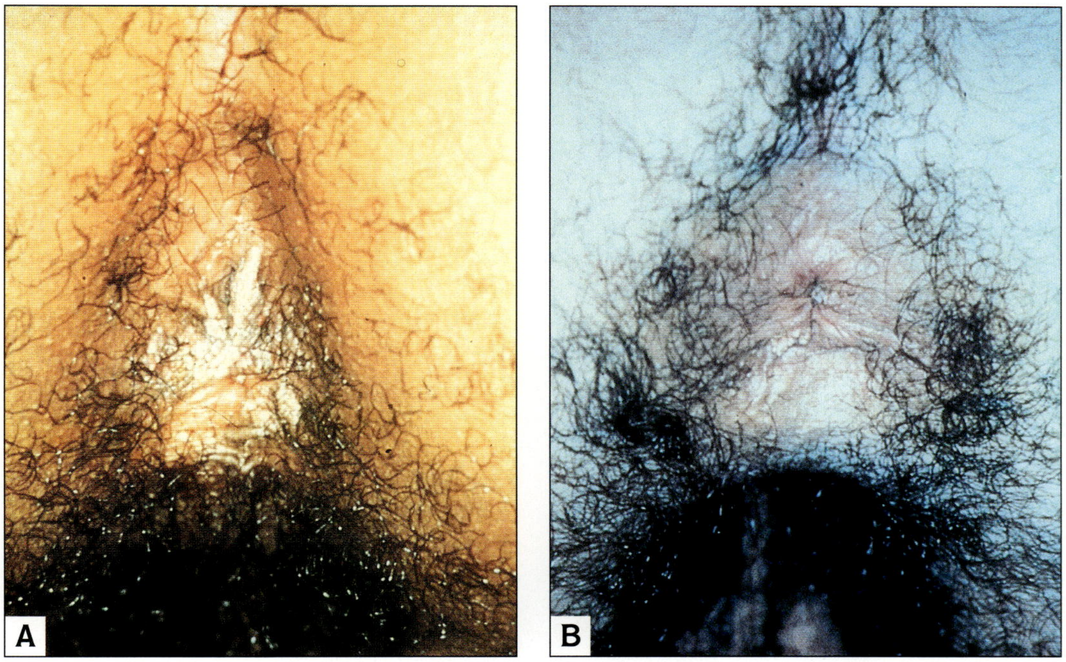

FIGURE 1-9.
Perianal warts. **A**, This patient was seen in 1977, before the identification of HIV, and was presumably immunologically intact. The presence of such perianal lesions in a man is possible evidence that the patient has engaged in receptive anal intercourse. Such patients should undergo anoscopy to look for internal lesions and should be evaluated for other anorectal sexually transmitted diseases, such as gonorrhea or chlamydial infection. They also should be strongly encouraged to undergo testing for HIV antibody. **B**, Perianal warts, in another homosexual man who practiced receptive anal intercourse, are seen to track into the anus. (*Courtesy of* M. F. Rein, MD.)

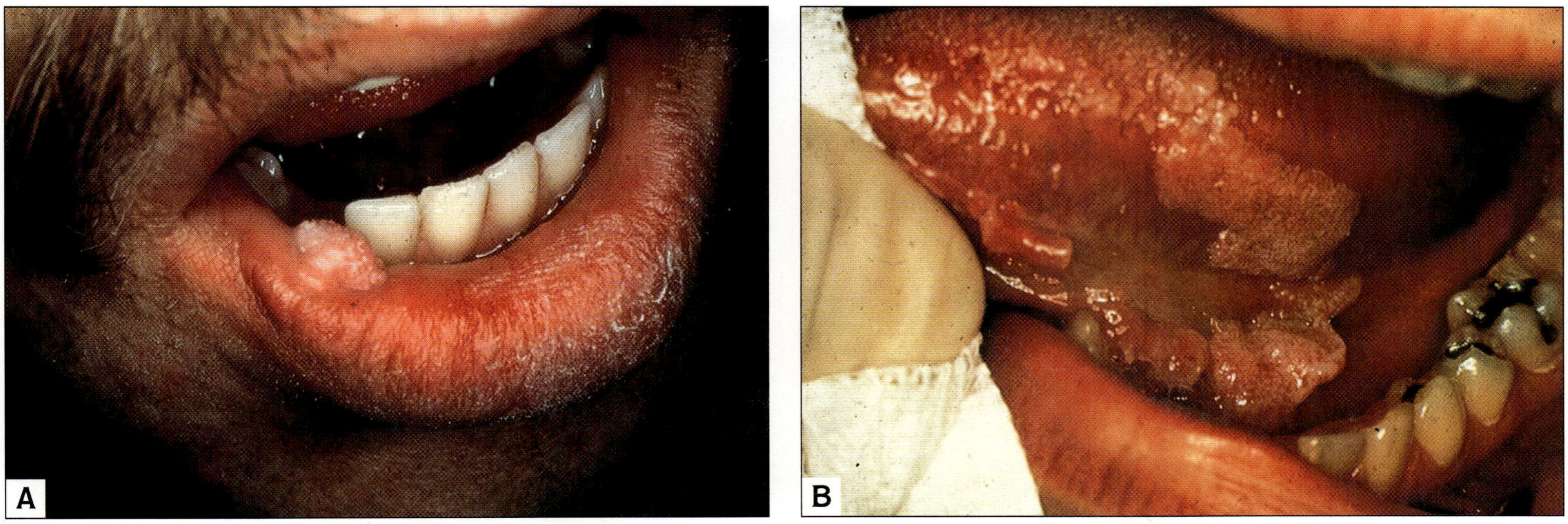

FIGURE 1-10.
Oral lesions. **A** and **B**, Condylomatous lesions affecting the lips (*A*) and oral mucosa (*B*) of an immunologically healthy homosexual man.

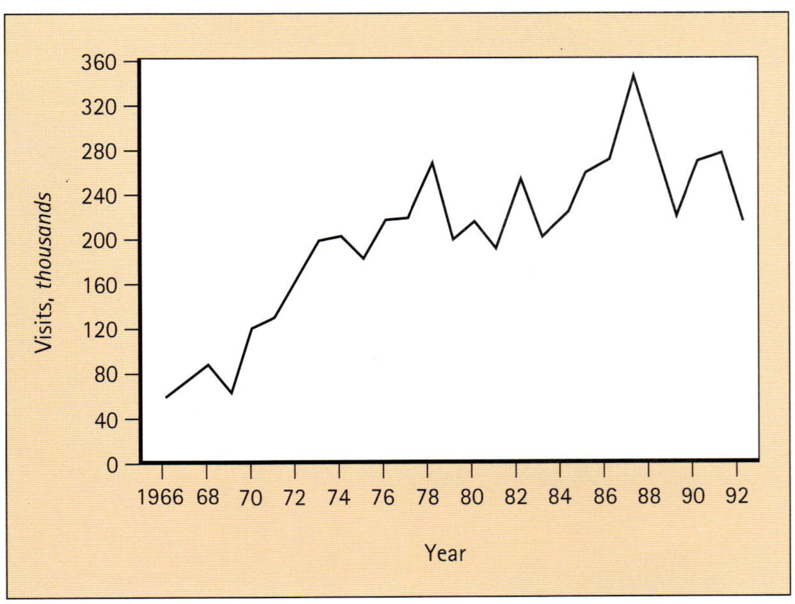

FIGURE 1-11.
Annual incidence of HPV-associated genital warts in the United States between 1966 and 1992. The incidence of genital warts has risen dramatically in the past 15 to 20 years. Using data collected by the National Disease and Therapeutic Index, the Centers for Disease Control and Prevention estimate that the number of physicians' office visits related to anogenital warts increased from 169,000 in 1966 to 1.1 million in 1984 in the United States. An estimated half million people each year acquire symptomatic genital warts [4]. (*From* Division of STD/HIV Prevention: *Sexually Transmitted Disease Surveilance, 1992*. Atlanta: Centers for Disease Control and Prevention; 1993:28.)

NATURAL HISTORY AND PATHOGENESIS

NATURAL HISTORY OF GENITAL HUMAN PAPILLOMAVIRUS INFECTIONS

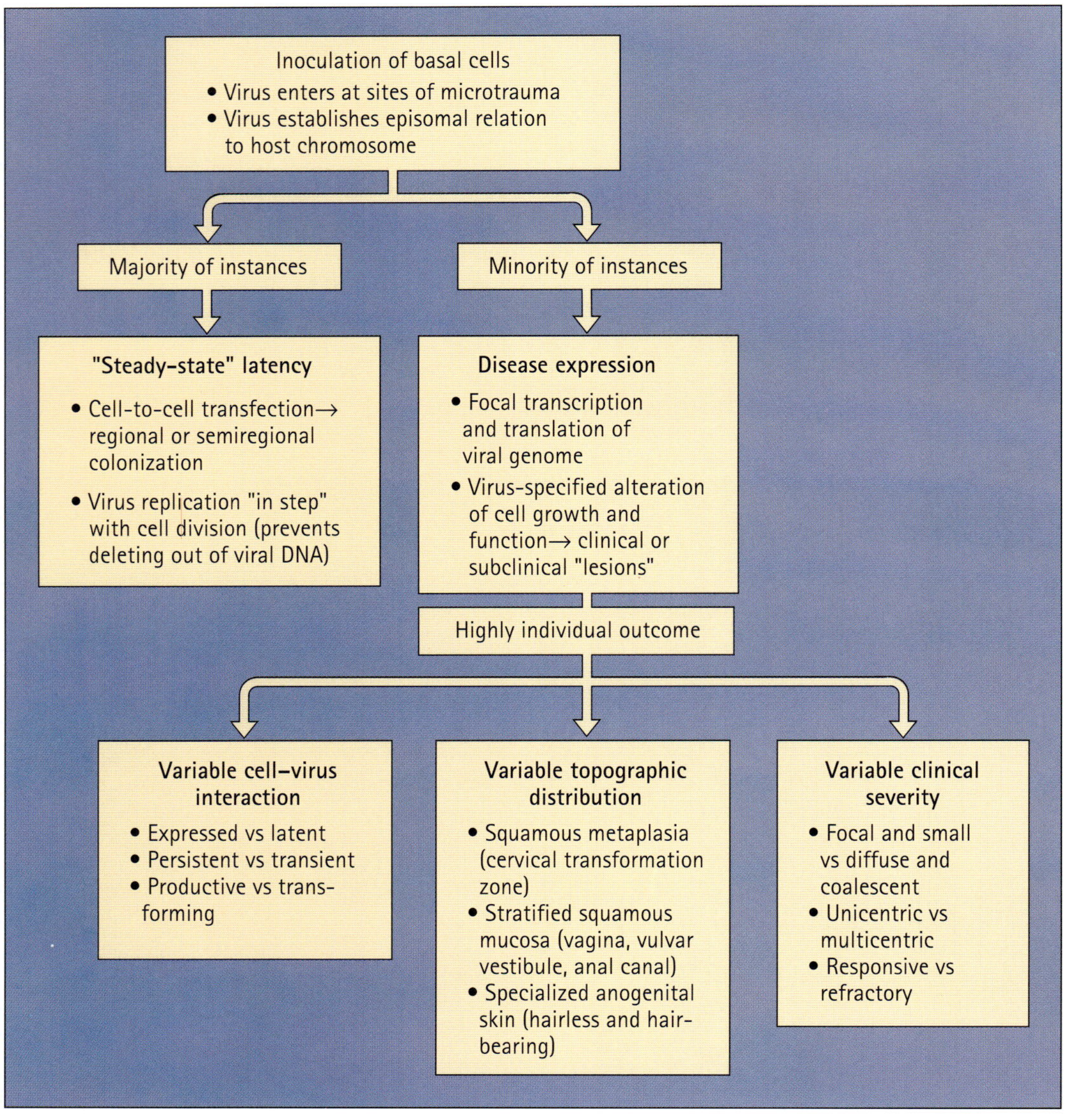

FIGURE 1-12.
Individual variation in the natural history of HPV infections. The viral life cycle begins with inoculation of the basal cells at sites of microtrauma. During the incubation phase, the virus establishes an episomal relationship to the host chromosome. In most instances, cell-to-cell transection produces a regional or semiregional colonization, in which there is no disease expression, and virus exposure can only be detected by molecular hybridization of exfoliated cells. The latency is maintained by the mechanism of virus replication in step with cell division Conversely, in a minority of instances, focal transcription and translation lead to disease expression. The outcome is highly individual, depending on variations in cell-virus interaction, topographic distribution, and clinical severity.

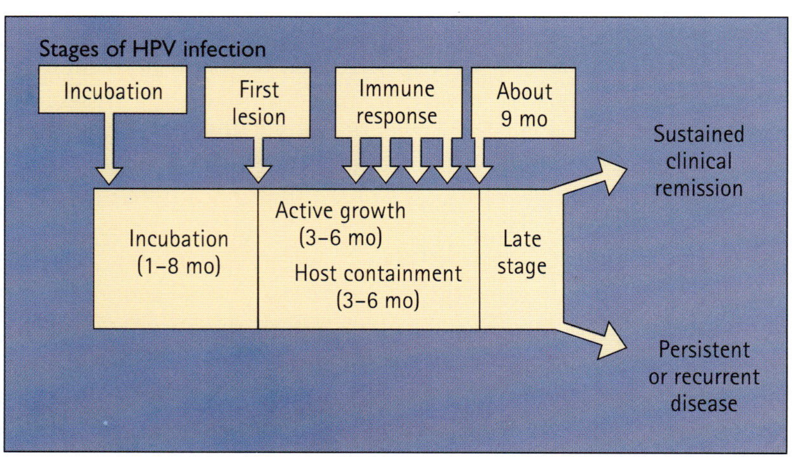

FIGURE 1-13.
Stages of HPV infection. After inoculation, there is an incubation period during which the virus establishes itself as a self-replicating, extrachromosomal plasmid throughout the lower genital tract. This is followed by a period of active lesion growth, which typically lasts 3 to 6 months. After a lag time of several months, there is a host-containment phase, during which lesion growth is slowed. In up to 20% of instances, spontaneous regression may occur, even of extensive disease. About 9 months from the time of the first lesion, the lesion growth and host containment come into essential equilibrium. At this point, patients diverge into two groups: those who remain in sustained clinical remission, and those who relapse into continued active disease expression. (*From* Reid and Dorsey [5]; with permission.)

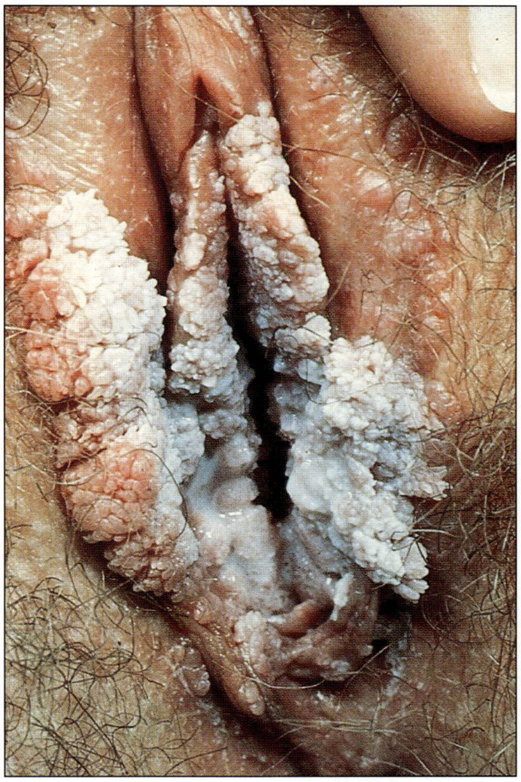

FIGURE 1-14.

Active lesion growth. Altered epithelial growth patterns and the proliferation of underlying capillaries produce a diffuse crop of symmetric soft papillomas. The associated vaginal discharge has produced maceration of some of the lesion of the nonglabrous skin. Accumulated clinical experience suggest that perhaps only 1 in 10 exposed individuals ever develop clinical disease. (*From* Reid and Campion [6]; with permission.)

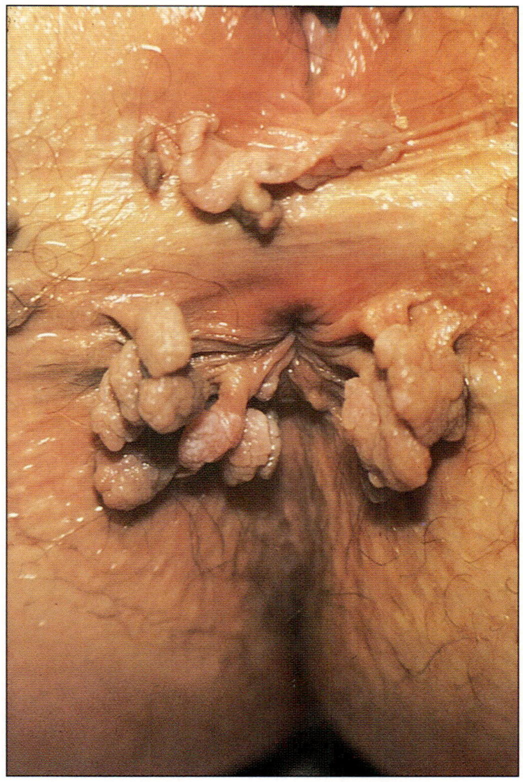

FIGURE 1-15.

Papular, pedunculated perianal warts of 4 years duration. (*From Reid [7]; with permission.)*

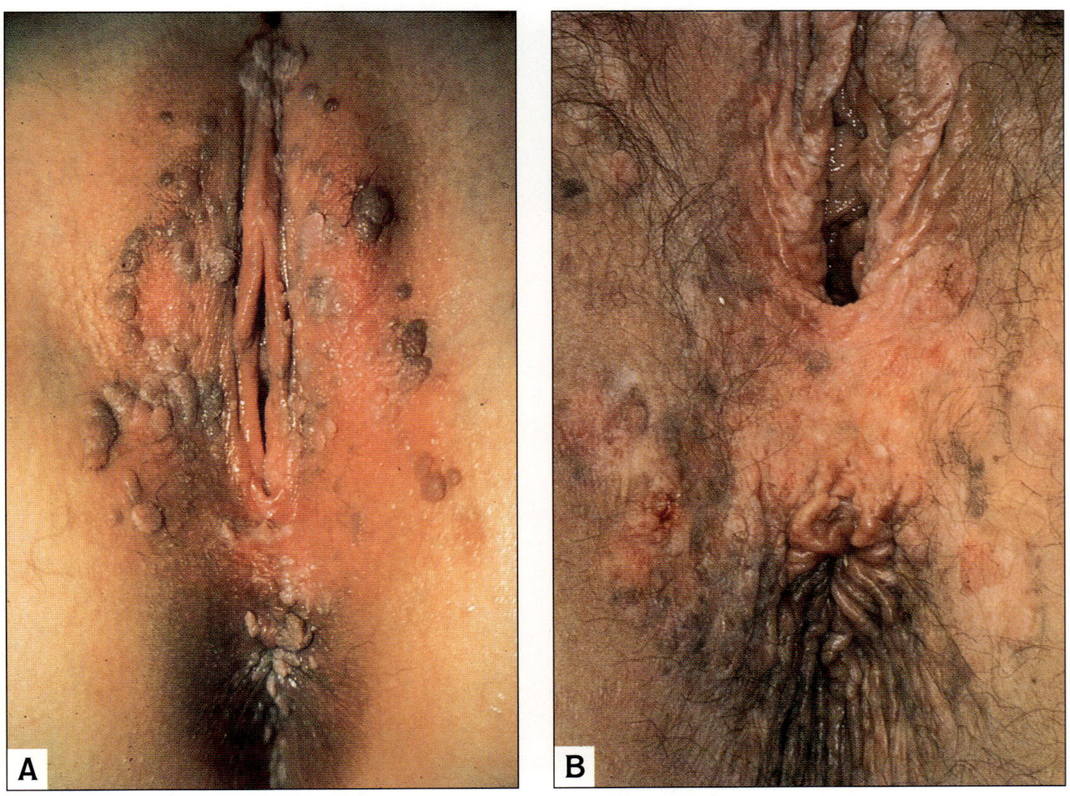

FIGURE 1-16.

Persistent of recurrent HPV infection **A**, Bowenoid papulosis. These pigmented peripheral papules recurred about 2 years after previously "cured" condylomas. Biopsy showed a premalignant epithelium, and virus testing detected HPV 16. Such cases traditionally are called *bowenoid papulosis* to distinguish these peripheral papules from the central macules of classic Bowen's disease. However, both lesions are associated with HPV 16, both have similar histology, and either can progress to invasive cancer. Therefore, the distinction is discouraged and these terms should be abandoned. **B**, Bowen's disease, diffuse macular vulvar intrepithelial neoplasia, grade 3 (VIN 3). In contrast with (*A*), this patient shows the classic macular lesion of Bowen's disease.

Cell-Virus Interactions

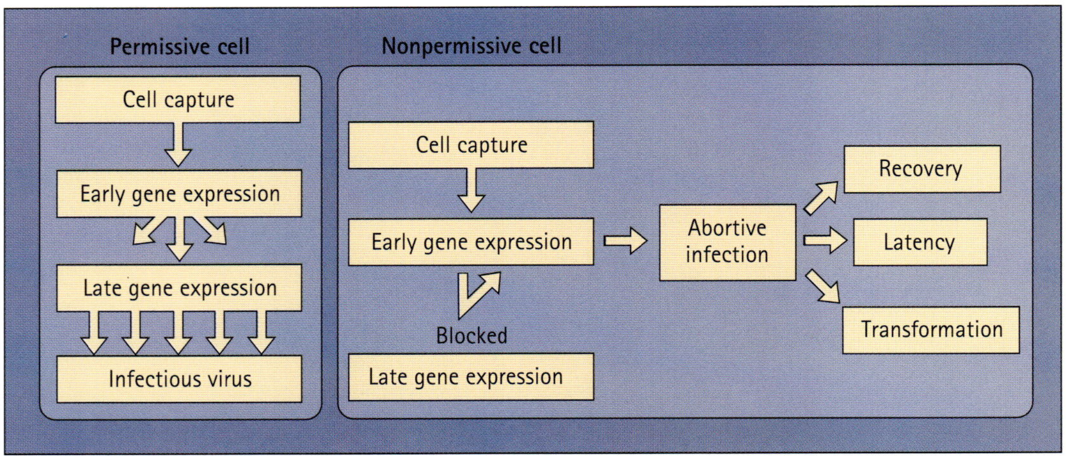

FIGURE 1-17.
Outcome of HPV infection in permissive cell versus nonpermissive cell. In the permissive cell, expression of the early viral genes produces cellular proliferation in the basal layers but leads to cell death and virion assembly in the upper layers. In nonpermissive cells, late gene expression fails, leading to an abortive infection from which recovery, persistent latency, or neoplastic transformation may result. (*From* Reid [8]; with permission.)

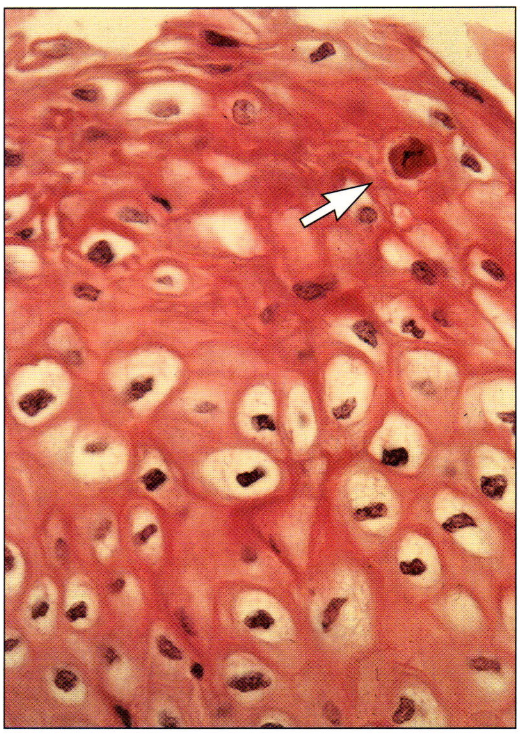

FIGURE 1-18.
Tissue micrograph of the upper layers of a productive cell-virus interaction in the cervical epithelium, showing koilocytotic atypia. There is prominent cytopathic effect producing a histologic picture termed *koilocytotic atypia*. The main features are hyperchromatism, nuclear shrinkage and collapse, and perinuclear cytoplasmic vacuolation, which are highly specific findings for HPV infection. One of the cells shows individual cell keratinization (*arrow*).

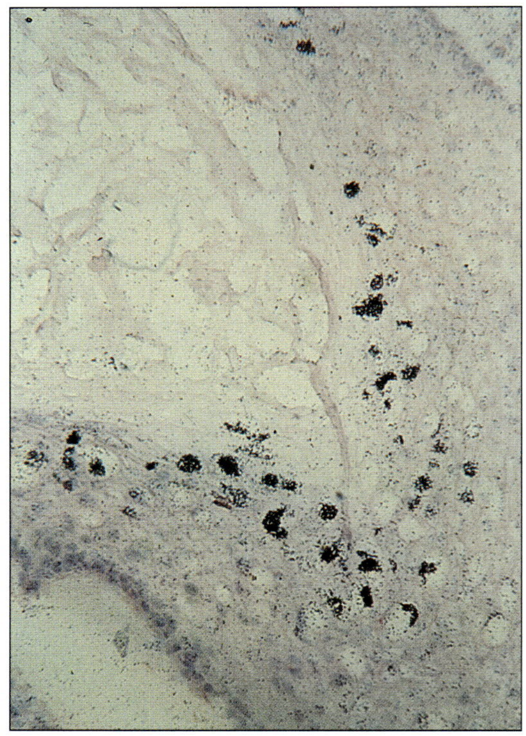

FIGURE 1-19.
In situ hybridization using ^{3}H-HPV-6 probe to identify replication of viral DNA within cells of a condyloma. Viral replication is indicated by the multiple intranuclear black granules, most prominent at the epithelial surface. (*Courtesy of* A. T. Lorincz, MD.)

Productive Viral Infection

EVENTS IN THE HPV LIFE CYCLE

Viral event	Histologic reflection
1. Cell capture (basal layer)	None
2. Early gene expression with "benign transformation" (parabasal layer)	Mitogenic effect (acanthosis, mitoses, hyperchromatism, delayed maturation) Viral DNA replication begins
3. Late gene expression begins in maturing cells (intermediate layer)	Initial viral cytopathic effect (mild koilocytosis)
4. Late gene expression in terminally differentiating cells (upper third)	Pronounced nuclear collapse and vacuolization Virion assembly begins

FIGURE 1-20.
Events in the HPV life cycle with associated histologic reflection. The synthesis of late proteins and production of intact viral particles occur in maturing cells within the intermediate and superficial layers.

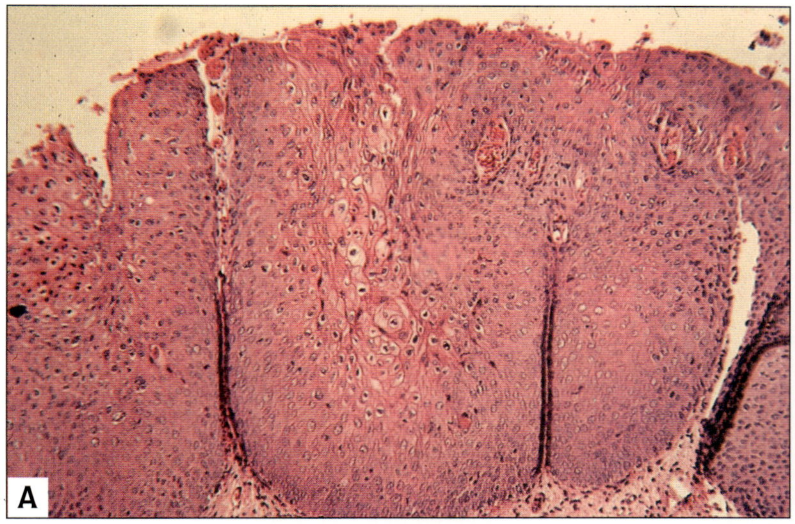

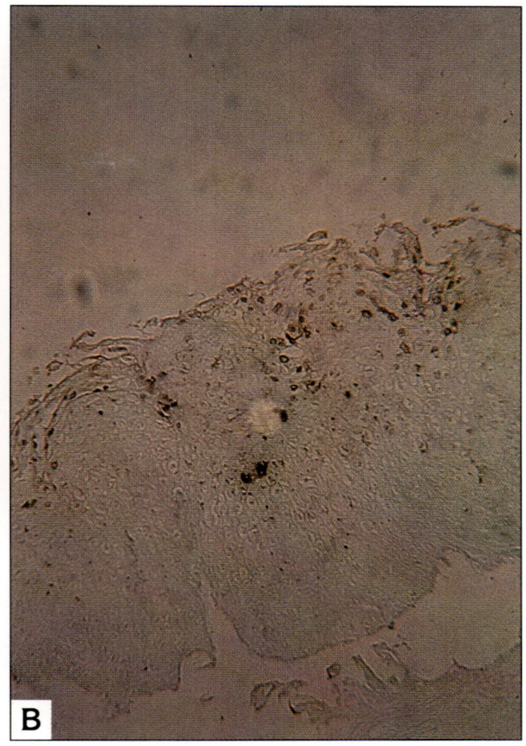

FIGURE 1-21.
Basal layer expression. **A** and **B**, Photomicrographs showing early gene expression in the basal layers (*A*) and late gene expression at the epithelial surface (*B*). Part (*A*) is stained with hematoxylin-eosin and part (*B*) is an unstained immunoperoxidase preparation of an adjacent section. Cells containing virus-specified capsid protein show intranuclear aggregations of brown staining, seen only in the intermediate and superficial layers.

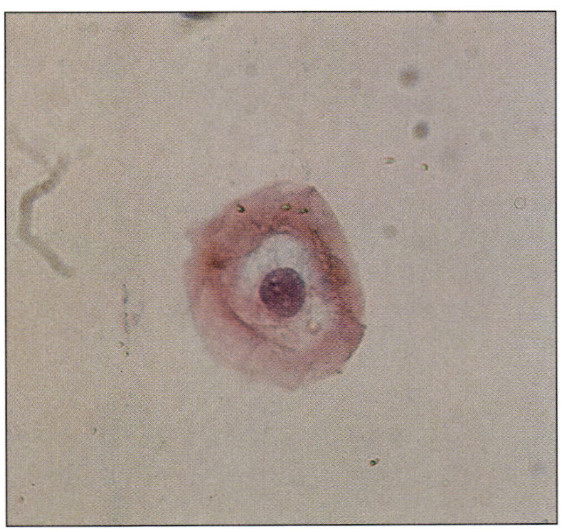

FIGURE 1-22.
Classic cytopathic effect seen on Papanicolaou staining of single exfoliated koilocyte. One can see nuclear condensation and the perinuclear clear zone, changes that are highly specific for HPV infection.

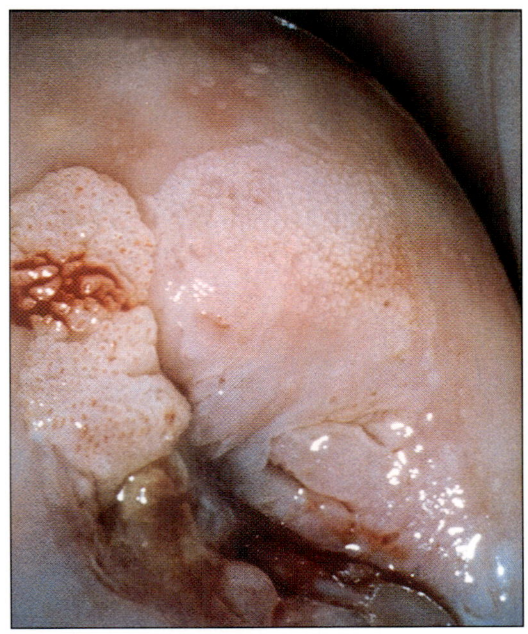

FIGURE 1-23.
Colpophotograph showing the prominent upgrowth of HPV-induced capillary proliferation, producing a macroscopically visible condyloma (*left*) and a subclinical acetowhite lesion visible only through the colposcope (*right*).

HUMAN PAPILLOMAVIRUS–INDUCED MALIGNANT TRANSFORMATION

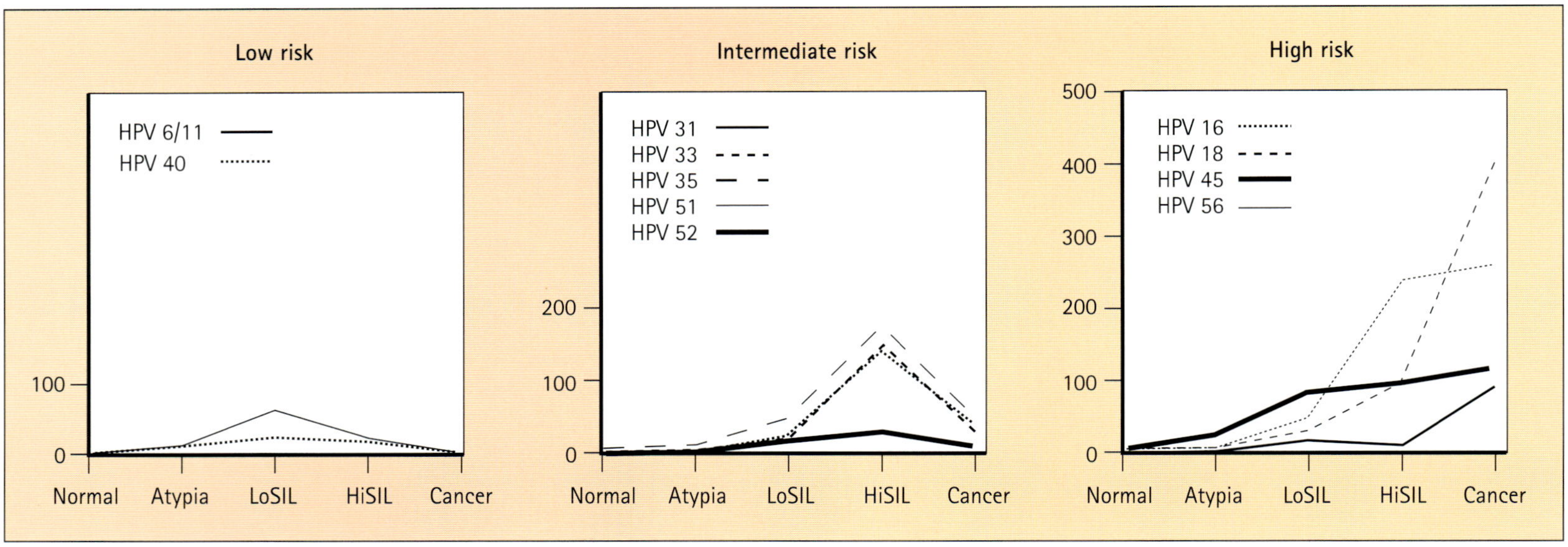

FIGURE 1-24.

Odds ratios for low-risk, intermediate-risk, and high-risk HPV types and malignancy. Among the more than 70 types of HPVs that have been identified, certain types, such as 6 and 11, are associated primarily with benign genital warts, but other types, such as 16, 18, and, less frequently, 31, 35, 39, 42 to 45, and 51 to 52, are associated with malignancy of various grades. These graphs display the relative risk of malignancy found in genital infections with various HPV types. Odds ratios were calculated from a series of 2 X 2 contingency tables comparing type-specific virus testing results with histology in a case-control analysis of 2627 women. To test the hypothesis that HPV type was related to histologic grade, contingency tables for atypia of uncertain significance (*n*=270), low-grade squamous intrapithelial lesion (LoSIL, *n*=377), high-grade SIL (HiSIL, *n*=261), and cancer (*n*=153) were profiled against the table for the control group (*n*=1566). Numerically, HPV 16 is the most important type, being represented in 47% of high-grade SILs and 47% of invasive cancers. HPVs 18, 45, and 56 are overrepresented in invasive cancers and underrepresented in high-grade SILs (27% vs 7%). Conversely, HPVs 31, 33, 35, 39, 51, 52, and 52 are overrepresented in HiSIL but underrepresented invasive cancer (24% vs 11%). (*From* Lorincz and coworkers [9]; with permission.)

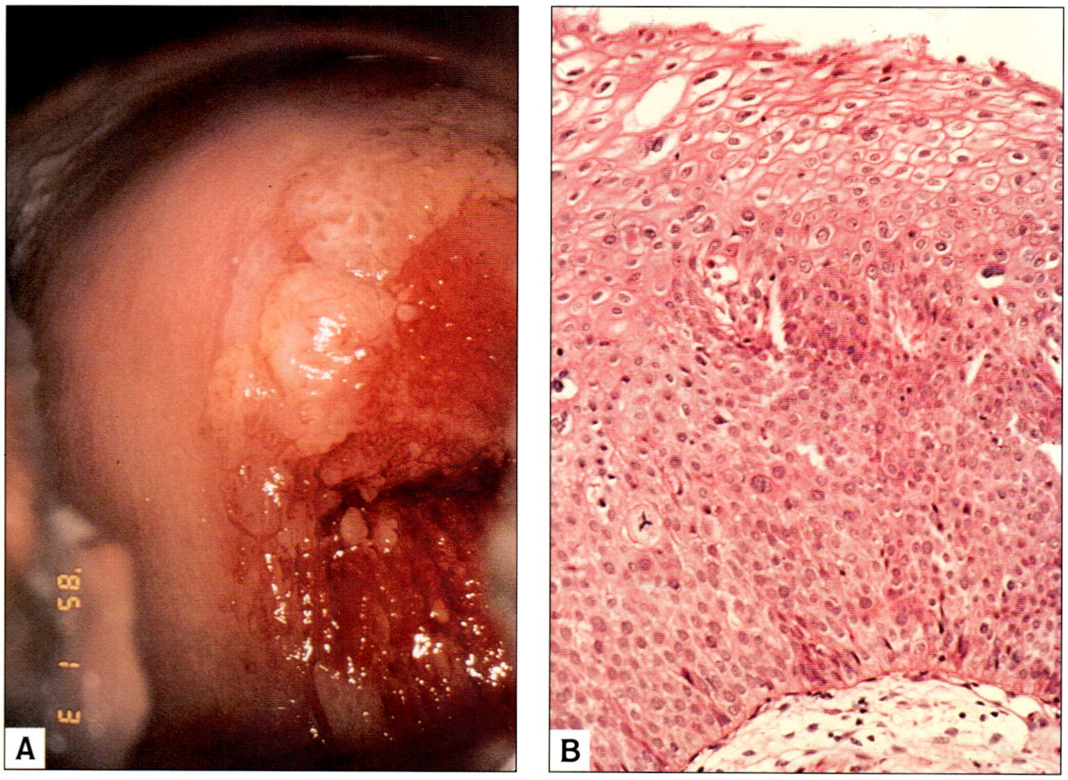

FIGURE 1-25.

Low-grade cervical squamous intraepithelial lesion (LoSIL) of doubtful neoplastic potential. **A**, Colpophotograph shows a definite LoSIL at the edge of an extensive immature transformation zone. **B**, Cervical biopsy specimen shows proliferation of atypical basal cells, giving way to partial viral cytopathic effect at the surface. A prominent tripolar atypical mitotic figure is seen in the *lower left*. (Hematoxylin-eosin stain). Ploidy analysis showed this lesion to be polyploid, reflecting potentially reversible cellular proliferation without definite genetic alteration within the infected epithelium. (Part B *from* Reid and Fu [10]; with permission.)

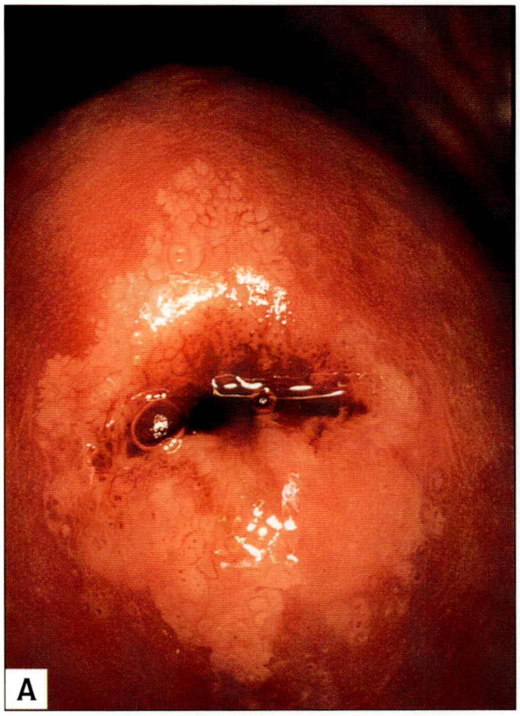

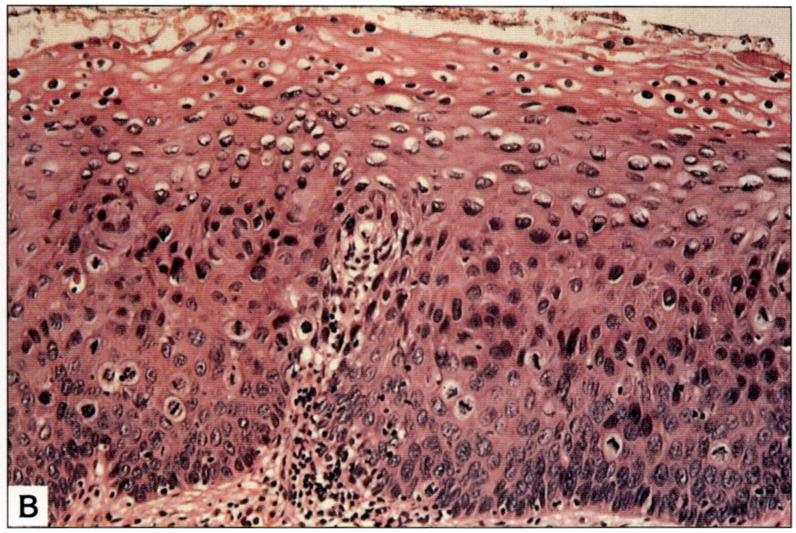

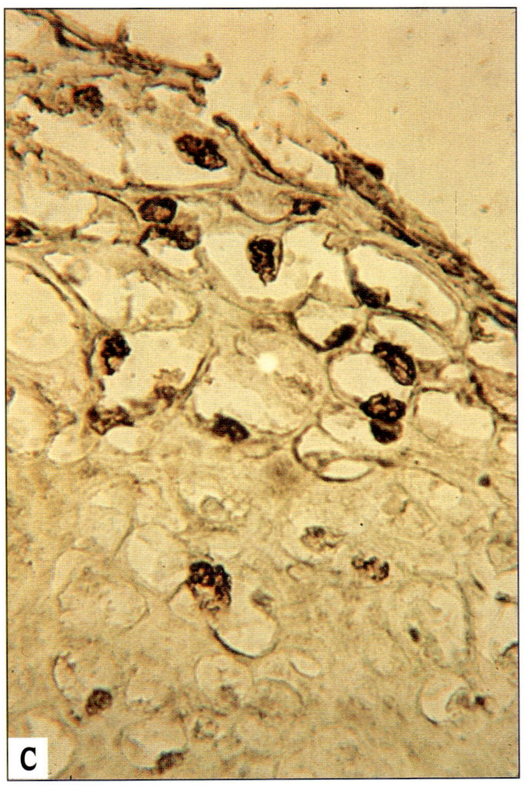

FIGURE 1-26.

Low-grade squamous intraepithelial lesion (LoSIL) with undoubted potential for malignant progression. **A**, Colpophotograph shows a flat acetowhite lesion with an irregular peripheral margin, shiny gray color, and a diffuse, fine mosaic pattern. The cervix has been soaked with 5% acetic acid for several minutes, causing HPV-infected areas to become white. On the anterior lip of the cervix, there is an internal demarcation just above the new squamo-columnar juction. Below this demarcation, colposcopic characteristics change, epithelial color changes from a shiny gray to dull white, and the vascular pattern changes from fine to coarse. This transition indicates that the lesion is undergoing progression from LoSIL to high-grade SIL (HiSIL). **B**, Directed biopsy shows that the lesion still has the tissue architectural pattern of a low-grade lesion, but within it are prominent cytologic features of developing HiSIL. Cells show hyperchromatism and pleomorphism. Multiple, highly abnormal mitotic figures can be seen throughout the lower half of the epithelium. Surface maturation of these abnormal basal cells results in prominent viral cytopathic effect, showing greater nuclear atypia than seen in most minor-gade lesions. The coarse punctuation seen in the colpophotograph (*A*) is reflected by the prominent intraepithelial capillary shown in this tissue section. (Hematoxylin-eosin stain.) **C**, Immunoperoxidase preparation shows late gene expression, as manifested by the brown intranuclear staining of virus-specified capsid protein within the nuclei of some surface koilocytes. Ploidy analysis indicates that this epithelium has undergone permanent premalignant transformation.

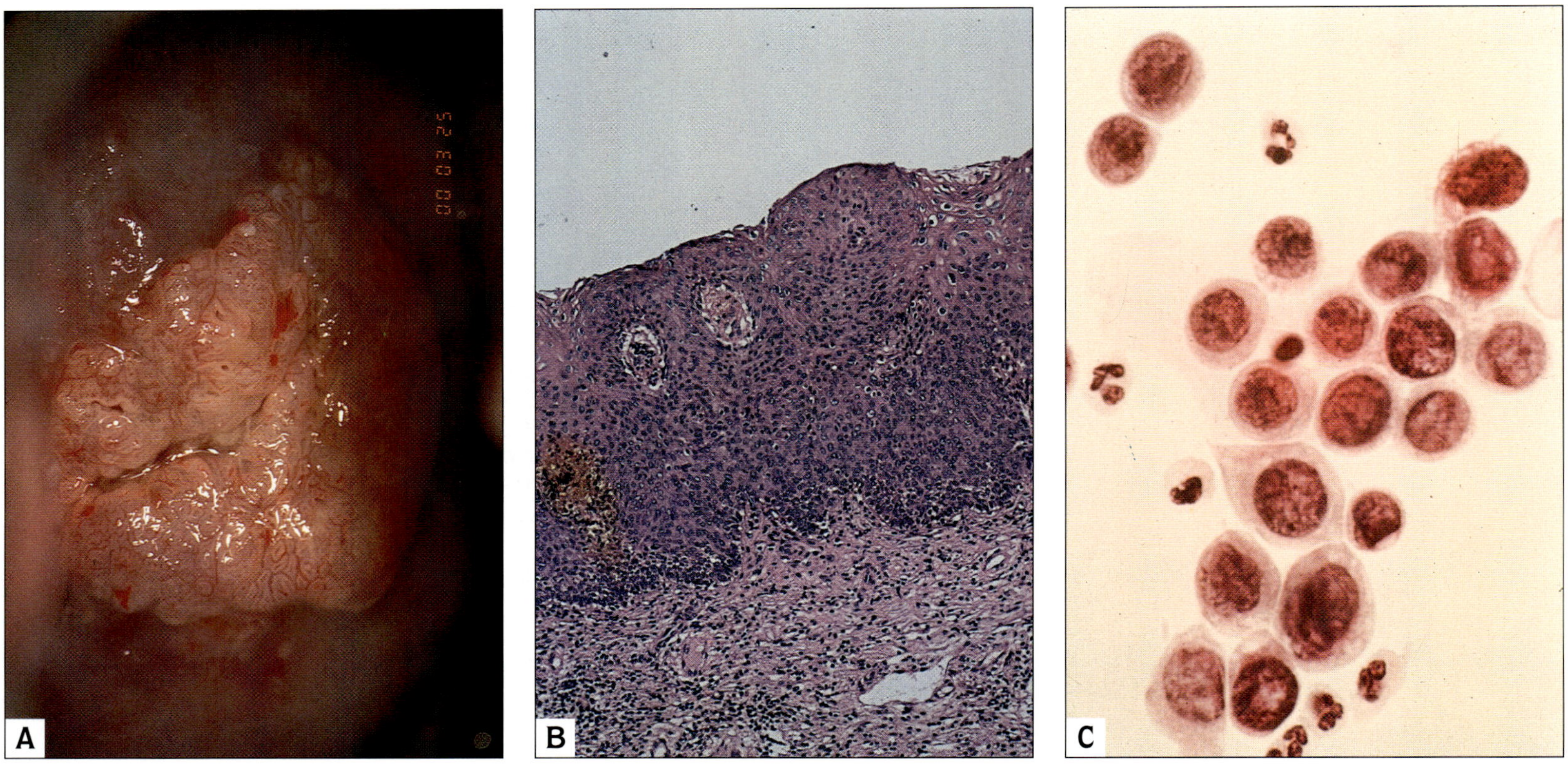

FIGURE 1–27.

Diagnostic features of high-grade squamous intraepithelial lesion (HiSIL). **A**, Colpophotograph, following acetic acid soaking of a large abnormal transformation zone, shows a dull premalignant epithelium traversed by a mixture of coarse mosaic and coarse punctuation. **B**, Directed biopsy confirms the presence of a HiSIL, as manifested by full thickness proliferation of primitive basaloid cells. Minimal focal koilocytotic atypia is seen at the *top left* and *top right*. Also, the mosaic pattern seen at colposcopy is reflected by the horizontal intraepithelial capillaries seen on the tissue section. (Hematolylin-eosin stain.) **C**, Papanicolaou smear shows a clump of highly abnormal basal cells with increased nuclear-cytoplasmic ratio.

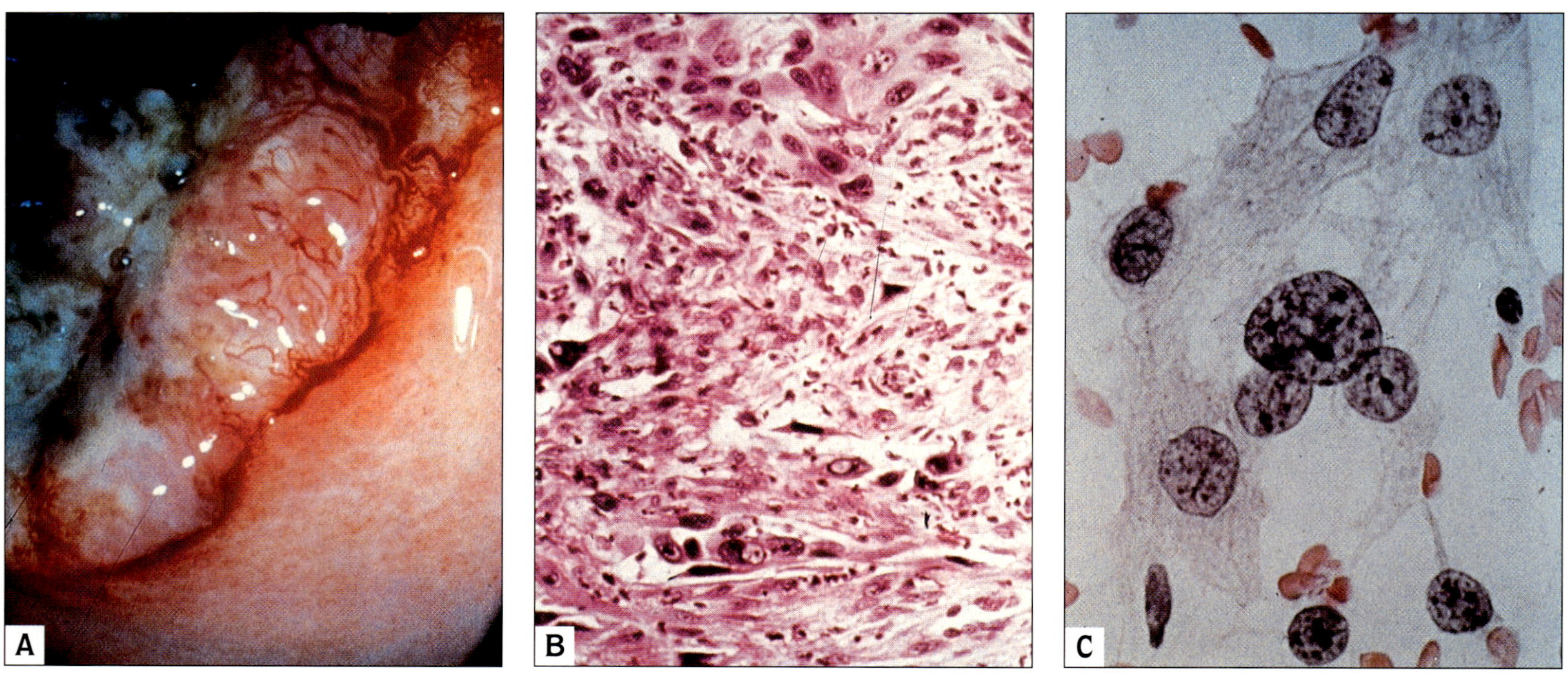

FIGURE 1–28.

Diagnostic features of invasive squamous carcinoma of cervix. **A**, Colpophotograph of the right posterior cervical lip shows a rolled epithelial edge, covered by partly necrotic epithelium. Angiogenic factor produced by these metabolically active cells results in prominent neovascularization, as evidenced by the multiple, horizontal atypical vessels growing from the lesion edge toward the necrotic ulcer crater. **B**, Photomicrograph shows bizarre epithelial cells invading the lamina propria of the cervix. Toward the bottom, tumor cells have infiltrated a "capillary-like space" **C**, In a Pap smear from the same patient, similar bizarre, pleomorphic cells with prominent nucleoli are seen against a "dirty background" (fibrin deposition and erythrocytes). (A *courtesy of* E. Pixley, MD.)

Mechanisms of Human Papillomavirus–Induced Malignant Transformation

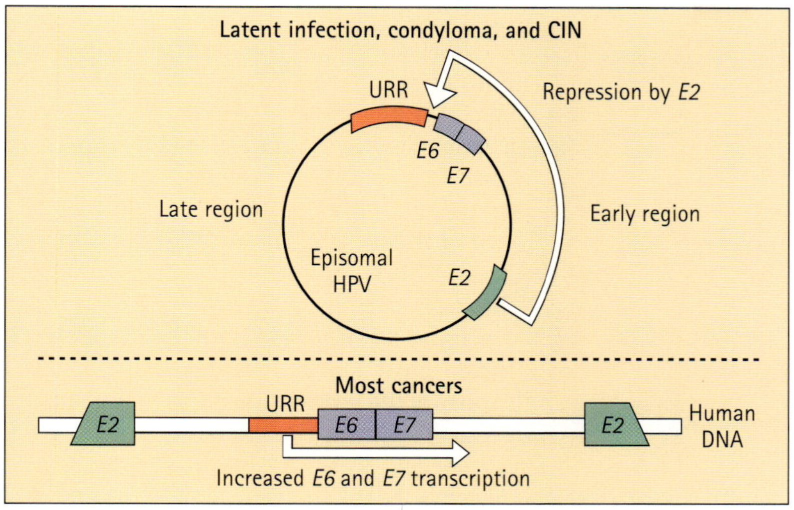

FIGURE 1-29.

Integration of HPV DNA into host genome. The diagram contrasts the episomal relationship seen in latent infection, condyloma, and cervical intraepithelial neoplasia (CIN) (*top part*) with integrated pattern of HPV DNA seen in invasive cancers (*bottom part*). In the nonintegrated form, the viral DNA exists as a circular plasmid, in which the two transforming genes (*E6* and *E7*) are located just downstream of the "viral brain." In the nonintegrated form, products of the E2 gene down-modulate expression of the *E6* and *E7* genes. Conversely, as these lesions become invasive, the circular genome of the plasmid splits at about the middle of the *E2* gene, producing a linear fragment of viral chromosome in which the late genes and part of the *E2* gene are located upstream from the upstream regulatory region (and thus inoperative). However, linearization does preserve the normal function of the two transforming genes, *E6* and *E7*, leading to overexpression of oncogenic proteins. (URR—upstream regulatory region.)

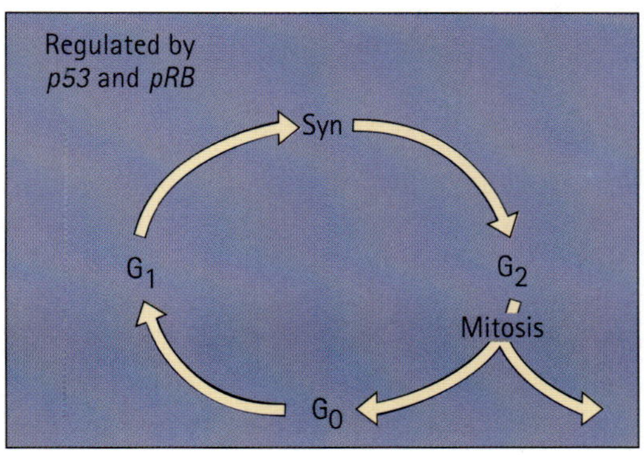

FIGURE 1-30.

Suspected mechanism by which oncogenic HPVs induce genetic mutation. Within the replicative cycle, cells are normally held in the G_1 phase by two important anti-oncogenes, *p53* and *pRB*, while chromosomal integrity is checked by endonucleases. However, in high-risk HPV infections, the protein specified by the HPV *E6* gene blocks *p53* and the protein specified by HPV *E7* blocks the retinoblastoma (RB) anti-oncogene. Thus, genetically damaged cells can undergo mitotic division. With time, these genetic errors can amplify to the point of producing the gross chromosomal distortions measured by DNA microspectrophotometry.

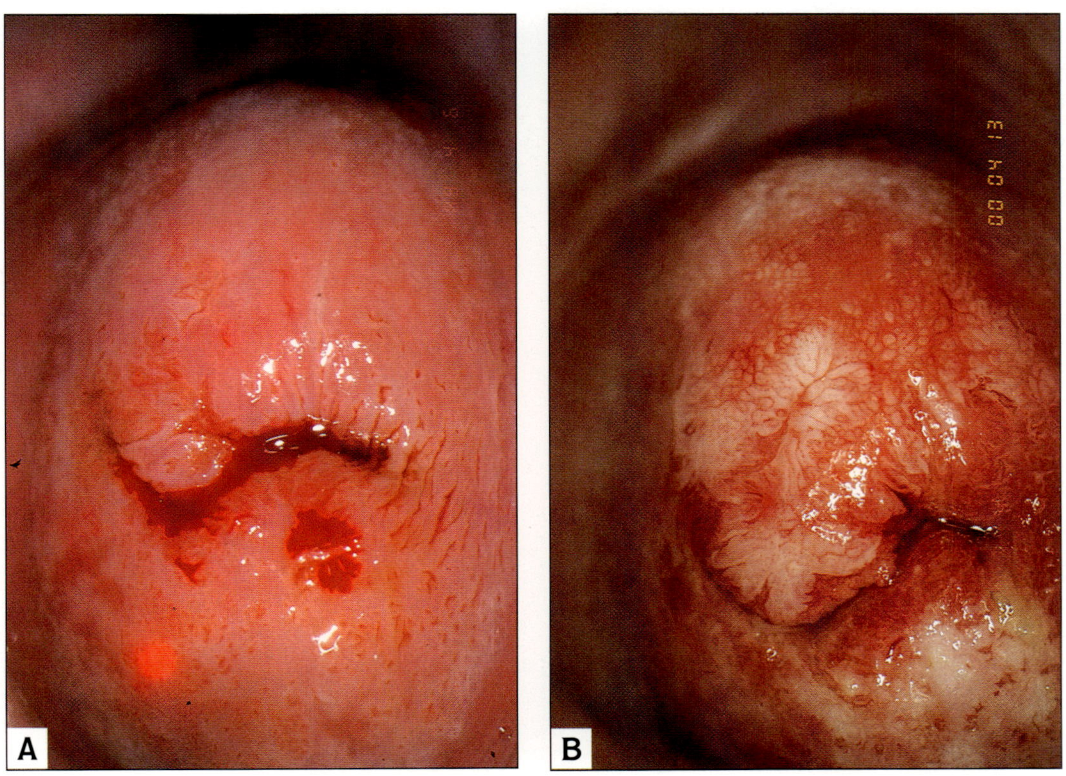

FIGURE 1-31.

Progressive potential depends on HPV type. **A**, Extensive minor-grade colposcopic change is seen in a patient at the enrollment visit of a 4-year natural-history study. Cervical cytology shows atypical squamous cells of uncertain significance. Virus testing isolated HPV 16 at this initial visit. **B**, Colposcopy 7 months later shows diffuse progression to cervical intraepithelial neoplasia, grade 3 (CIN 3), on both anterior and posterior cervical lips.

DISTINGUISHING EXPRESSED HUMAN PAPILLOMAVIRUS DISEASE FROM LATENT INFECTION OR NONSPECIFIC MIMICRY

HPV INFECTION: SPECTRUM OF CLINICAL CHANGE

Well-developed	Erroneous diagnosis
Productive	Micropapillomatosis labialis
Transforming	Borderline koilocytosis
	Clinically apparent
Latent	Subclinical acetowhitening
HPV genomes in normal cells	

FIGURE 1-32.

Spectrum of clinical changes seen in HPV infection. Transcription and translation of viral genetic information produces virus-specified proteins that disrupt tissue growth and maturation. In permissive cells, cell-virus interaction results in prolific DNA replication and variable virion assembly, to reinitiate the cycle of infectivity. Conversely, transforming cell-virus interactions lead to premalignant tissue changes, usually associated with cumulative genetic errors within the host chromosome. Both productive and transforming infections can be either clinically apparent (visible to the naked eye) or subclinical (seen through the colposcope as acetowhite change, with or without prominent vascular patterns). In other patients, HPV genomic material can be isolated from morphologically normal keratinocytes; such latent infections presumably represent a cell-virus interaction in which there is insufficient expression of viral genes to disrupt cell growth and maturation. Finally, there is rampant clinical misdiagnosis of nonspecific acetowhitening and micropapillary epithelial change as low-grade HPV infection. Multiple studies have clearly demonstrated that such tissues contain viral genetic material at about the same rate as the normal population.

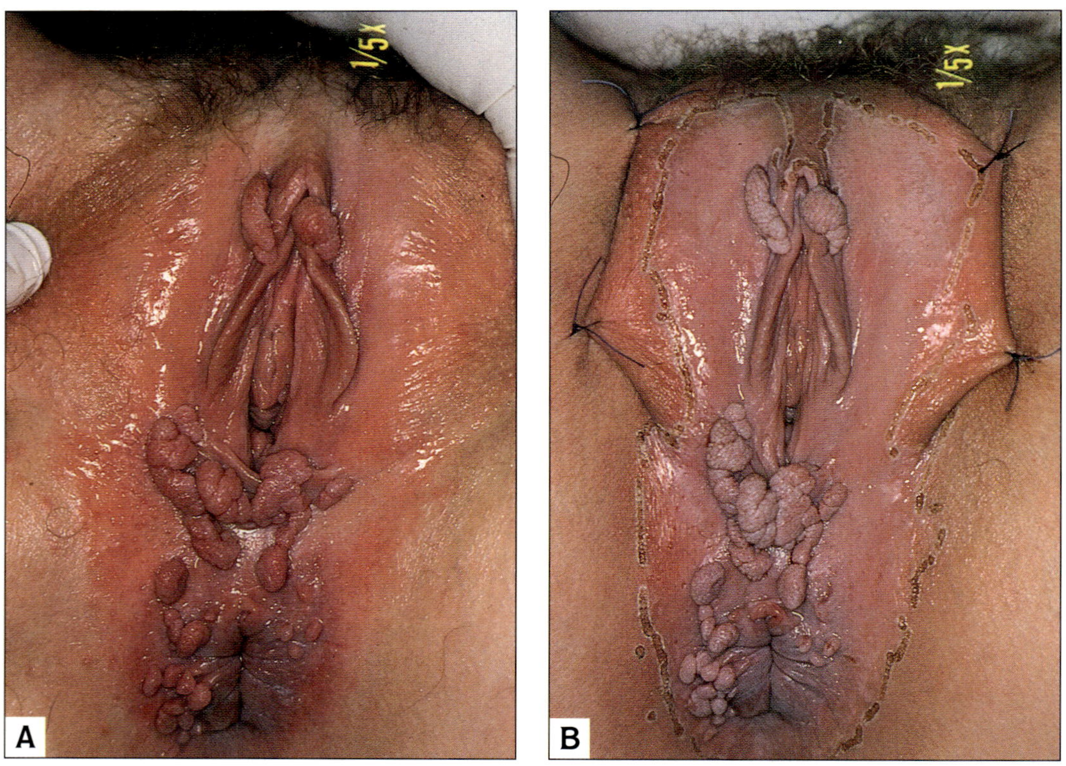

FIGURE 1-33.

Acetic acid testing. Application of a 3% to 5% acetic acid solution for up to 3 minutes causes HPV-infected areas to become white, which is a useful diagnostic indicator of infection. **A**, Prior to acetic acid application, multiple exophytic (clinically apparent) condylomas are visible. Surrounding skin is slightly erythematous but appears to be unaffected. **B**, After application of acetic acid, the surrounding skin shows a diffuse acetowhite change indicating HPV infection. Histologic changes within the exophytic and subclinical lesions were similar, both showing an equivalent degree of basal proliferation and surface koilocytosis. Southern blot hybridization detected the same type of viral DNA in both the exophytic and subclinical lesions. Both represent productive cell-virus interactions, and both may contain infectious virus particles.

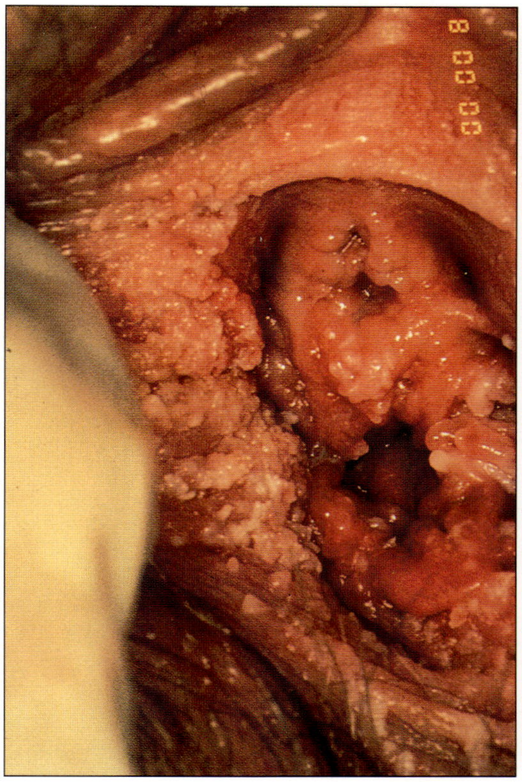

FIGURE 1-34.
Micropapillomatosis labialis. Despite the superficial resemblance to condylomas, such micropapillary changes are common in normal women. Whether these appearances represent individual anatomic variation of whether they arise as a result of nonspecific irritation is uncertain. Multiple studies have demonstrated that such patients test negative with HPV DNA hybridization.

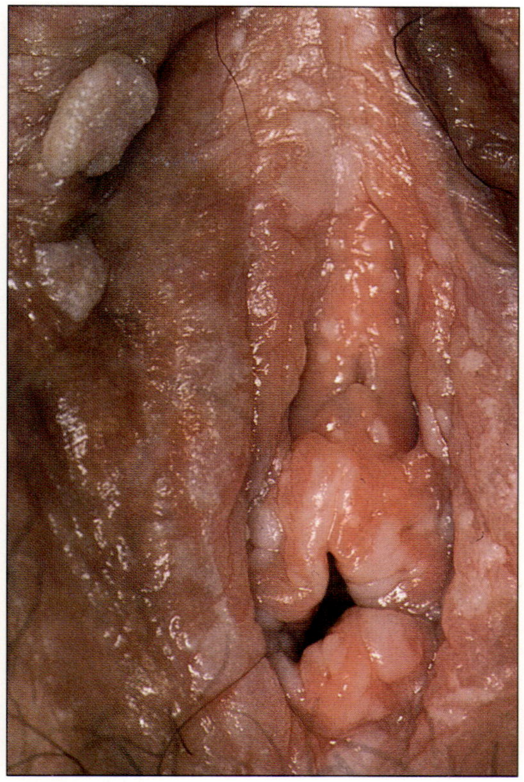

FIGURE 1-35.
Multiple, slightly elevated, sharply marginated acetowhite lesions with accompanying vascular pattern. Lesions show an asymmetric distribution that crosses anatomic subdivisions of the vulvar epithelium. The patient also has two exophytic condylomas. These appearances contrast sharply with the symmetric, anatomically confined, micropapillomatous change shown in Fig. 1-34.

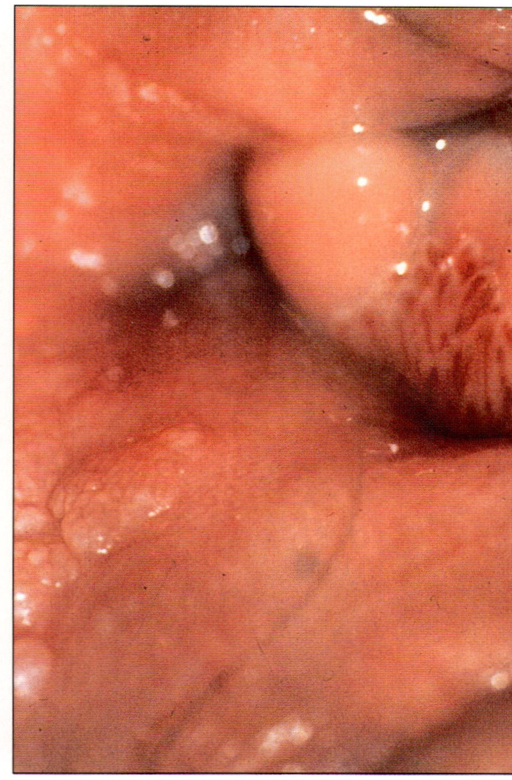

FIGURE 1-36.
Subtle but genuine condylomas of the vulvar vestibule. One micropapilliferous lesion is growing out of a minor vestibular gland at the hymenal edge. Other lesions are more sessile and show minimal variation in surface contour. In contrast to the pattern of diffuse single papillae seen in micropapillomatosis labialis, the fingerlike extensions on genuine condylomas arise from a central core.

REFERENCES

1. Bonnez W, Reichman RC: Papillomaviruses. In *Principles and Practice of Infectious Diseases*, edn 4. Edited by Mandell GL, Bennett JE, Dolin R. New York: Churchill Livingstone; 1995:1387–1400.
2. Pfister H: Relationship of papillomaviruses to anogenital cancer. *Obstet Gynecol Clin North Am*, 4:349–351.
3. Oriel D: Genital human papillomavirus infection. In *Sexually Transmitted Disease*, edn 2. Edited by Holmes KK, Mardh P-A, Sparling PF, *et al*. New York: McGraw-Hill; 1990:435.
4. *Division of STD/HIV Prevention: Sexually Transmitted Disease Surveillance, 1992*. Atlanta: Centers for Disease Control and Prevention; 1993:28.
5. Reid R, Dorsey JH: Physical and surgical principles of carbon dioxide laser surgery in the lower genital tract. In *Gynecologic Oncology*, edn 2. Edited by Coppelson M. Edinburgh: Churchill Livingstone; 1992:1087–1131.
6. Reid R, Campion M: HPV-associated lesions of the cervix: biology and colposcopic features. *Clin Obstet Gynecol* 1989, 32:157–179.
7. Reid R: Human papillomavirus–associated diseases of the lower genital tract. In *Laser Surgery in Gynecology and Obstetrics*, edn 2. Edited by Keys WR. Chicago: Year Book; 1990:46–99.
8. Reid R: Papillomavirus and cervical neoplasia: modern implications and future prospects. *Colposc Gynecol Laser Surg* 1984, 1:3–34.
9. Lorincz AT, Reid R, Jenson AB: Human papillomavirus infection of the cervix: relative risk associations of 15 common anogenital types. *Obstet Gynecol* 1992, 79:328–337.
10. Reid R, Fu YS: Is there a morphologic spectrum linking condyloma to cervical cancer? In *Banbury Report No. 21: Viral Etiology of Cervical Cancer*. Cold Spring Harbor, NY: Cold Spring Harbor Laboratory, 1986.

SELECTED BIBLIOGRAPHY

Campion MJ: Clinical manifestations and natural history of genital human papillomavirus infection. *Obstet Gynecol Clin North Am* 1987, 14:363–388.

Reid R: Biology and colposcopic features of human papillomavirus–associated cervical disease. *Obstet Gynecol Clin North Am* 1993, 20:123–151.

Reid R: Laser therapy of human papillomavirus infections. In *Laser Surgery in Gynecology and Obstetrics*, edn 2. Edited by Keye W. Chicago: Year Book Publishers; 1989:46–99.

Reid R, Absten G: Lasers I gynecology: why pragmatic surgeons have not abandoned this valuable technology. *Lasers Surg Med* 1995 (in press).

CHAPTER 2

Vulvar Disease

Raymond H. Kaufman and Dale Brown, Jr

The topic of this chapter is the wide variety of pathologic disease involving the vulva. These include common infections (bacterial and viral), benign tumors, non-neoplastic epithelial disorders, invasive lesions, and invasive neoplasms. Paramount in the management of vulvar disease is correct diagnosis. Unfortunately, by the time many individuals with vulvar disease are seen by a gynecologist, they have already visited multiple physicians and have had a variety of treatment. Often in the patient with chronic symptoms, the medications are the cause of the problem, and discontinuation of all medication will result in the slow disappearance of symptoms.

Frequently, clinicians neglect to perform biopsies before initiating treatment. As a general rule, however, all lesions that cannot be readily diagnosed on the basis of history and physical examination should be biopsied. Many vulvar diseases cannot be diagnosed without histologic evaluation. Vulvar biopsy is an easily performed office procedure done under local anesthesia using a dermal punch. In the presence of bullous disease or persistent erosions, immunofluorescent staining of a tissue specimen is of value in establishing the diagnosis. If this is to be done, the biopsies should be taken just adjacent to the lesion so that an epithelial lining is present for examination. The specimen must be placed in special carrier solution and then brought to the laboratory for immediate examination in the fresh state.

This chapter is divided into seven sections consisting of benign solid tumors, benign cystic tymors, red lesions, white lesions, pigmented lesions, viral diseases, and miscellaneous diseases.

BENIGN SOLID TUMORS

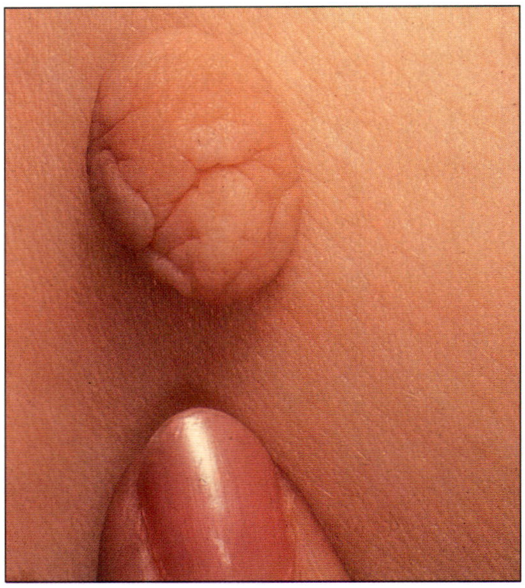

FIGURE 2-1.

Acrochordon. The acrochordon is a fleshy, polypoid tumor that is most often found on the upper, inner thighs, lateral labia majora, or mons pubis. It is often referred to as a fibroepitheial polyp or squamous papilloma. Microscopic examination reveals a covering of mature, slightly hyperkeratotic squamous epithelium. The underlying fibrous stroma is often slightly edematous. In most instances it is not necessary to remove the acrochordon unless it becomes irritated or inflamed secondary to friction.

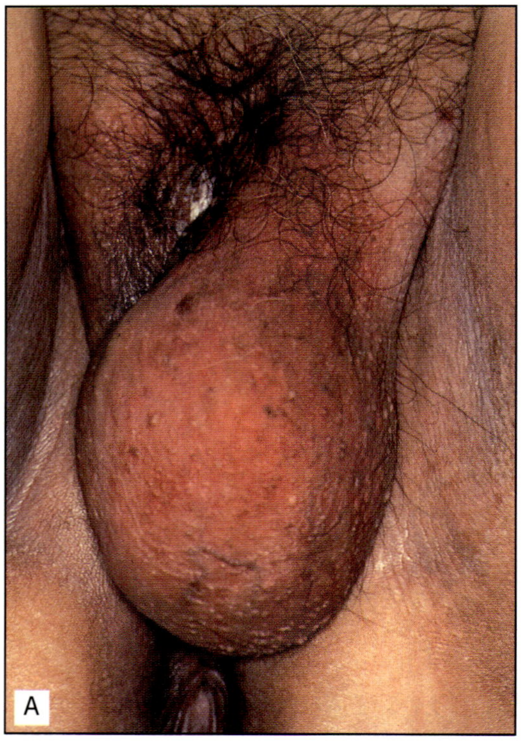

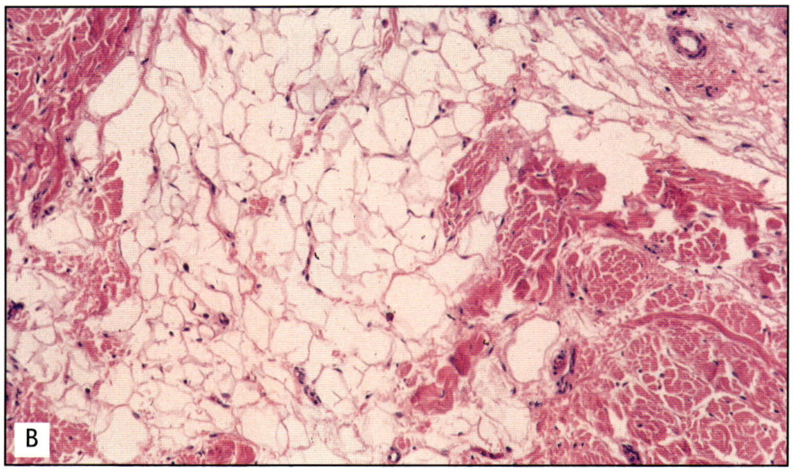

FIGURE 2-2.

Lipoma. **A**, A lipoma is a soft, polypoid structure that may be pedunculated or sessile and may vary in size. Because of their soft consistency on palpation, lipomas may often be confused with a vulvar cyst. **B**, A lipoma is composed of mature fat cells with strands of fibrous tissue dispersed between lobules of fat. Excision is the appropriate treatment for a large symptomatic lipoma. However, the majority of lipomas do not require removal.

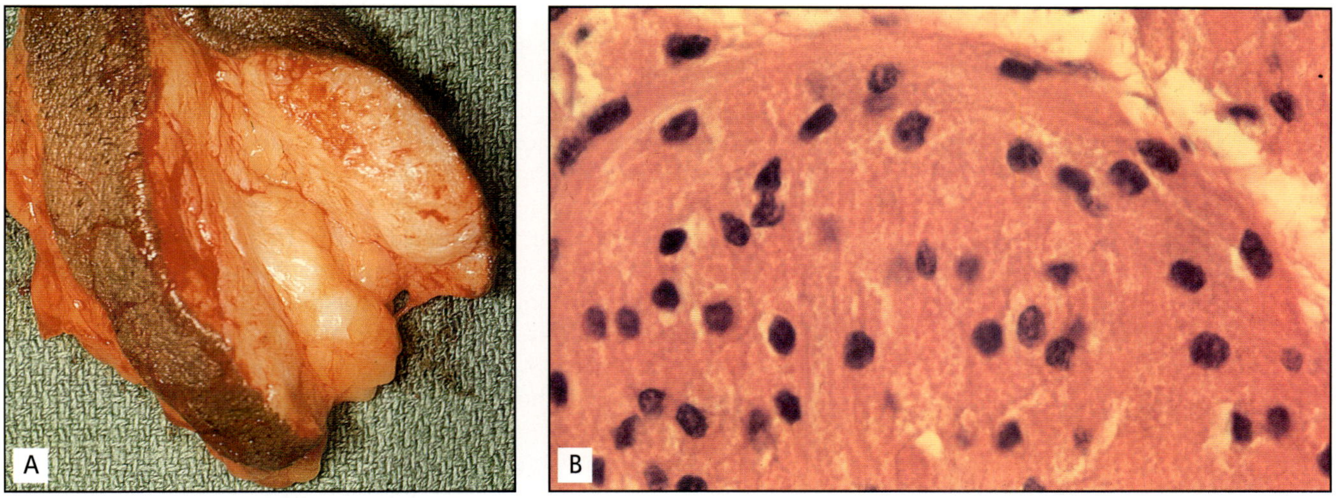

FIGURE 2-3.

Granular cell tumor. The granular cell tumor, often known as a granular cell myoblastoma is a relatively uncommon tumor that involves the vulva. It is a benign neoplasm with cells that tend to follow the course of nerve fibers, thus it frequently tends to recur if not adequately excised. The tumor usually lies deep within the subcutaneous tissue, but often encroaches on the overlying squamous epithelium (**A**). In this circumstance, there is often a response of the squamous epithelium leading to a pronounced pseudoepitheliomatous hyperplasia. Microscopically, this may give the appearance of an invasive squamous cell carcinoma which, in fact, it is not. When small, it is asymptomatic, but as it enlarges, it may encroach on the overlying squamous epithelium with ulceration and bleeding. The tumor is firm in consistency and on cross section has a yellow, white, fibrous appearance. Microscopic examination (**B**) reveals bundles of large eosinophilic-staining, round to polyhedral cells with indistinct cell borders. These clusters of cells are separated by bands of collagen fibers. The cytoplasm of the cells contains numerous small eosinophilic granules. The nuclei vary from small to large, are dark-staining, and centrally placed. The margins of the tumor are irregular and often one can see strands of tumor cells extending out into the adjacent tissue, especially following the pathway of nerve fibers. Treatment consists of wide local excision of the tumor. This should include at least 2 cm of normal-appearing skin and subcutaneous tissue surrounding the mass.

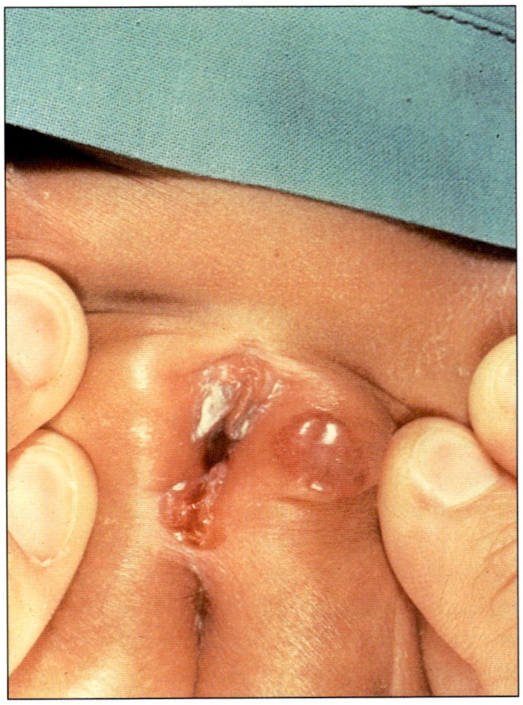

FIGURE 2-4.

Strawberry hemangioma. A variety of different types of hemangiomas may involve the vulva. The strawberry hemangioma is most commonly found in the infant. This is an elevated, red, soft tumor that may vary in diameter from a few millimeters to several centimeters. In early infancy it may rapidly grow and subsequently undergo spontaneous involution over several years. It often tends to ulcerate and bleed secondary to trauma. Microscopic examination reveals the presence of dilated, normal-appearing capillaries located in the upper dermis. Many newly formed vessels are also seen. Cryotherapy is an efficient form of treatment.

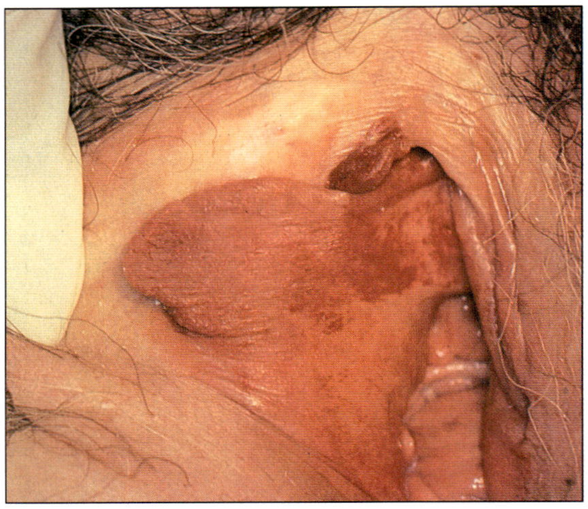

FIGURE 2-5.

Cavernous hemangioma. Cavernous hemangioma most often occurs during the first few months of life and increases in size until the child is 18 to 24 months of age. Thereafter, it usually remains static or begins to regress and even almost completely disappears. Those that tend to rapidly increase during the first few months of life are more likely to spontaneously involute. Cavernous hemangiomas involving the vulva are often multilobular and purple in color. They may vary significantly in size. The hemangioma may extend up into the vagina and the paravaginal tissues. Although these tumors are often quite extensive, in most instances they are asymptomatic. Microscopic examination reveals the presence of large, irregular, blood-filled spaces lined by a single layer of endothelial cells. The blood vessel walls are thickened by an overgrowth of adventitial cells. The vessels tend to ramify into the subcutaneous fat, underlying fascia, and muscle. In most cases, treatment should be expectant since attempted surgical removal can often be met with disastrous blood loss. The argon laser has proved to be effective in treating selected hemangiomas.

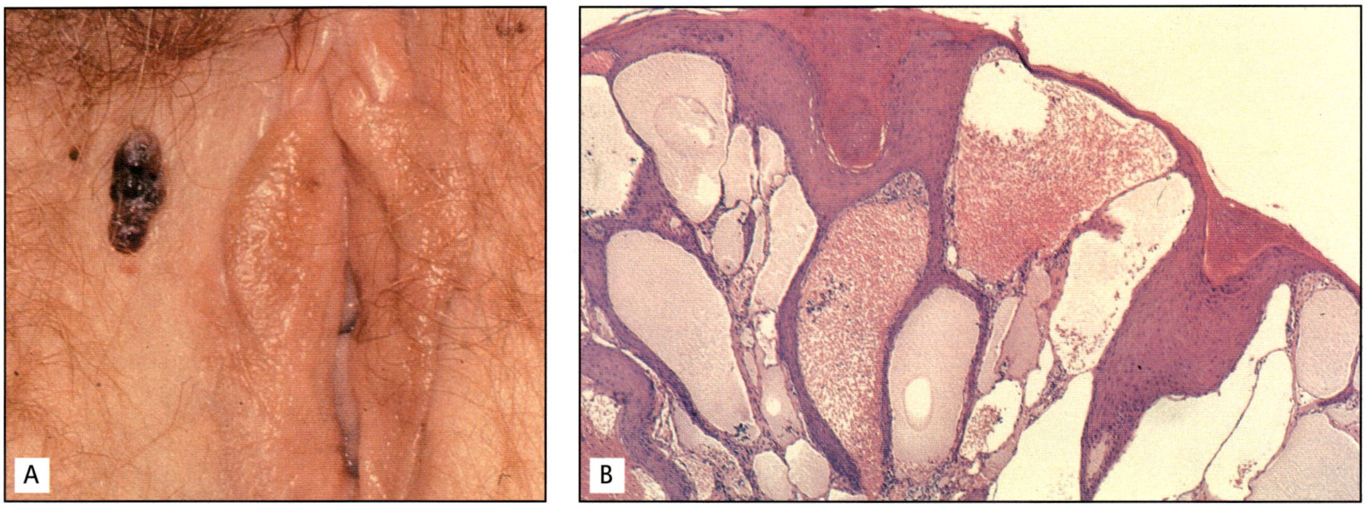

FIGURE 2-6.

Angiokeratoma. Angiokeratoma frequently involves the vulva. These tumors are usually single, but may be multiple, dark red to black, irregular, lobulated, papular structures (**A**). They seldom cause symptoms, however, when they are irritated or ulcerate, they may bleed. Microscopic examination reveals an epidermis thrown into irregular folds with hyperkeratosis and parakeratosis. There is irregular elongation of the rete pegs. The upper dermis contains dilated irregular capillaries very often located in the papillae and surrounded by a downward extension of the epidermis (**B**). The treatment consists of local excision. Often, this is done to establish the correct diagnosis.

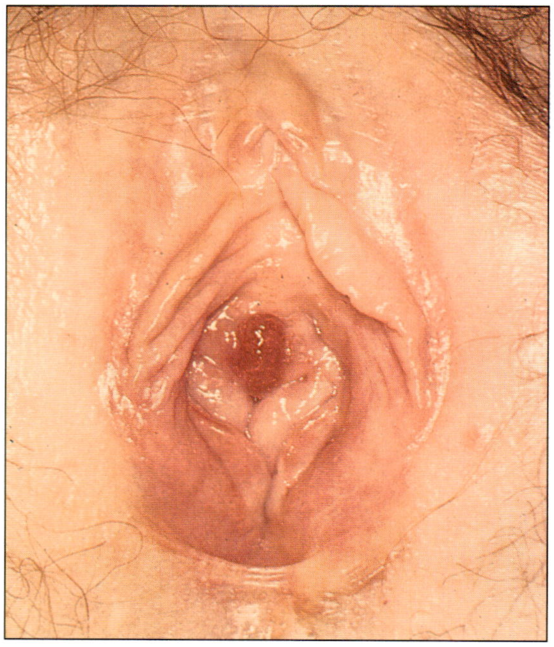

FIGURE 2-7.

Urethral caruncle. The urethral caruncle is found almost exclusively in the post menopausal woman. These tumors develop secondary to atrophy of vulvovaginal tissue with an ectropion of the posterior urethral wall. They usually present as red, fleshy, sometimes friable tumors located on the distal portion of the urethral orifice, as seen in the figure. They may vary in size from a few millimeters to as large as 1 cm in diameter. Although asymptomatic in most cases, occasionally they may be a source of postmenopausal bloody spotting. Biopsy is rarely indicated unless they do not regress with appropriate therapy or they continue to be symptomatic. In most instances, subjective complaints and bloody spotting can be controlled by the topical application of an estrogen cream to the vagina and urethra. Systemic estrogen may also be effective. If this therapy is not effective, the caruncle can be removed by local excision or cryocautery. Microscopic examination reveals loose connective tissue containing many dilated capillaries and inflammatory cells. The tumor is covered by a layer of either squamous or transitional epithelial cells. No treatment is required for small asymptomatic caruncles. If the patient is symptomatic, complaining of bleeding or discomfort, they can usually be adequately contolled, as noted above.

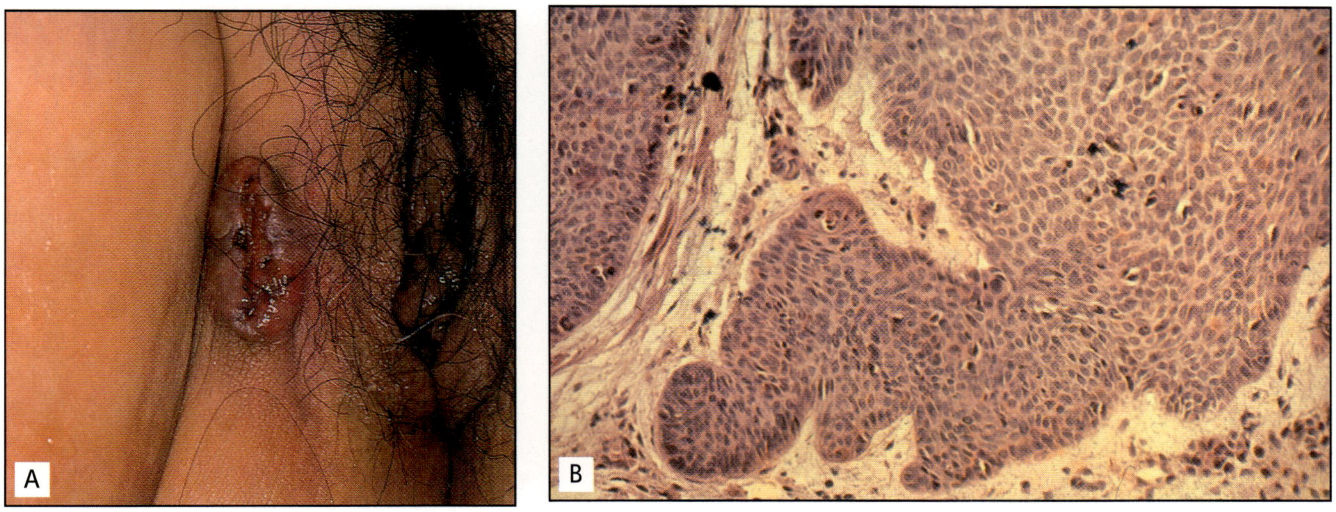

FIGURE 2-8.
Basal cell tumor. There are many who would place the basal cell tumor within the category of malignant diseases involving the vulva; however, this tumor rarely, if ever, metastasizes and is characterized by local extension of cells into the tissues adjacent to the tumor. Basal cell tumors constitute approximately 3% of neoplasms involving the vulva. They are most often seen in the postmenopausal woman and present as a slightly raised, slowly growing nodule which eventually develops central ulceration and a pearly, rolled border (**A**). Occasionally, they are nodular or polypoid. Microscopic examination reveals nests of closely packed, uniform, oval formed cells. These cells appear to arise from the basal layer of the epidermis or from a hair shaft. The masses of cells appear to be pushing into the underlying dermis and the advancing edge is usually lined by a layer of cells arranged in a radial fashion (peripheral palisading). The nuclei are deeply basophilic surrounded by a rim of cytoplasm (**B**). Basal cell tumors must be distinguished from squamous cell carcinoma, which can usually easily be done on the basis of the histopathology and the fact that the basal cell tumor cells appear to be pushing into the underlying dermis. There is retraction of the dermal tissue from the advancing cells, in contrast to invasive carcinoma in which the cells appear to be infiltrating into the stroma. Treatment consists of wide local excision.

BENIGN CYSTIC TUMORS

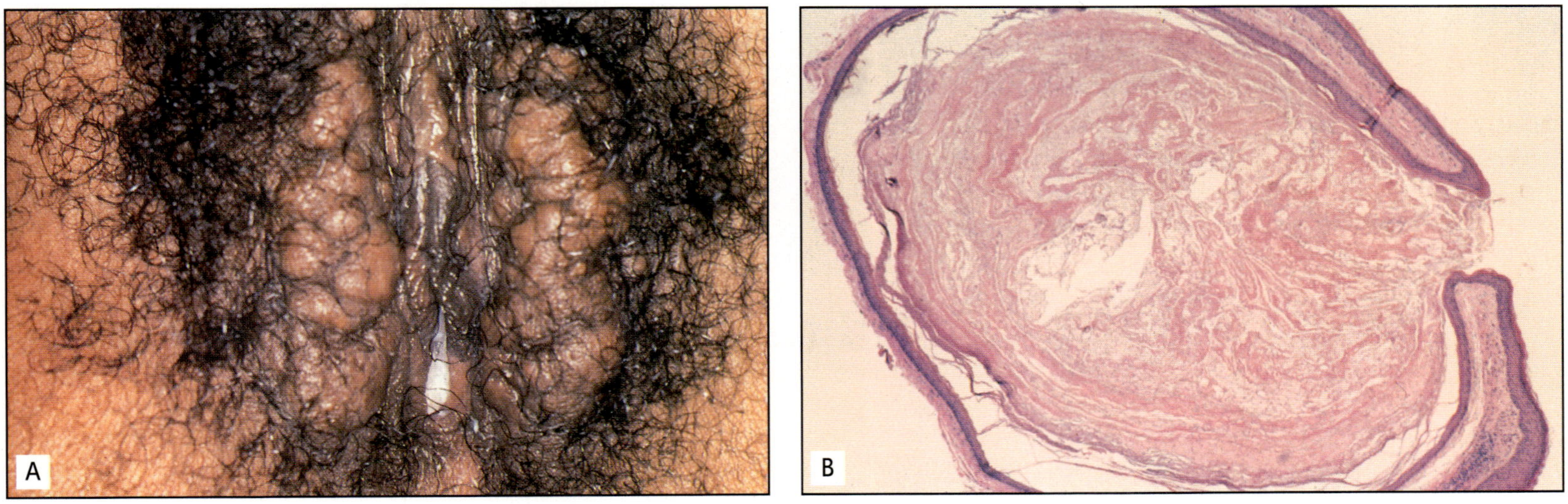

FIGURE 2-9.
Epidermal inclusion cyst. The epidermal inclusion cyst is probably the most common tumor found on the vulva. In the past, these cysts have often erroneously been referred to as sebaceous cysts. They arise most often from obstruction of a hair follicle with gradual distention and enlargement of the hair shaft. Occasionally, they arise secondary to trauma (*eg*, after an episiotomy). They may be seen as single or multiple cystic structures involving the vulvar skin (**A**). Microscopic examination reveals a lining of squamous epithelium (**B**). The cyst cavity frequently contains abundant desquamated squamous cells. In most instances, epidermal inclusion cysts of the vulva are asymptomatic and thus require no treatment. Occasionally, they become infected, and when this repeatedly occurs, they should be surgically excised. Likewise, if their presence is causing discomfort or the patient would like the cyst removed because of cosmetic reasons, they can usually be excised under local anesthesia in the office.

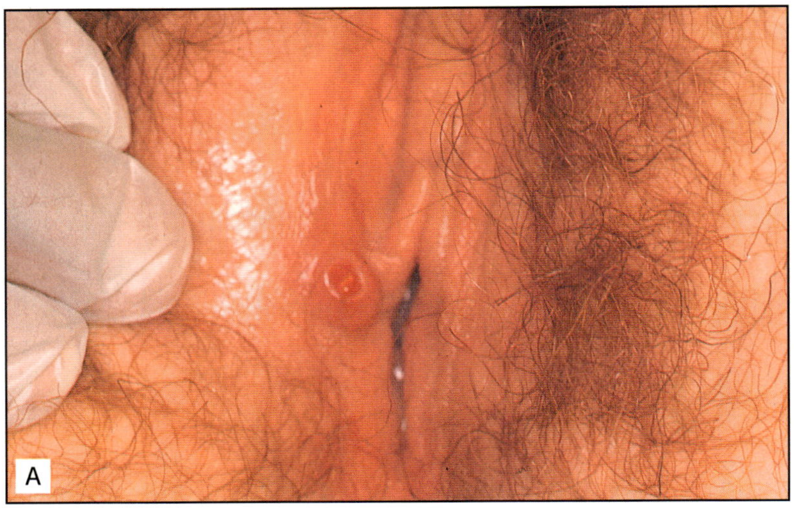

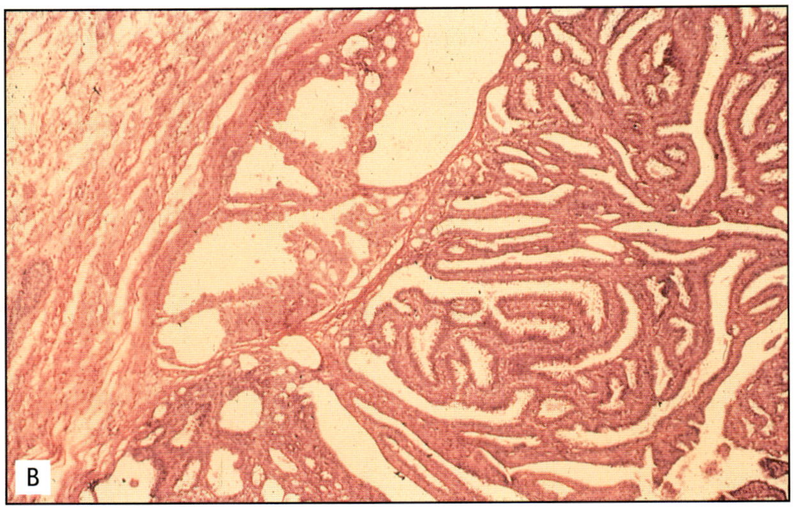

FIGURE 2-10.

Hydradenoma. Hydradenomas are believed to arise from apocrine sweat glands. However, there is some evidence to suggest that they may also arise from the eccrine glands. They are usually seen as sharply circumscribed, elevated nodules that most often are localized in the sulcus between the labium majus and minus. Rapid growth of the tumor may result in umbilication or even protrusion of the contents of the cyst onto the surface (**A**). Microscopic examination reveals an adenomatous pattern comprised of irregular tubules with papillary projections covered by a single layer of epithelial cells separated by fine connective tissue septi (**B**). Because of the pronounced glandular proliferation, the tumor may be mistaken for adenocarcinoma. The hydradenoma should easily be distinguished from carcinoma on the basis of the morphology. Local excision is adequate treatment.

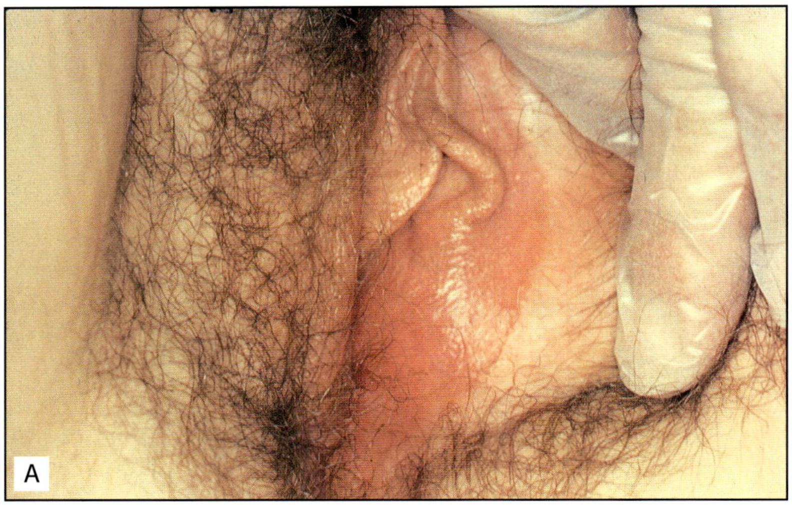

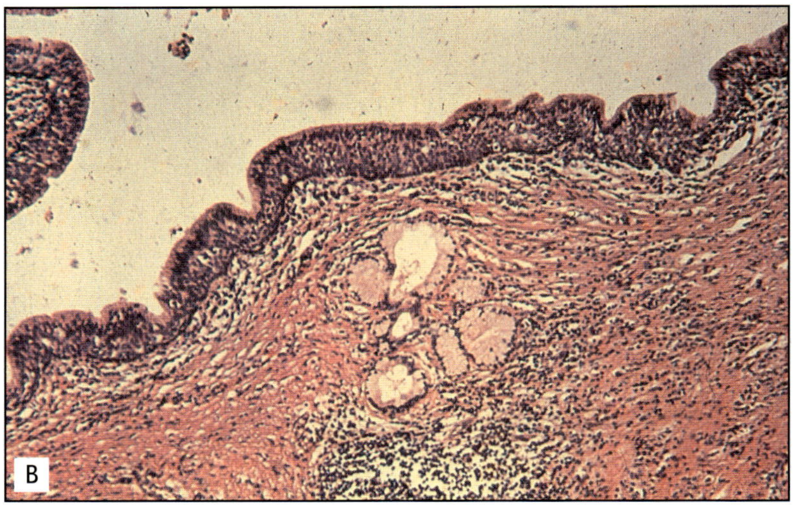

FIGURE 2-11.

Bartholin's duct cyst. This presents as a cystic mass that usually arises as a result of obstruction of Bartholin's duct. By extending a line down from the labia minora one can usually bisect the cyst (**A**). They are usually asymptomatic and require no treatment. Transitional epithelium lines the cyst (**B**). Marsupialization is performed when the patient is symptomatic or when treatment is required.

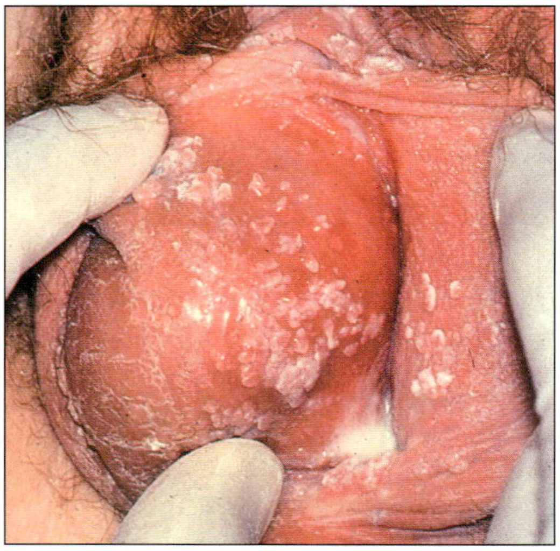

FIGURE 2-12.

Bartholin abscess. A Bartholin abscess presents as swelling with edema and redness located in the lower medial portion of the vulva near the insertion of Bartholin's duct into the vestibule. The abscess may become very large and cause associated cellulitis. Culture of the abscess contents usually reveals a mixed flora with *Escherichia coli* the predominant organism. They are infrequently related to gonococcal infection. Treatment involves incision and drainage with insertion of a Word catheter for approximately 6 weeks. This results in the formation of a new "os" for the Bartholin gland.

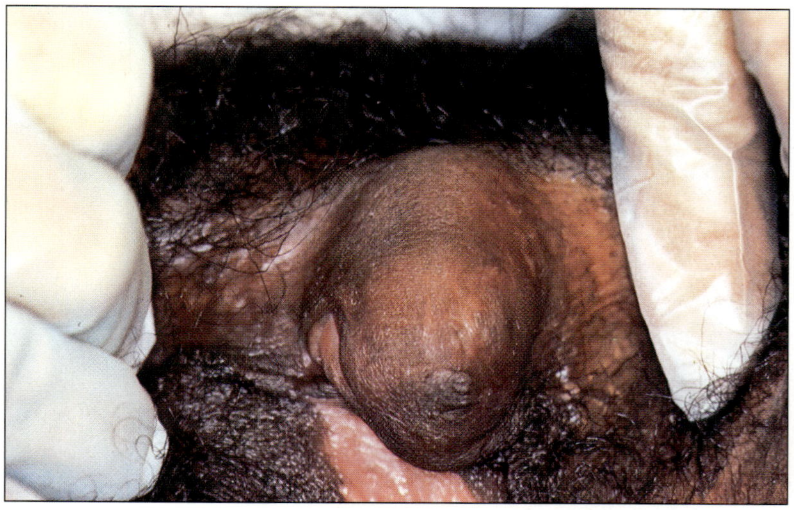

FIGURE 2-13.

Pilonidal cyst. The pilonidal cyst is usually found in the sacrococcygeal area. However, on occasion, it may be found involving the vulva. The cysts are most commonly located in the midline in the region of the clitoris and should be suspected in a patient with recurrent abscesses of the clitoris and periclitoral tissues. They usually present as swelling and pain in the region of the clitoris associated with erythema, induration, and tenderness when they become infected. The abscesses may spontaneously drain and occasionally a chronic draining sinus may be associated with a pilonidal cyst. The sinus tract is usually lined by squamous epithelium near the surface, but at a deeper level it may be lined by granulation tissue. The tract usually opens into an abscess with purulent exudate and hair. In the presence of an acute abscess and surrounding cellulitis, incision and drainage with associated antiobiotic coverage is adequate but only temporary treatment. Complete excision of the cyst and sinus tract must be carried out. If the entire sinus tract is not removed, recurrent enlargement and infection will occur.

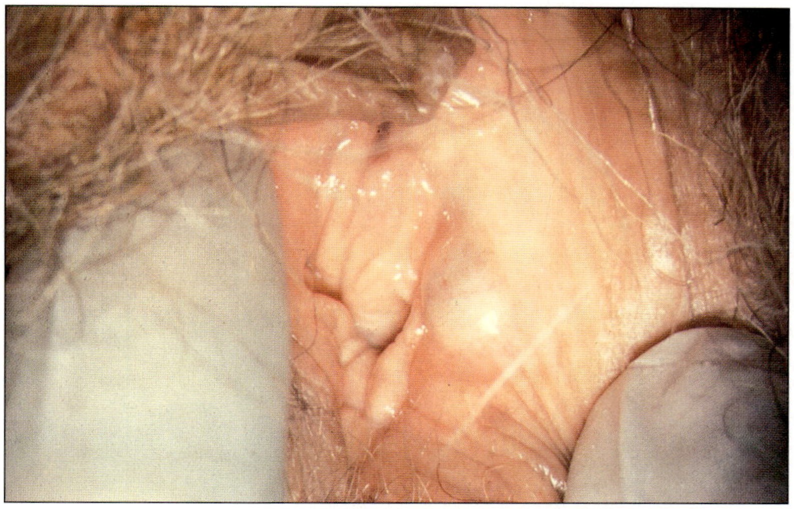

FIGURE 2-14.

Mucus cyst of the vestibule. Mucus cysts of urogenital sinus origin are usually found in the region of the vestibule including the inner labia minora. They are lined by a single layer of columnar epithelial cells that morphologically resemble the cells of the endocervix. Occasionally, metaplastic squamous epithelium is found lining portions of the cyst wall. Small asymptomatic cysts require no treatment. If they are large enough to cause discomfort to the patient they can be surgically excised.

RED LESIONS

INTRAEPITHELIAL NEOPLASTIC DISORDERS OF VULVAR SKIN AND MUCOSA

A. Squamous (may include HPV change)
  1. Vulvar intraepithelial neoplasia, (VIN) 1 (dysplasia, mild)
  2. VIN 2 (dysplasia, moderate)
  3. VIN 3 (dysplasia, severe; carcinoma *in situ*)

B. Other
  1. Paget's disease (intraepithelial)
  2. Melanoma *in situ* (level 1)

FIGURE 2-15.

Classification of vulvar intraepithelial neoplasia (VIN). Vulvar intraepithelial neoplasia has been classified by the Nomenclature Committee of the International Society for the Study of Vulvo-vaginal Diseases as shown in the table. HPV—human papillomavirus. (From Kaufman RH, Faro S. Benign Diseases of the Vulva and Vagina. Mosby Yearbook, St. Louis, 1994.)

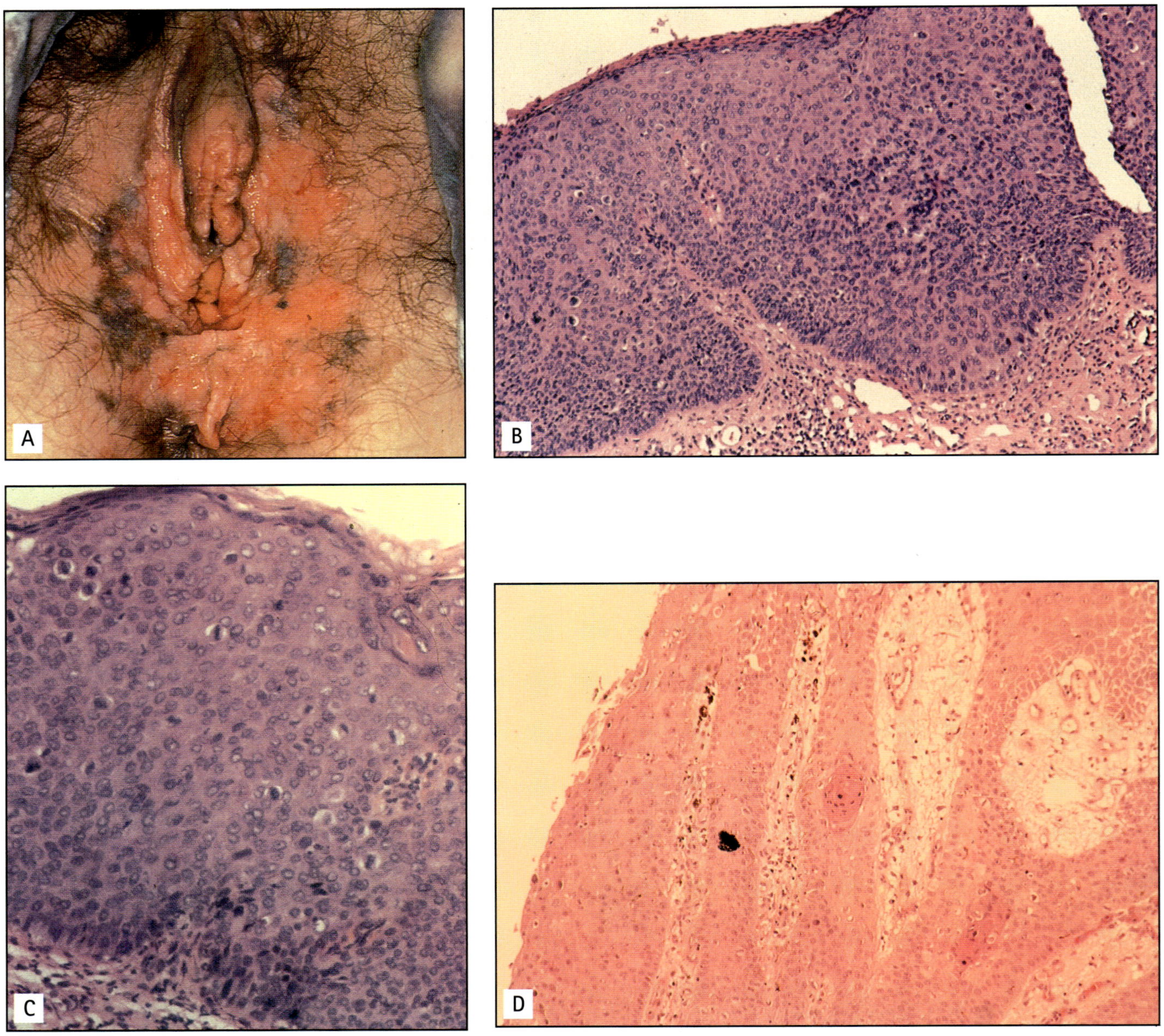

FIGURE 2-16.

Vulvar intraepithelial neoplasia (VIN). The gross appearance of VIN is usually quite distinct and should arouse the suspicion of the clinician. It may present as a red, white, or pigmented lesion or as all three combined. This photograph depicts an example of VIN 3 presenting as a red, pigmented lesion (**A**). The morphology of VIN is usually quite distinct, but there are several subtle differences among three described varieties. The first two, basaloid and warty, are believed to be human papillomavirus (HPV) related (most often HPV 16, but other high-risk HPV types may also be associated with VIN 3). The basaloid type of VIN 3 consists of a proliferation of basal-type cells extending through the full thickness of epithelium associated with the presence of atypical mitoses and nuclear variability (**B**). The warty type consists of a proliferation of cells with significant variability in size and shape of nuclei: large, irregular nuclei, cor ronds, and often koilocytes occur within the more superficial cells. The epithelium is often thrown into "spinelike" projections (**C**). A third well-differentiated variety of VIN 3 consists of a proliferation of more mature-appearing squamous cells revealing the presence of abnormal keratinization within the cytoplasm and some nuclear variability (**D**). This is not usually associated with HPV infection. It appears to be a relatively aggressive form of VIN commonly leading rapidly to the development of invasive squamous cell carcinoma. The treatment of VIN 3 depends on the size and location of the lesion and whether or not it is multifocal. The latter is a frequent finding. Mucosal lesions can usually be treated effectively using the carbon dioxide laser. On the skin (hair bearing surface), small, single lesions (less than 1 cm in diameter) can also usually be treated adequately with the laser; however those larger than 1 cm are best managed by wide local excision.

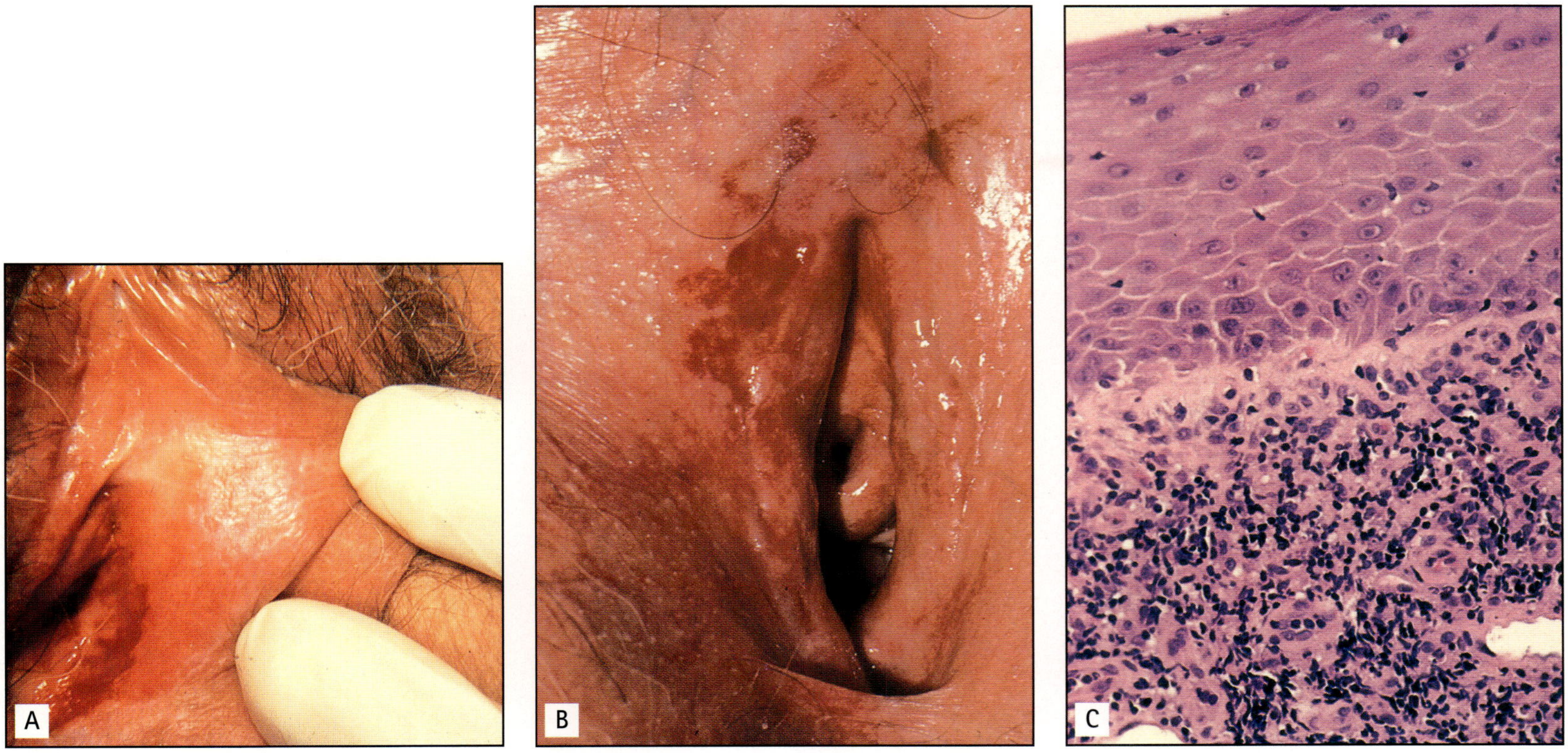

FIGURE 2–17.

Erosive lichen planus. Erosive lichen planus is an unusual variant of lichen planus, but is a relatively common papulosquamous disorder of unknown etiology. It presents as erosive or desquamative lesions that may involve some combination of the vulva, vaginal, or gingival surfaces. Fine, very subtle white lacy papules represent mild lichen planus of the vulva. The white lacy-curtain appearance is the result of reticulated Wickham's striae. Erosive disease in the vestibule or the introitus may be surrounded by white epithelium that may or may not be classically reticulated or lacy (**A**). Erythroplakic areas with varying degrees of epithelial desquamation or frank erosion are seen (**B**). Vulvar adhesions seen as anterior and posterior vestibular bands may contribute to stenosis of the introitus. Additionally, marked resorption of the labia minora and atrophy including obliteration of the clitoral hood may be seen, as also occurs in lichen sclerosus. The etiology is unknown. It is presumed to be a cell-mediated autoimmune phenomenon. The histopathology reveals the presence of an irregular epithelial hyperplasia and a bandlike lymphocytic infiltrate at the interface between the epithelium and the dermis (**C**). "Saw-tooth" elongation of the rete pegs may be seen. Civatte bodies that represent necrotic keratinocytes may be present in the epidermis or upper dermis. Acanthosis with a hyperkeratosis is usual. However, epithelial erosion may be present. The diagnosis is made by biopsy which should be performed in an area where the white reticulated border is observed if present.

Treatment of mild disease is a low midpotency topical steroid, *eg* hydrocortisone 1% (Hytone). For widespread desquamative, erosive vulvovaginal lichen planus, prednisone at a dosage of 40 to 70 mg daily for 2 to 6 weeks with an abrupt discontinuation may provide the patient with much needed relief. The daily use of intravaginal hydrocortisone suppositories (25 mg) is often effective. Treatment must be continued for a prolonged period of time (3 to 4 months) and then gradually decreased. Cytotoxic agents are reserved for extreme refractory cases.

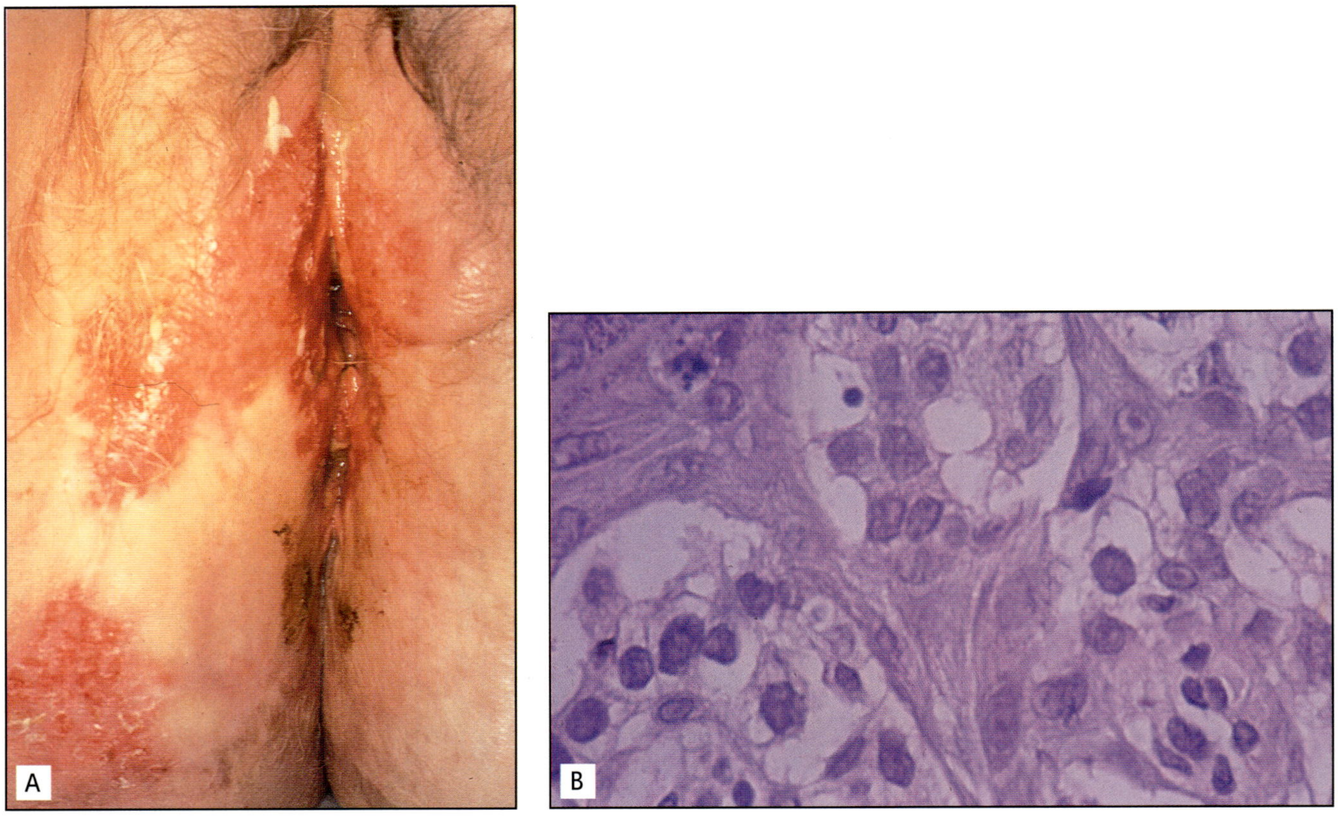

FIGURE 2-18.
Paget's disease. Paget's disease of the vulva is believed to arise from cells of apocrine derivation. It arises within the epidermis from epidermal cells having the potential to form apocrine glands. The appearance of Paget's disease is variable, but most typically is seen as an erythematous, exematoid lesion having a crusted or scaly surface (**A**). The microscopic appearance is characteristic consisting of the presence of large, irregular Paget cells which contain a clear vacuolated cytoplasm. The nuclei are vesicular and vary only slightly in size and shape. The cells are often seen in groups especially around the tips of epithelial folds (**B**) and may also be seen in adjacent skin appendages such as a hair shaft. Histochemical staining usually confirms the diagnosis of Paget's disease. The cells contain mucopolysaccarides which can be identified. The treatment of Paget's disease consists of wide local excision. It is important that an adequate amount of subcutaneous tissue be removed and thus underlying skin appendages are taken with the specimen. There is often intraepidermal migration of Paget cells beyond the visible lesion. Thus, even though excision may appear to be adequate (with free margins), local recurrences frequently occur.

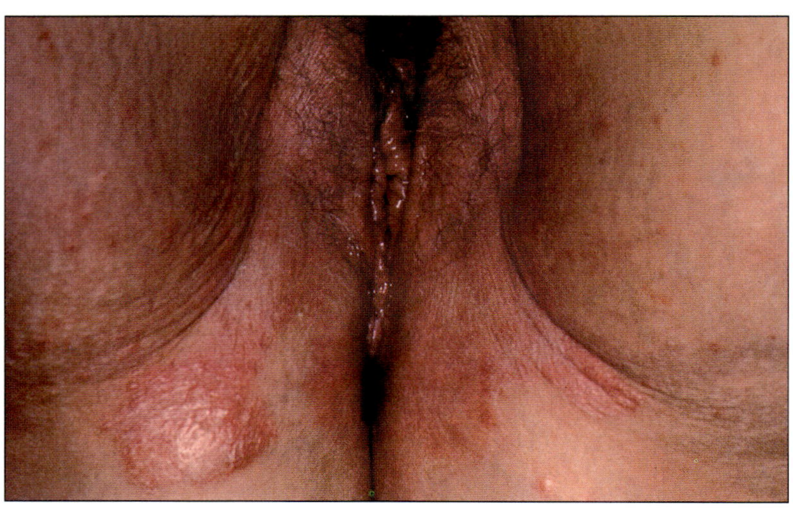

FIGURE 2-19.
Psoriasis. This is an inflammatory disease characterized by red scaling plaques covered with a dense silvery scale, as seen in the figure. Lesions have a predilection for areas of the scalp, elbows and knees, and gluteal cleft. They may appear well circumscribed, or plaques may become confluent and be less well demarcated. When located on the vulva they usually occur on the hair-bearing portion. As a result of heat, moisture and friction, lesions may resemble a fungal infection, such as cutaneous candidiasis. Patients may complain of pruritus or be asymptomatic.

Etiology is felt to be a multifactorial genetic disorder in which there appears to be some disordered immunity. Both environmental and genetic factors are apparently required to influence clinical expression of the disease. The course of psoriasis exhibits waxing and waning of activity. Local care of the genital area is necessary because of the maceration, erosion, and supraimposed infection that can occur as the result of incompletely removed fecal material and urine. The vulva should be kept dry allowing good aeration of the skin folds. Involvement of the genital area is usually controlled by topical corticosteroid therapy.

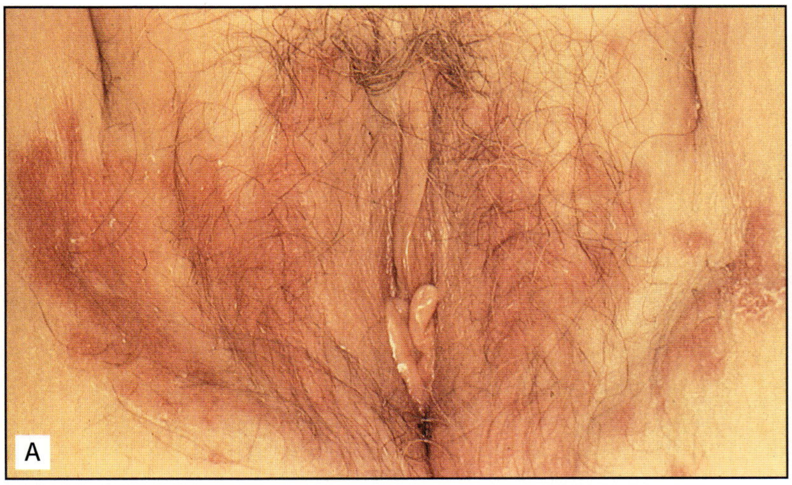

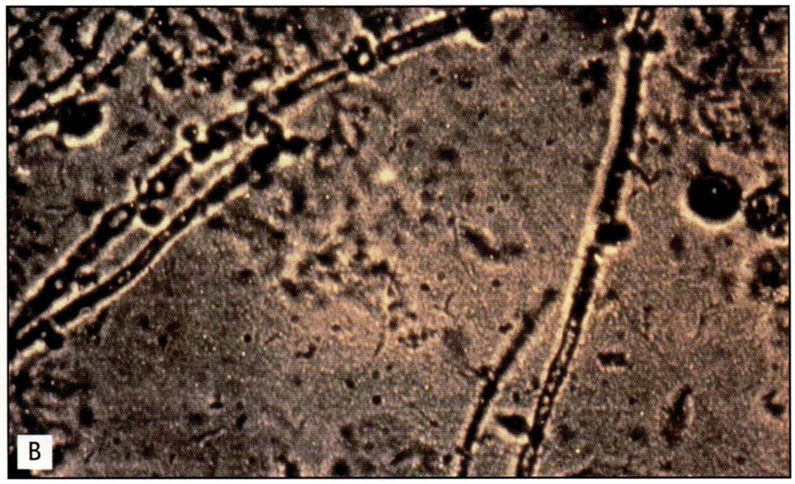

FIGURE 2-20.

Cutaneous candidiasis. Cutaneous candidiasis may be seen with or without an associated vaginal candidiasis. The patient most commonly presents with a complaint of vulvar pruritus but burning may occasionally be the symptom that brings the patient to the physician. Diffuse hyperemia involving the outer labia minora and labia majora is seen. This may extend to the crural folds. The presence of "satellite" lesions —small pustules surrounded by hyperemia—is often a clue to the nature of the problem (**A**). Diagnosis is confirmed by taking a scraping from the lesion that is placed in 15% to 20% potassium hydroxide and then examined under the microscope (**B**). Treatment with a topical antifungal cream twice daily for 2 weeks associated with the use of an oral anitfungal agent is usually very effective.

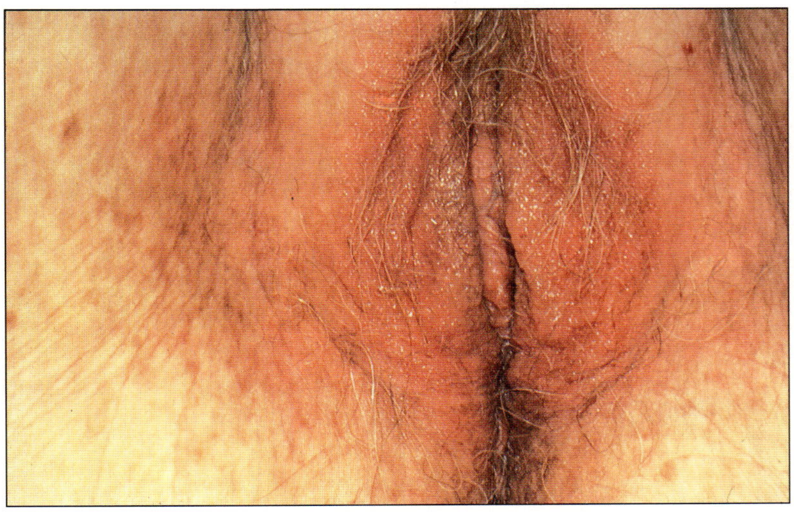

FIGURE 2-21.

Contact dermatitis. This is an eruption or erosion that occurs from direct contact with a substance that is either irritating or specifically allergenic. Symptoms are soreness or burning if on the basis of an irritant exposure. Itching is more associated with an allergic contact. Acute contact dermatitis manifests by blistering due to an intense edema. When the contact is an irritant there exists a chemical or thermal burn. When the contact is allergenic, the result is vesiculation as seen in poison ivy or poison oak. Chronic contact dermatis is manifested by redness, scaling, and often thickening or lichenification, as seen in the figure. Treatment consists of the discontinuation of all irritants. The use of wet soaks of 15% to 20% Burow's solution for immediate relief of symptoms followed by the application of a topical 0.1% corticosteroid ointment, *eg*, triamcinolone twice daily, is usually effective . If the contact reaction is allergic in nature the above approach will often be successful, but occasionally systemic steroids are required. Nighttime sedation for itching or pain may be needed (*eg*, hydroxyzine [Atarax] 25–50 mg every night at bedtime).

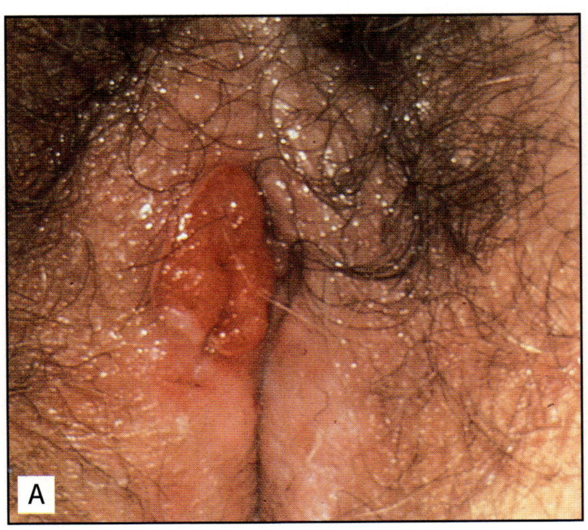

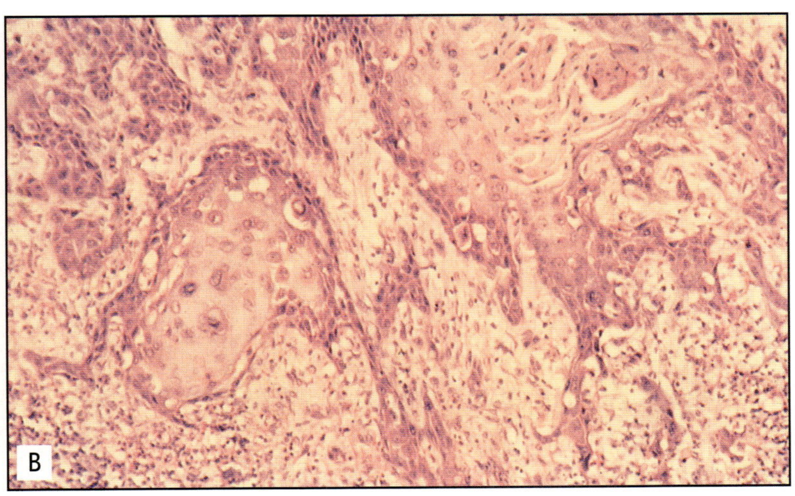

FIGURE 2-22.

Squamous cell carcinoma. Squamous cell carcinoma often presents as a raised, granular, red, firm lesion. The gross appearance (**A**) should immediately arouse the clinician's suspicion and a biopsy should be taken immediately from the edge of the lesion. It frequently is seen in association with lichen sclerosus as depicted in this photograph. Histopathology reveals sheets of squamous cells infiltrating the dermis (**B**). Usually, the cells are well differentiated with abnormal keratinization seen within the cell cytoplasm often leading to the formation of "keratin pearls." Less well differentiated lesions demonstrate the presence of neoplastic cells with nuclei that vary significantly in size and shape and show little, if any, cellular keratinization. Treatment of squamous cell carcinoma of the vulva should be performed by a gynecologic oncologist.

CLASSIFICATION OF NON-NEOPLASTIC EPITHELIAL DISORDERS OF THE VULVA

Lichen sclerosus

Squamous cell hyperplasia (formerly hyperplastic dystrophy)

Other dermatoses

FIGURE 2-23.

Classification of non-neoplastic vulvar epithelial disorders. The non-neoplastic epithelial disorders of the vulva have been recently classified by the Nomenclature Committee of The International Society for the Study of Vulvo-vaginal Disease as shown in the table. Since lichen sclerosus and squamous cell hyperplasia most often present as white lesions, they are listed under this category.

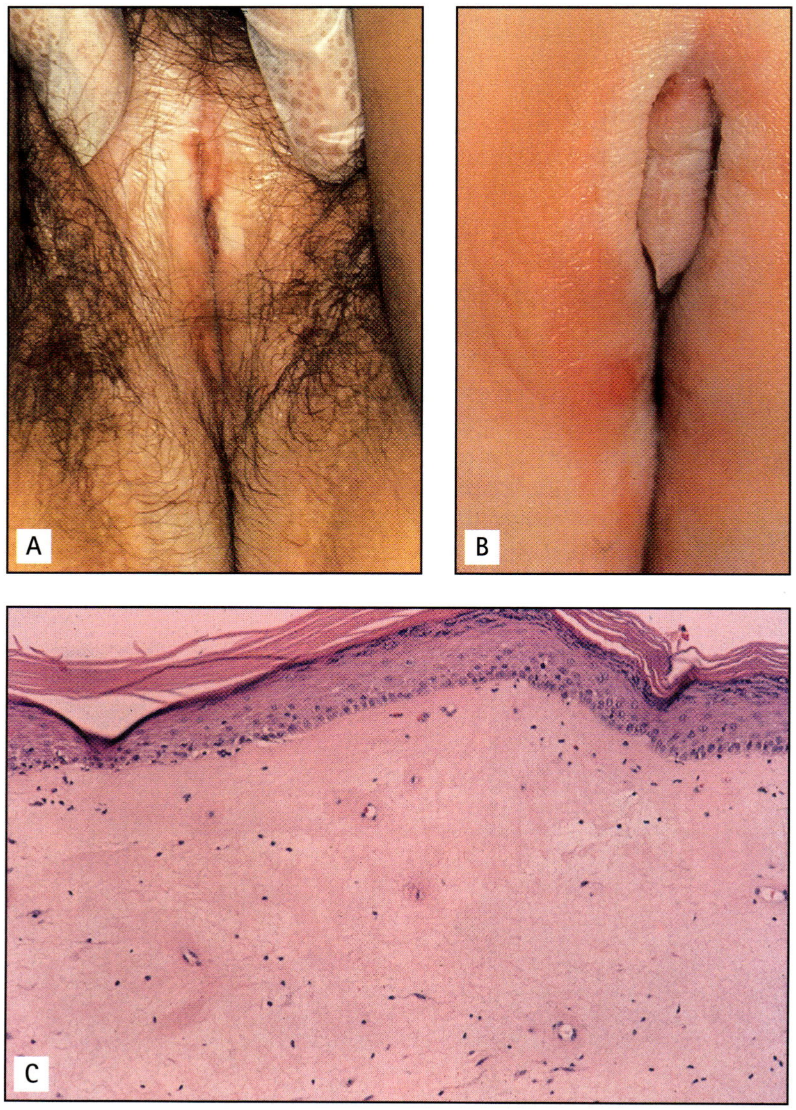

FIGURE 2-24.

Lichen sclerosus. Lichen sclerosus is usually found in women older than 50 years of age. It has a strong predilection for genital skin. The majority of patients complain of itching (greater than 95%), irritation, burning, dyspareunia, tearing, bleeding, fissuring, and discharge. Pruritus is most likely the result of degeneration and inflammation of terminal nerve endings. Dyspareunia may be a result of shrinkage of the introitus. The classic appearance is well-demarcated white plaques of thin, fragile skin that may appear smooth without skin regularities, having a "cigarette-paper" or parchment-like appearance. Extension may be in a figure-of-8 configuration involving the clitoris, labia majora, labia minora, perineum, and perianal area (**A**). Resorption of the labia minora may occur. The irregular keratotic papules appear white as a result of hydration. Lichen sclerosus is occasionally seen in children (**B**). It may regress as the child becomes older, but the majority continue to demonstrate changes until adulthood. Remission may occur in pregnancy. Microscopic findings reveal epithelial thinning with flattening of the rete pegs. Beneath the epidermis is a relatively acellular zone of homogenized pink-staining, collagenous-appearing tissue, in which edema is occasionally seen (**C**).

Treatment of lichen sclerosus is clobetasol (a synthetic fluorinated corticosteroid) 0.05% applied twice daily for 1 month, once daily for 2 months, then twice weekly for 3 months. Thereafter it may be used on an as-needed basis, but not more often than once or twice a week. Those patients who have phimosis or fissuring may gain relief with the use of 2% testosterone ointment applied once or twice daily for 2 to 4 weeks. Antihistamines may be needed to control nighttime itching.

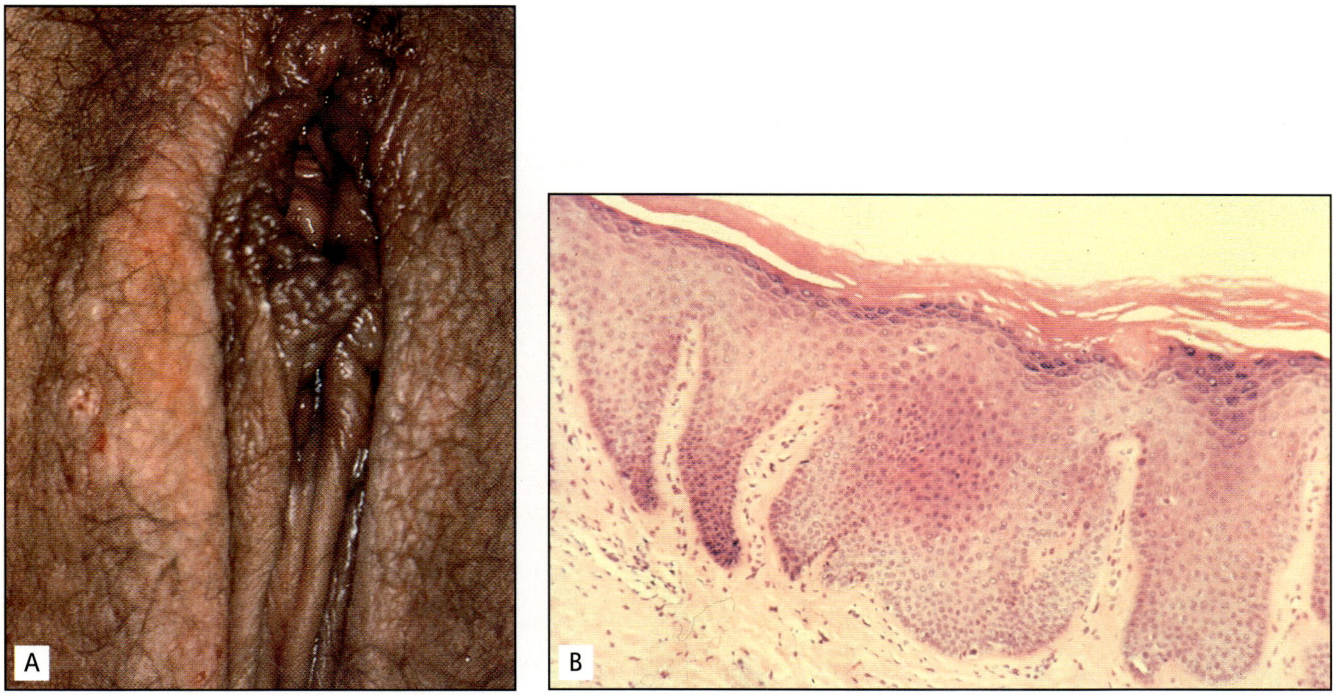

FIGURE 2-25.

Squamous cell hyperplasia. Squamous cell hyperplasia probably represents lichen simplex chronicus. Primary symptoms are that of itching, which may worsen at night. Inspection may reveal localized, elevated, well-defined or poorly defined white or even red plaques with superimposed features of epithelial disruption. Evidence of weeping, crust formation, or yellow scale may be seen. Margination between diseased and nondiseased skin tends to be *indistinct*. Lichenification is often present and is recognized as a palpable thickness with accentuation of the normal cross-hatch-type skin markings (**A**). Microscopic findings reveal a variable increase in the thickening of the horny layer (hyperkeratosis) with irregular thickening of the malpighian layer (acanthosis). Lengthening and the distortion of the rete pegs are present. A variable inflammatory reaction may be seen in the dermis consisting of lymphocytes and plasma cells (**B**). Diagnosis is confirmed by biopsy.

Treatment of squamous cell hyperplasia consists of topical therapy, generally clobetasol propionate .05% (Temovate) applied twice daily until symptoms resolve, then fluocinolone acetonide 0.025% or 0.01% daily or as needed. Antihistamines usually are needed to control nighttime itching. Squamous cell carcinoma has been found to develop in association with either lichen sclerosus or squamous cell hyperplasia in about 3% to 5% of cases. Patients should be followed on a 6-month basis, and whenever any unusual thickness, granularity, or discoloration occurs biopsy should be obtained.

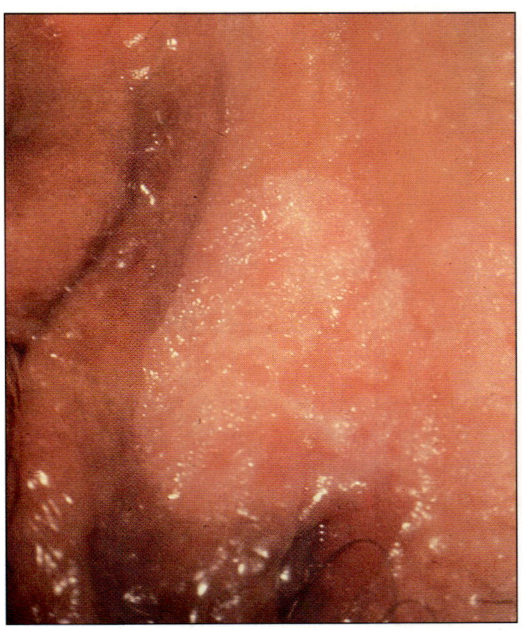

FIGURE 2-26.

Vulvar intraepithelial neoplasia (VIN-3)—white lesion. VIN can also present as a white lesion. The discussion regarding etiology, histopathology, and treatment has been presented earlier in the section on red lesions.

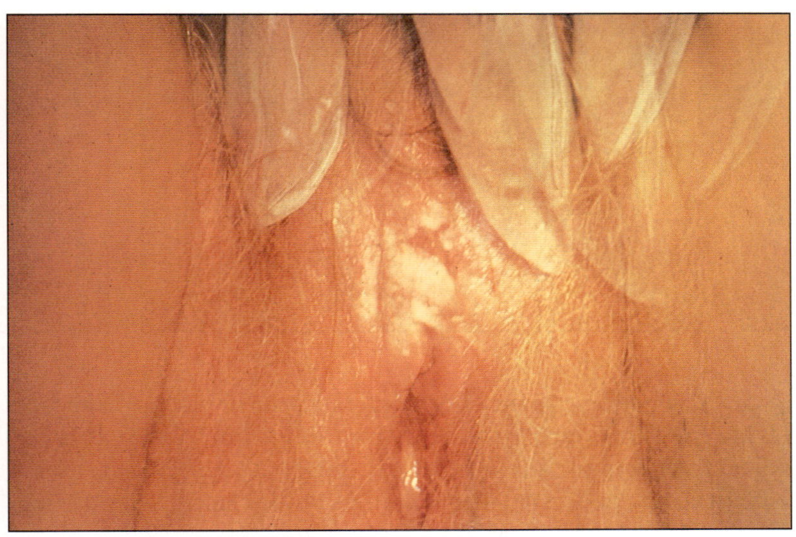

FIGURE 2-27.

Squamous cell carcinoma. Although invasive squamous cell carcinoma of the vulva usually is seen as a red, granular, firm lesion involving the vulva, it may also present as a white lesion. This is especially true when seen in association with vulvar intraepithelial neoplasia presenting as a white lesion. The figure demonstrates a diffuse, thickened white apearance to the vulvar tissue. On biopsy, this revealed invasive squamous cell carcinoma.

PIGMENTED LESIONS

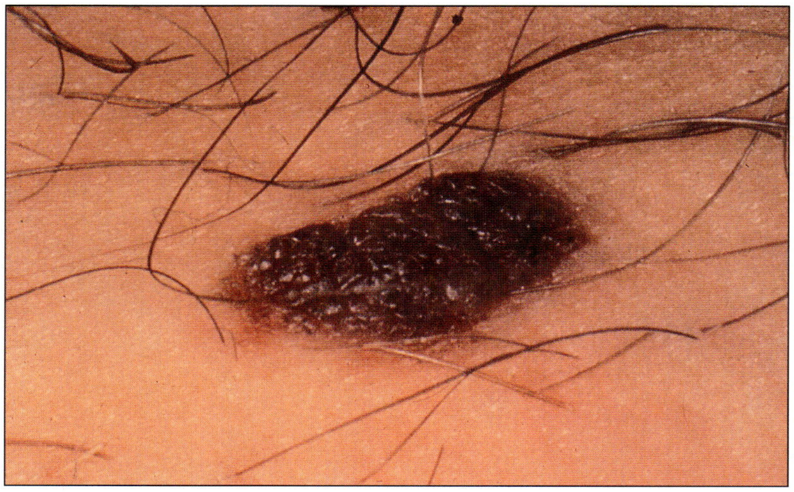

FIGURE 2-28.
Nevus. A variety of pigmented lesions involve the vulva. These include the nevus (shown in this figure), vulvar intraepithelial neoplasia, seborrheic keratosis, melanosis, and melanoma. As a general principle, it is probably wise to biopsy all pigmented lesions one sees on the vulva unless the clinician is absolutely sure of the diagnosis—which is rarely the case.

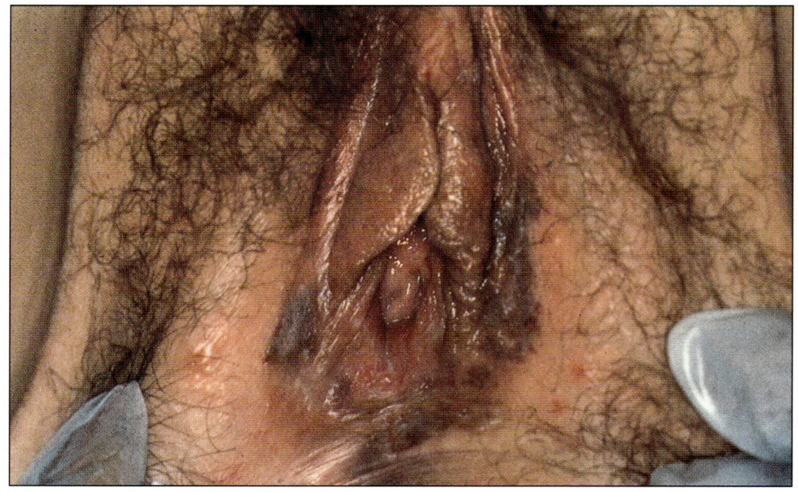

FIGURE 2-29.
Vulvar intraepithelial neoplasia (VIN-3)—pigmented lesion. As already discussed, VIN 3 may present as a pigmented (shown in the figure), red, or white lesion. The pigmented form of VIN frequently presents as isolated, slightly elevated, rounded papules and many dermatologists use the term *bowenoid papulosis* to describe this lesion. In the male, this lesion frequently develops rapidly and spontaneously regresses. In our experience, however, this rarely occurs in the female. Biopsy confirms the diagnosis. The cause is almost invariably human papillomavirus related. The histopathology and management of VIN has been discussed in the earlier section on red lesions.

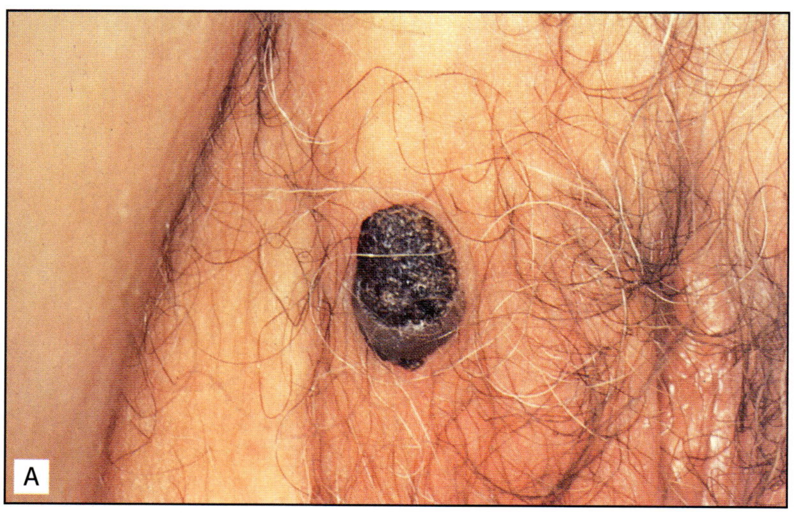

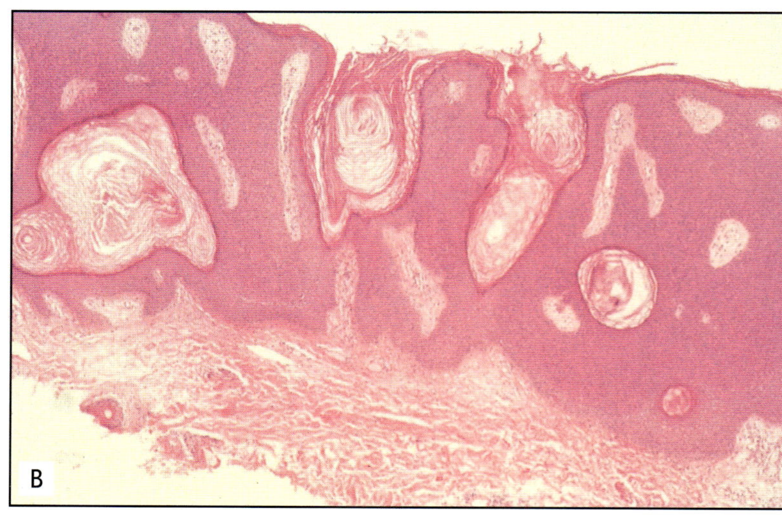

FIGURE 2-30.
Seborrheic keratosis. Seborrheic keratosis is most often seen in older women involving the trunk, face, neck, and arms. Occasionally, a lesion appears on the vulva usually as a solitary, raised, sharply circumscribed verrucous lesion (**A**). The lesions may vary from flesh-colored to black, although most are dark brown and have a greasy appearance. They have the appearance of being pasted to the skin surface. Microscopic examination reveals marked hyperkeratosis, acanthosis, and papillomatosis. The epidermal cells appear to grow upward with the lower borders of the tumor lying above a line drawn between the normal skin on each side of the tumor. The tumor usually consists of solid sheets of epithelial cells surrounding connective tissue. The keratin often invaginates into the lesion forming cystic inclusions of keratinized material (**B**). If the diagnosis is apparent, no treatment is required, however, excision biopsy is usually warranted primarily to establish the diagnosis. This can usually be done in the office under local anesthesia.

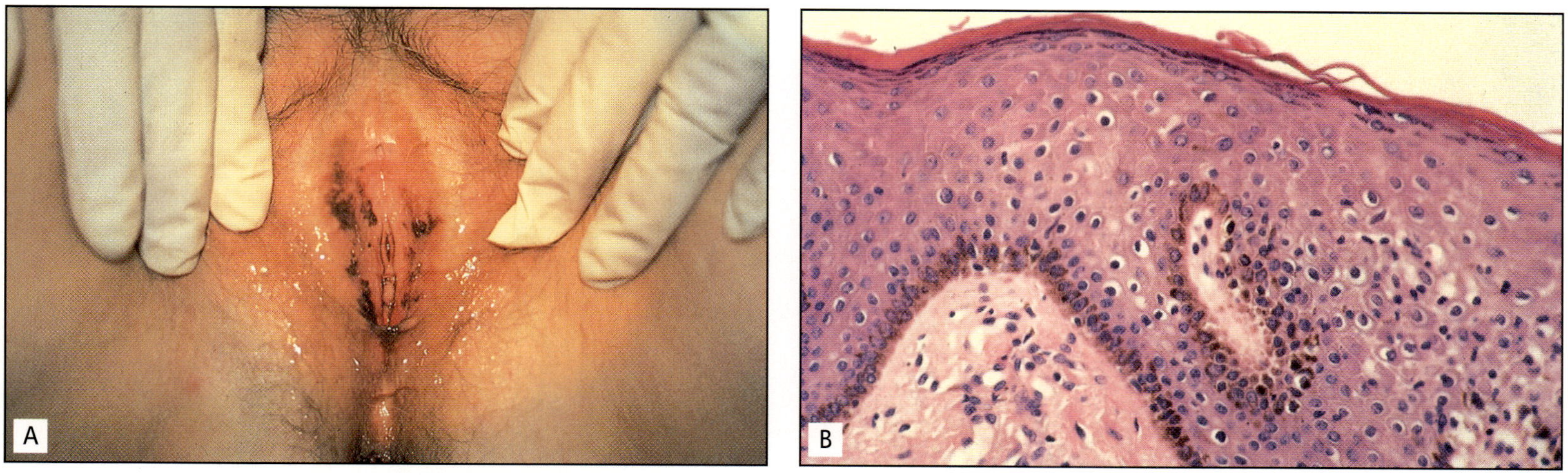

FIGURE 2-31.

Melanosis. Melanosis of the vulva is frequently confused with a junctional nevus or melanoma. It presents as a pigmented patch that is flat and smooth (**A**). It may be seen as small, focal areas or as a large macular, pigmented area. Similiar findings may occasionally be noted in the vagina. Microscopic examination reveals an increased number of typical melanocytes arranged at the dermal-epidermal junction of a hyperpigmented epidermis (**B**). They are perfectly benign and have no relationship to melanoma.

BRESLOW STAGING SYSTEM FOR MELANOMA

Level	Thickness, *mm*
1	0–0.75
2	0.76–1.5
3	1.6–3
4	3.1–4
5	Over 4

FIGURE 2-32.

Melanoma—Breslow staging. Of critical importance is the depth of invasion of the melanoma and currently most pathologists use the Breslow staging system (as shown in the figure) or a modification of it. Survival is directly related to the depth of invasion. Level 1 and 2 melanomas have an excellent prognosis, whereas level 4 and 5 melanomas have an extremely poor outlook.

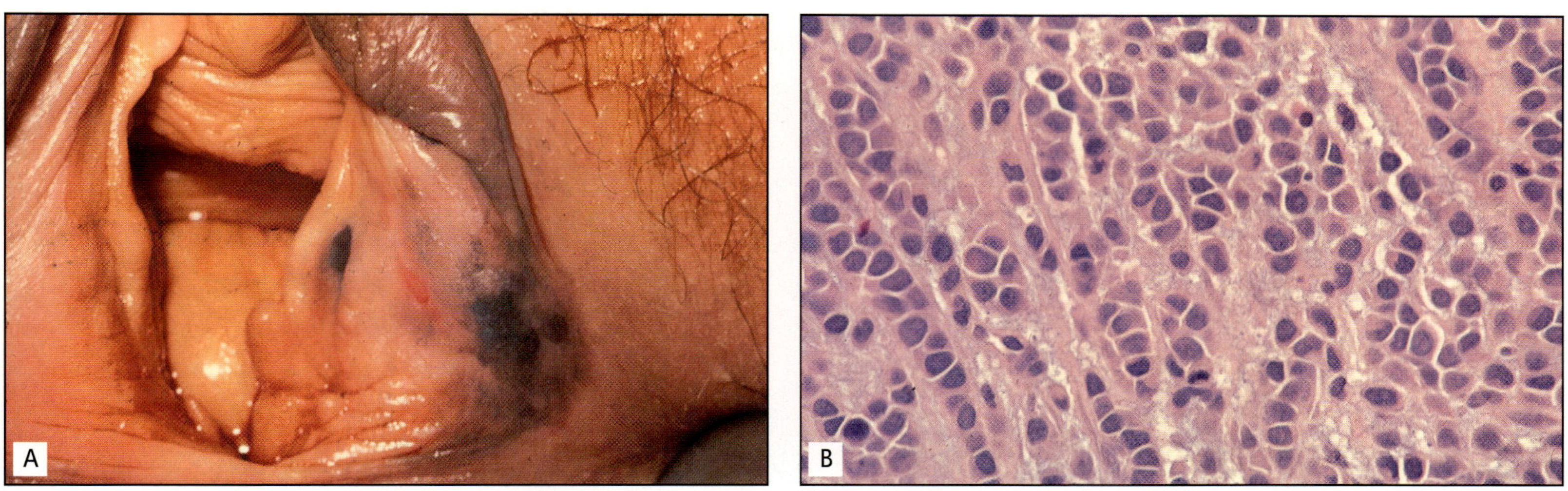

FIGURE 2-33.

Melanoma. Melanoma of the vulva occurs infrequently and constitutes from 1% to 3% of malignant vulvar tumors. It usually presents as a darkly pigmented, asymmetric, irregular lesion and may take one of two forms: the nodular melanoma which extends rapidly and deeply into the underlying tissue, or the superficial spreading melanoma which tends to spread peripherally and invades the underlying tissue in a slower fashion than does the nodular variety. Melanoma often tends to be multifocal; multiple pigmented areas may be seen on the vulva, which reveal melanoma on biopsy (**A**). Microscopic examination demonstrates the presence of sheets of neoplastic cells with nuclei that are large and irregular and that occasionally contain melanin pigment (**B**). If these changes are limited strictly to the epithelium, they are considered the equivalent of melanoma *in situ* (level 1). Another term occasionally used for this is atypical melanocytic hyperplasia. Therapy of melanoma has changed significantly in the past several years. Whereas ultraradical surgery was used in the past, this is no longer the case. Wide local excision of the tumor removing adequate margins (up to 3 cm of normal tissue), as well as subcutaneous tissue down to the fascia, is appropriate treatment. The regional lymph nodes on the side of the tumor should also be removed primarily for prognostic reasons, since once lymph node metastases have occurred, the prognosis is extremely poor.

VIRAL DISEASES

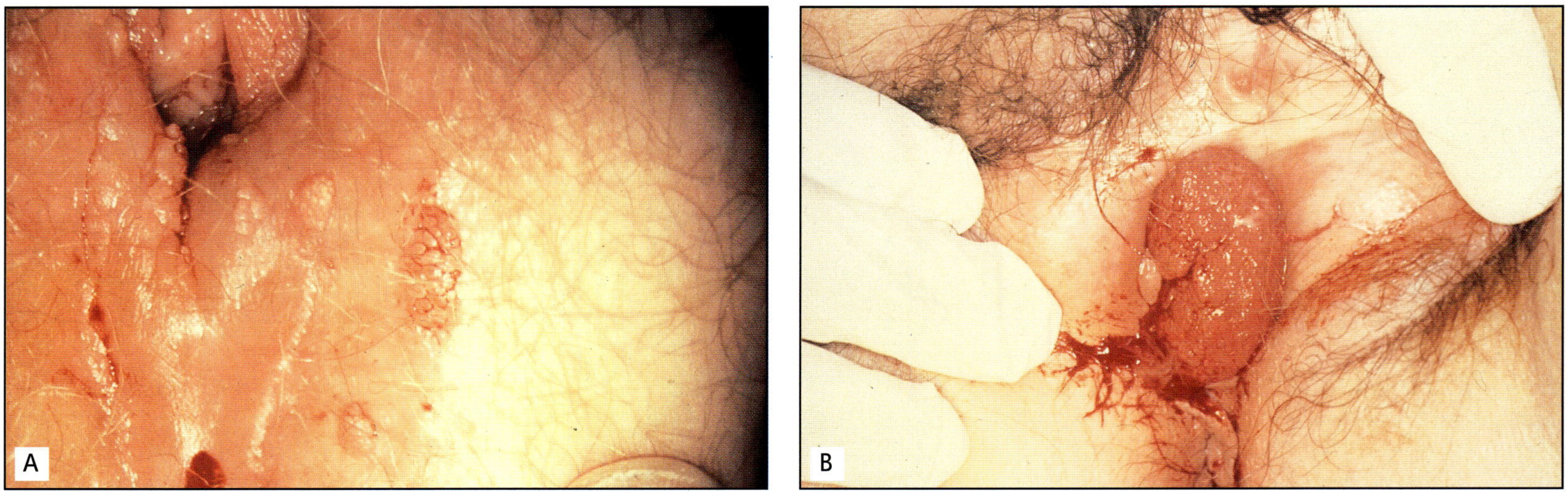

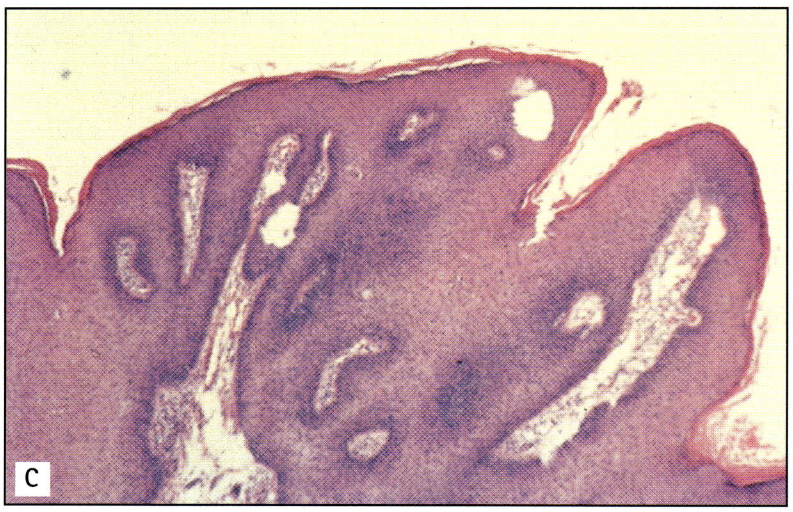

FIGURE 2-34.

Condylomata acuminata. Condylomata acuminata are caused by the human papillomavirus (HPV)—usually HPV 6 or 11. The gross appearance of a condyloma acuminatum varies significantly from a solitary, raised, irregular papillary lesion to multiple lesions (**A**).

The condyloma of Buschke and Lowenstein (verrucous carcinoma) is also a form of condyloma associated with HPV 6. This presents as a large, single, sessile, cauliflower-like lesion that may involve extensive areas of the vulva and may resemble an invasive carcinoma although it does not metastisize (**B**). The histopathology of condyloma acuminatum reveals a markedly thickened squamous epithelium forming numerous papillary folds around stalks of connective tissue. Acanthosis, elongation of the epithelial folds, papillomatosis, a variable degree of parakeratosis and hyperkeratosis, and an inflammatory infiltrate within the dermis are seen (**C**). The more superficial cells may demonstrate the presence of koilocytes. Treatment of condylomata acuminata is discussed in Chapter 1.

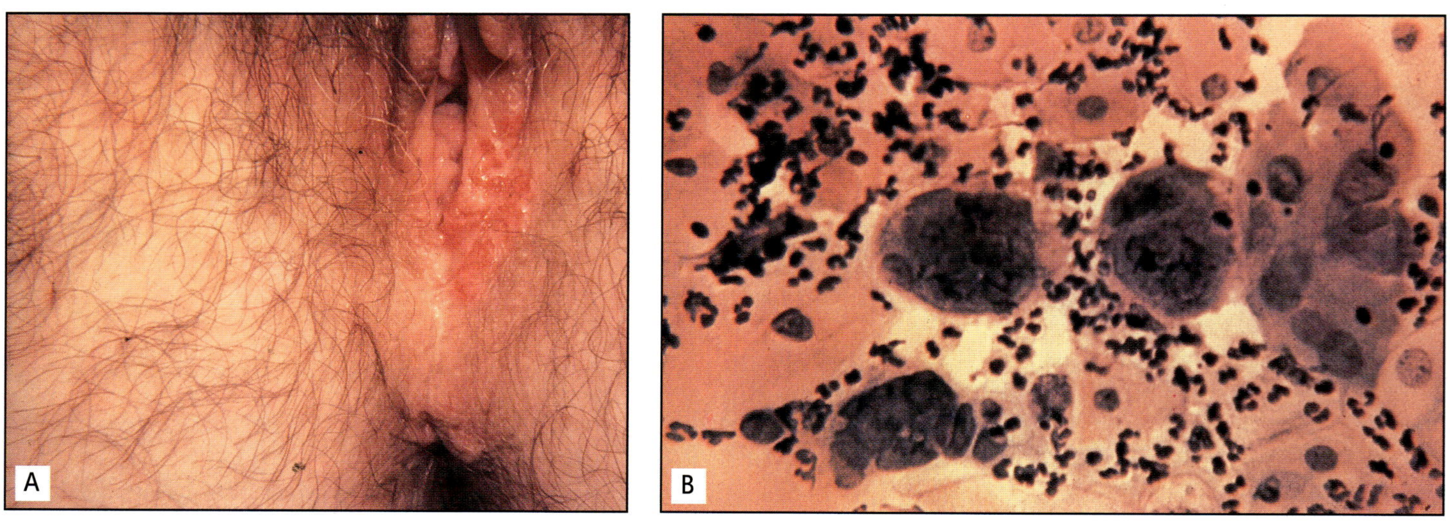

FIGURE 2-35.

Genital herpes. Diagnosis is made by the observation of the presence of shallow, painful ulcers (**A**). Culture identification of the herpes simplex virus is necessary, however, for verification. Viral cultures should be obtained as soon as clinical manifestations occur. Maximum excretion of the virus in recurrent disease occurs about 48 hours after onset of symptoms. Smears taken directly from lesions may reveal characteristic multinucleated giant cells. The nuclei have a ground-glass appearance, and nuclear inclusion bodies may occasionally be visualized (**B**). Treatment consists of acyclovir, valacyclovir or famciclovir. Treatment of acute infection consists of acyclovir 200 gm 5 times daily or longer as needed for primary disease. For suppressive therapy, 400 mg twice daily of acyclovir is effective. Valacyclovir is taken as 500 mg twice daily for 5 or more days in the acute phase. For suppressive therapy, 500 mg to 1 g daily is also effective.

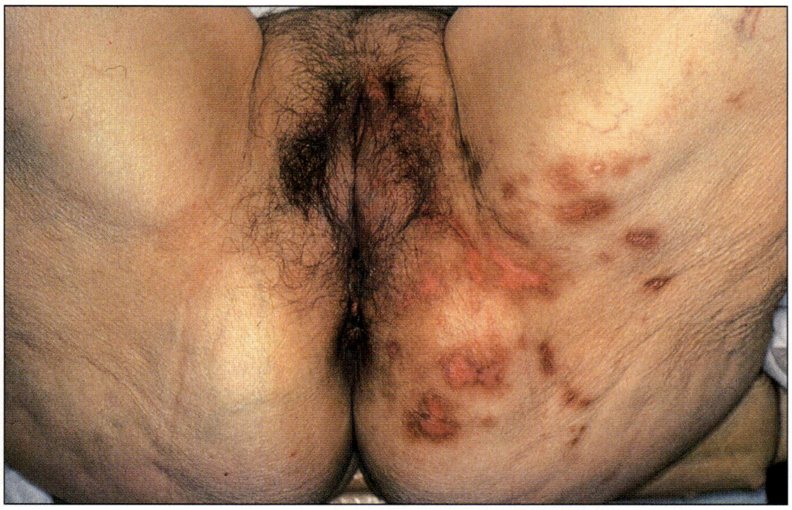

FIGURE 2-36.

Herpes zoster. Herpes zoster is manifested as acute vesiculations that occur localized to a single cutaneous dermatome. Symptoms are usually intense pain in the affected area several days before eruptions present. Vesicles and small bullae appear over erythematous plaques that may coalesce and become hemorrhagic. Vesiculations in herpes zoster are unilateral (as seen in the figure) and are usually larger than those in herpes simplex. Herpes zoster is more likely to be seen in elderly or immunosuppressed patients. The approximate time of healing is 2 to 4 weeks, but postherpetic neuralgia is a frequent complaint. Diagnosis can be made by the presence of giant multinucleated cells on biopsy or Zanck smear. Culture of the vesicle fluid differentiates it from herpes simplex. The etiologic agent is the varicella zoster virus. Treatment with valacyclovir in high dose (1 g three times daily) is effective in decreasing the duration of viral shedding and symptoms.

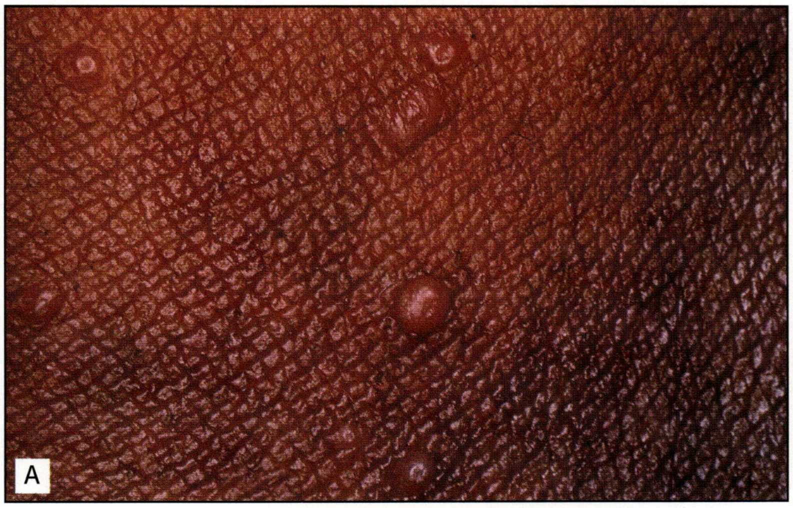

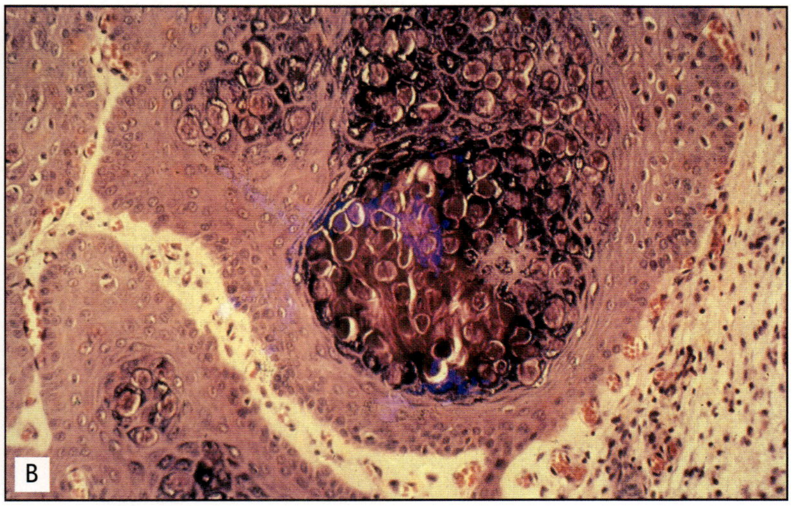

FIGURE 2-37.

Molluscum contagiosum. Seen in the adult, this is a sexually transmitted infection caused by a poxvirus. There are two major subtypes of the virus, both of which result in similar-appearing lesions. Lesions produced by the virus are small, smooth nodules that often have central umbilication (**A**). They are usually asymptomatic but may be associated with mild pruritus. Molluscum contagiosum is frequently found in human immunodeficiency virus–positive individuals, in which it may occasionally present as large nodular tumors. Microscopic examination reveals a mass of acanthotic epithelium that extends down and compresses the corium. Cytoplasmic inclusion bodies (molluscum bodies) are found within the cells (**B**). Lesions are easily removed with a sharp dermal curette.

MISCELLANEOUS LESIONS

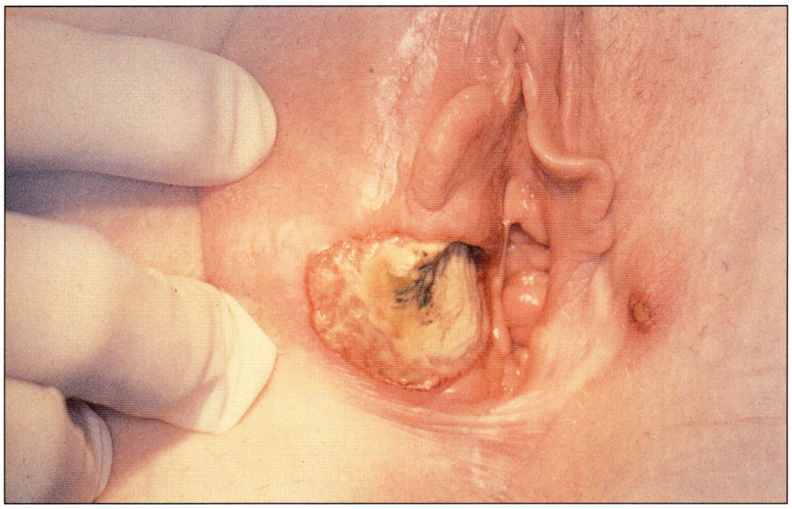

FIGURE 2-38.

Beçhet's disease. Beçhet's disease is rarely seen in the United States. It is characterized by the presence of genital and oral ulcers, as well as inflammation of the eye. Individuals with Beçhet's disease may occasionally develop disturbance of the central nervous system, nephritis, arthritis, and thrombophlebitis. They may also manifest other skin diseases such as erythema multiforme. The etiology has not been determined. The disease on the vulva usually begins as small vesicles or papules that ulcerate, enlarge, become craterous, and often are covered by necrotic debris (as seen in the figure). The ulcers may vary in size from several millimeters to centimeters, and at times they may spontaneously heal and recur, although in most instances, they persist. Healing is usually followed by fibrosis and scarring. Most individuals with Beçhet's disease complain of incapacitating vulvar pain, as well as dyspareunia. Occasionally, they complain of a foul discharge. Biopsy of such an ulcer should be obtained to exclude other problems such as carcinoma or tuberculosis. No specific findings are noted on biopsy, however, an intense inflammatory infiltrate of lymphocytes and plasma cells are noted especially around the blood vessel walls and perivascular tissues. The endothelial cells within the blood vessels demonstrate swelling. Topical treatment is usually unsuccessful and many different approaches have been used. We have obtained the best results with triamcinalone 40 mg given intramuscularly and then repeated again in 10 days. This has resulted in disappearance of both vulvar and oral lesions in most of the patients so treated, however recurrences are not uncommon.

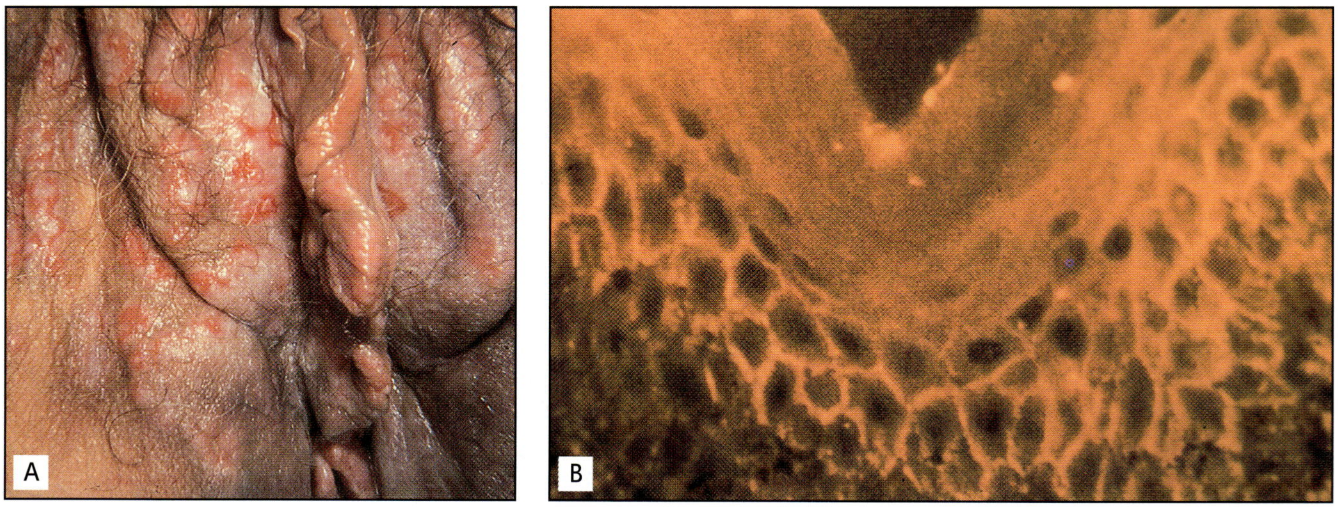

FIGURE 2-39.

Pemphigus vulgaris. This is an autoimmune disease that usually occurs between the fourth and sixth decade with a predilection for Jewish women. Initially, genital lesions appear as nonspecific erosions which are fragile and may or may not develop bullae (**A**). Symptoms are burning, itching, rawness, and stinging. Large erosions may produce extensive pain, which are associated with secondary infection. Genital lesions are usually associated with mucous membrane lesions, especially of the mouth. The diagnosis is confirmed by biopsy (best taken from normal-appearing skin or mucosa just adjacent to a lesion) with immunofluorescent staining which reveals characteristic intercellular fluorescence (**B**). Treatment consists of systemic corticosteroids with possible use of antimetabolites (*eg*, cyclophosphamide, azathioprine). In refractive cases gold has been used and recently cyclosporine has been found to be beneficial.

SELECTED BIBLIOGRAPHY

Kaufman RH, Faro S: Benign Diseases of the Vulva and Vagina. St. Louis: Mosby-Year Book; 1994.

Lynch PJ, Edwards L: Genital Dermatology. New York: Churchill Livingstone; 1994.

CHAPTER 3

Vagina

Mark Spitzer and Melinda Mann

As a portion of the female genital tract, the vagina is most enigmatic. It is often the site of some of the most common and least common of gynecologic conditions. Furthermore, although vaginal disorders are responsible for more gynecologic complaints than any other gynecologic disorder and although the vagina is easily accessible, it is the least understood of any of the portions of the female genital tract. As a whole, clinicians know very little about it and treat it merely as a passageway or access point to the upper genital tract. An understanding of the conditions (both common and rare) that are found in the vagina requires an understanding of microbiology, endocrinology, and developmental anatomy, as well as pathology and oncology.

Vaginitis accounts for up to 10% of all office visits to gynecologists. The estimated annual cost for the evaluation and treatment of vaginitis is as high as $600 million, and the loss of productivity may be double this figure, yet the microbiology of the normal vaginal flora that is altered in these infections is only superficially understood by most clinicians, and their treatment is often empiric and uses a shotgun approach.

Congenital anomalies and diethylstilbestrol-related lesions are clinically important and yet are infrequently encountered by most clinicians. They are often viewed as unrelated, rare, sporadic events that are difficult to conceptualize. Vaginal cancers are the rarest of the female genital tract neoplasms. Primary squamous cell vaginal cancer is so rare compared with its cervical and vulvar counterparts that its diagnosis can only be confirmed after excluding other squamous cell etiologies. Other benign and malignant vaginal neoplasms are even rarer. Careful observation, awareness of these conditions, and a willingness to biopsy liberally in most cases is necessary to making the diagnosis of these rare conditions. Finally, there are several unusual vaginal findings whose recognition is difficult simply because they are rare. The aim of this chapter is to show images of the vagina in disease and in health and to explore some of the underlying pathophysiology related to these conditions to enhance the reader's understanding.

THE NORMAL VAGINA THROUGHOUT LIFE

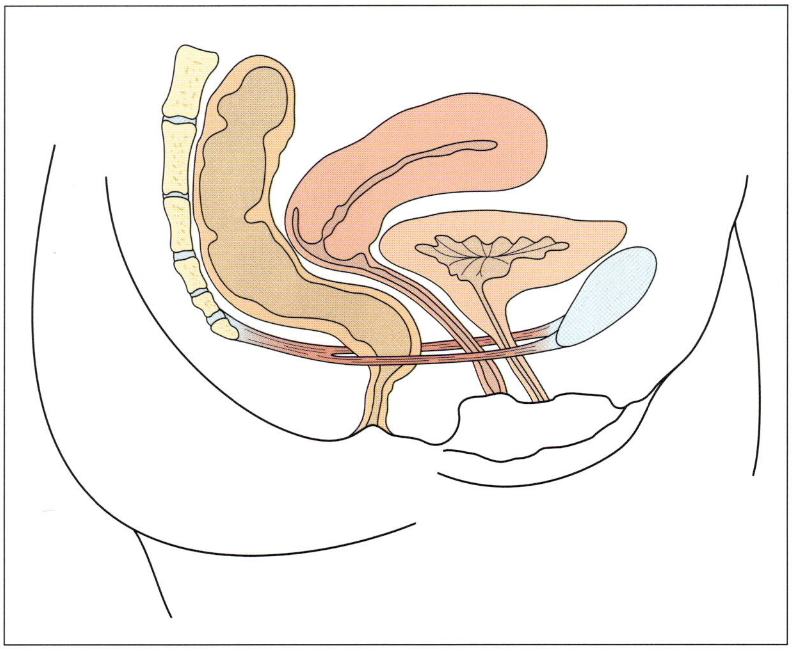

FIGURE 3-1.

Normal anatomy. The vagina is a fibromuscular tube lined by a mucous membrane that connects the vulva and introitus to the cervix and uterus. The vagina is approximately 10 cm long. Because the cervix enters the vagina through the anterior wall, it is usually about 2.5 cm shorter than the posterior wall. In the upright healthy female, the vagina arcs posteriorly until the upper vagina lies in an almost horizontal position on top of the rectum and the levator plate. When the uterus is retroverted, the vaginal axis may be rotated slightly more anteriorly. The vagina is further supported by the pelvic diaphgram, urogenital diaphgram and perineal body in the lower third, and the middle third of the vagina receives support from the pelvic diaphgram and part of the cardinal ligaments.

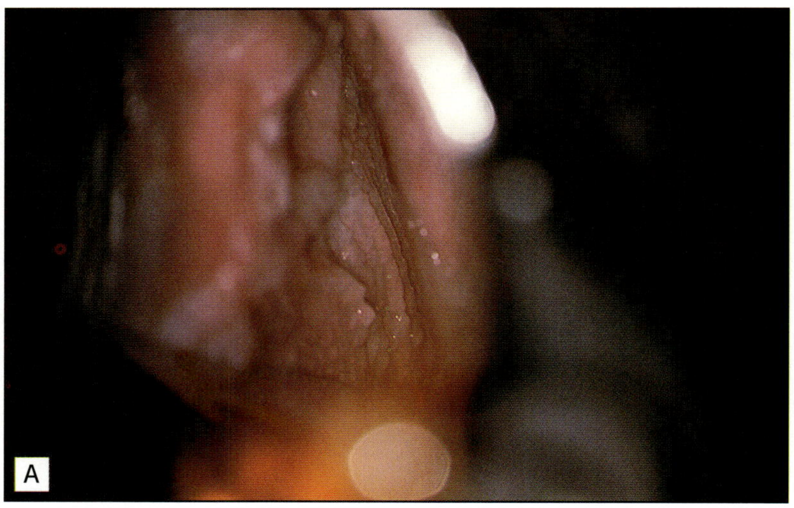

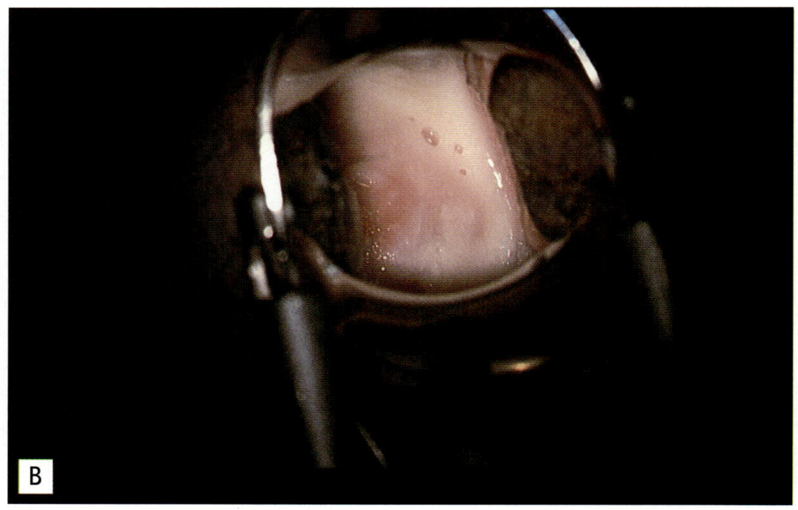

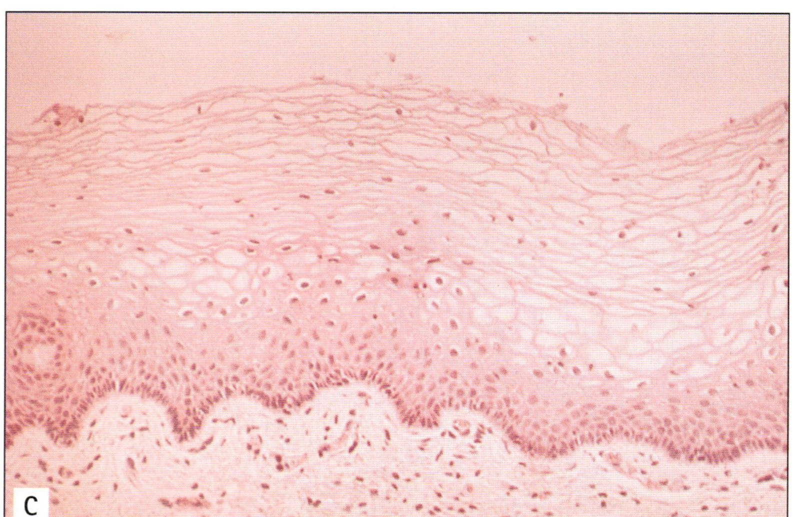

FIGURE 3-2.

Normal vagina—microscopic features. The vaginal mucosa in the normal adult is pale pink in color and has ill-defined circumferentially oriented folds called rugae. The rugae are 2 to 5 mm thick and vary by location and with varying hormonal stimulation. These rugae, along with the vagina's elasticity and tone, contribute to its ability to distend during coitus and the birthing process. **A**, Normal rugae in a reproductive age woman. **B**, Physiologic discharge made up of desquamated epithelial cells and normal vaginal flora. **C**, Histologically, the vaginal mucosa is lined by a stratified squamous epithelium that is glycogenated and nonkeratinizing in the mature adult. The vaginal epithelium is arbitrarily divided into layers. The basal layer consists of a single row of columnar cells perpendicular to the basement membrane. The parabasilar layer is 2 to 5 cells thick and consists of cuboidal cells. Mitoses rarely rise above the parabasilar layer in normal epithelium. The intermediate layer is of variable thickness, and its cells are somewhat flattened. The superficial layer also varies in thickness, and its cells are markedly flattened. As cells mature from the basilar through the superficial layer, the nuclei become progressively smaller and more pyknotic, and the nuclear to cytoplasmic ratio falls. A variable amount of glycogen is found in the vaginal epithelium of a mature adult, predominantly in the intermediate and superficial layers. Initially, glycogen accumulates in the perinuclear region in the intermediate layer, and it eventually occupies most of the cell. It is important to distinguish perinuclear glycogen found in the intermediate cell layer from perinuclear halos of koilocytes, which have irregular borders and are associated with nuclear abnormalities, and found predominantly in the superficial layer.

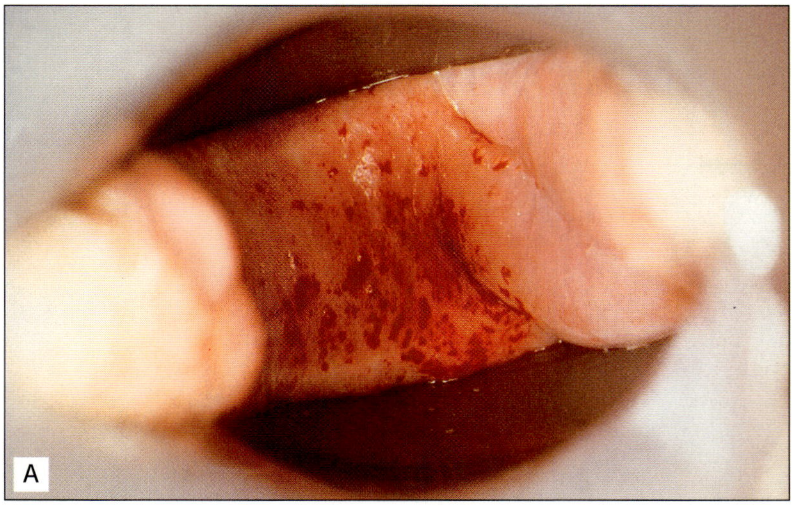

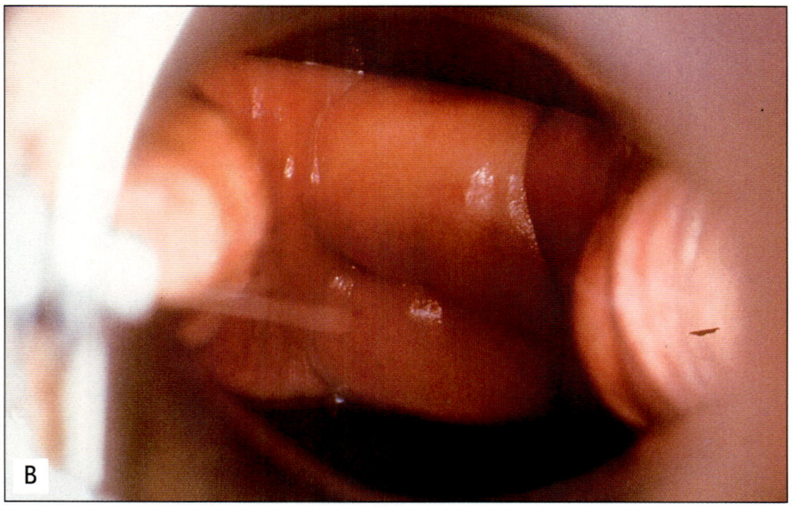

FIGURE 3-3.

Postmenopausal atrophy. In the postmenopausal woman, the fall in estrogen levels cause several changes. The vagina becomes shorter and narrower because of an increase in submucosal connective tissue. The rugae become flattened. Squamous epithelial cells do not mature, and the vagina is eventually lined predominantly by parabasilar cells. Because the epithelium is so thin, its color takes on a redder appearance. Vaginal secretions diminish, and the vagina becomes dry and fragile. Petechial hemorrhages are common, and the vagina is very subject to trauma and inflammation. **A**, A markedly atrophic vagina with petechial hemorrhages. **B**, Same patient after therapy with vaginal estrogen cream.

At birth, the vagina is under the influence of maternal estrogen. Consequently, the vaginal epithelium is well cornified, and the pH is in the adult range (3.8–4.2). After birth, maternal estrogen is withdrawn, lactobacilli are gradually replaced by intestinal flora, the pH rises to 7.0 to 8.0, and the cornified, glycogen-rich mucosal epithelium is replaced by a thin atrophic epithelium. At puberty, the process is reversed again. Because of the hypoestrogenic state associated with lactation, atrophic changes can also be seen in nursing women. (*Courtesy of* B. A. Krumholz, MD.)

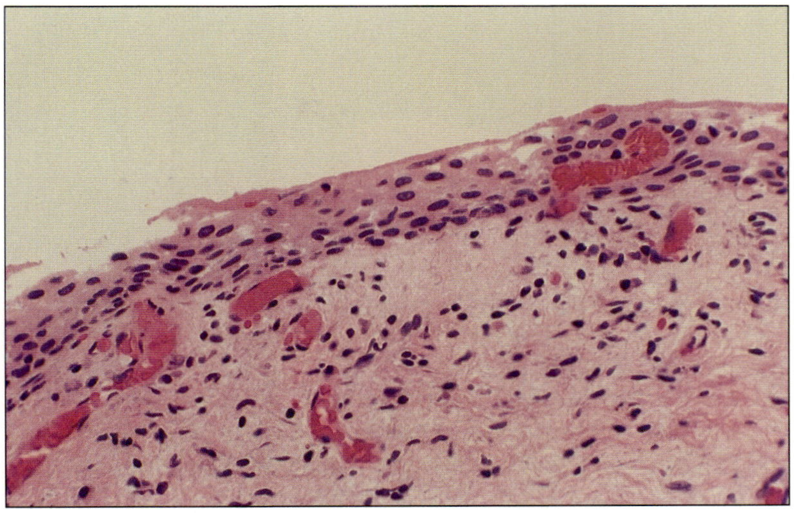

FIGURE 3-4.

Postmenopausal atrophy—microscopic features. In the late menopausal woman, because of the loss of superficial and intermediate cells, the vaginal epithelium may be only six to eight cells in depth. Although the cells have a high nuclear to cytoplasmic ratio, the fact that the nuclei are bland helps distinguish this atrophic epithelium from high grade dysplasia. The glycogen content of the epithelium decreases, which contributes to a drop in the number of lactobacilli and a rise in the vaginal pH. The shift in vaginal flora and pH increases the susceptibility to irritation, trauma, and infection. (*Courtesy of* P. Wasserman, MD)

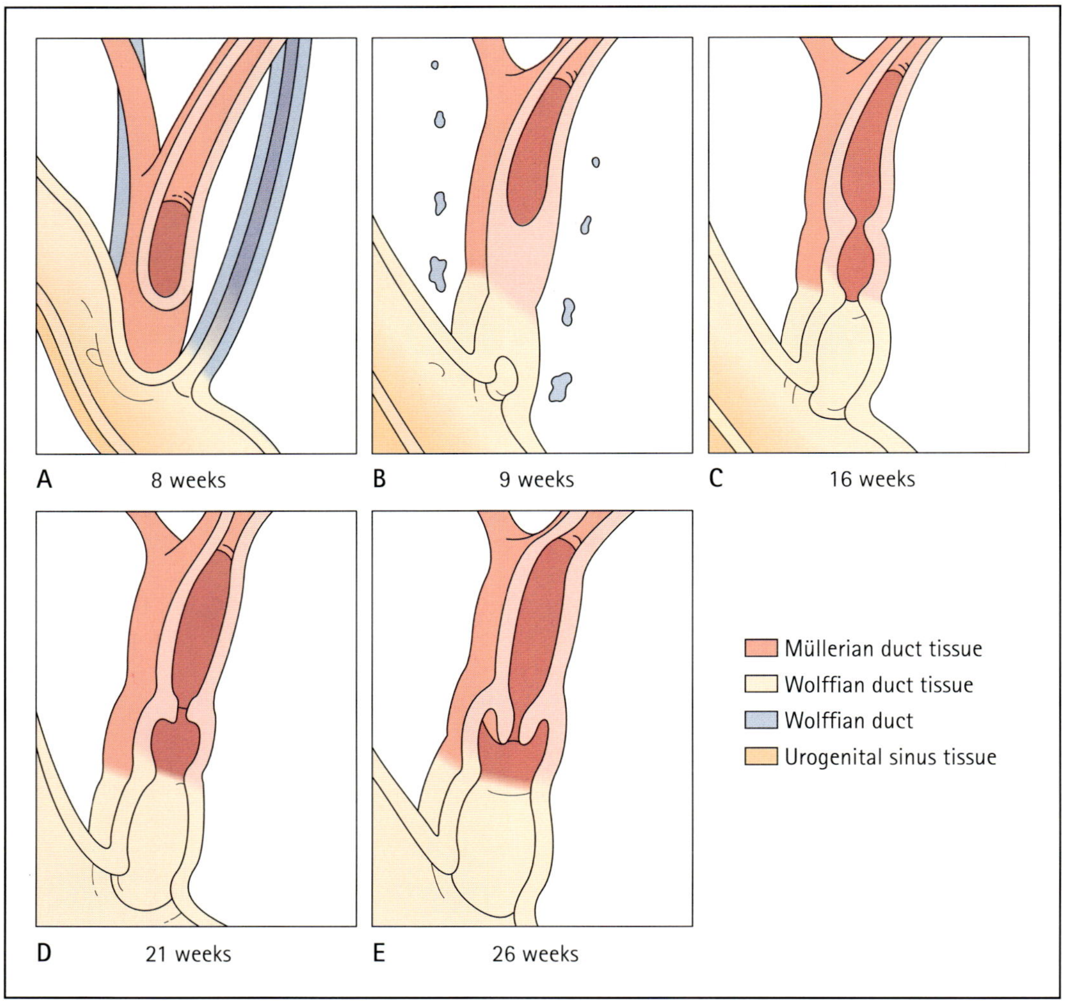

FIGURE 3-5.

Embryology. The upper vaginal epithelium is of mesodermal origin. The lower vagina is derived from the wall of the urogenital sinus, and the upper vagina is derived from the lining of the fused müllerian ducts. By the end of the eighth week, in the absence of a testes that secretes testosterone and müllerian inhibiting factor (MIF), the müllerian ducts fuse and meet the posterior wall of the urogenital sinus, which is mesoderm of wolffian origin (**A**). This contact induces the growth of the vaginal plate (**B**). By nine weeks, the septum between the vaginal plate and the müllerian duct breaks, resulting in a continuous vaginal canal (**C**). The vaginal canal is patent from early in development, which contributes to the conversion of the columnar müllerian epithelium to squamous epithelium via squamous metaplasia. The cervix begins developing at 21 weeks (**D**) and is formed at 26 weeks of age (**E**).

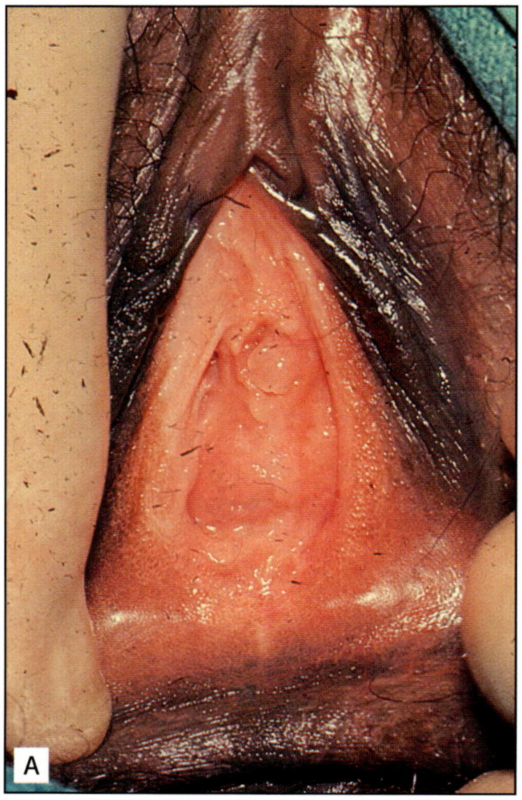

FIGURE 3-6.

Imperforate hymen. Partial or complete failure of the posterior wall of the urogenital sinus to cavitate results in a partial or complete imperforate hymen. Imperforate hymen is the most common significant congenital anomaly of the vagina and occurs in about 1 in 2000 female patients. At menarche, a completely imperforate hymen is associated with hematocolpos or hematometra and frequently results in endometriosis. Occasionally, hydrocolpos occurs in an infant with an imperforate hymen and excessive secretions of cervical glands owing to circulating maternal estrogen. An imperforate hymen is characterized by a tense, shiny membrane bulging between the labia. This helps distinguish it from partial or complete vaginal atresia, in which a blind pouch and no bulging membrane is seen. In extreme cases, the girl presents at puberty with primary amenorrhea and a suprapubic mass that does not disappear after the bladder is catheterized. There may also be partial rectal obstruction, urinary retention, and lower extremity edema caused by the mass effect. Treatment consists of resection of the membrane or cruciate incisions. **A**, An imperforate hymen in a postmenarcheal girl. Although the hymen is seen to be bulging somewhat, in more classic cases it is thinner and the bulge is more prominent.

(Continued on next page)

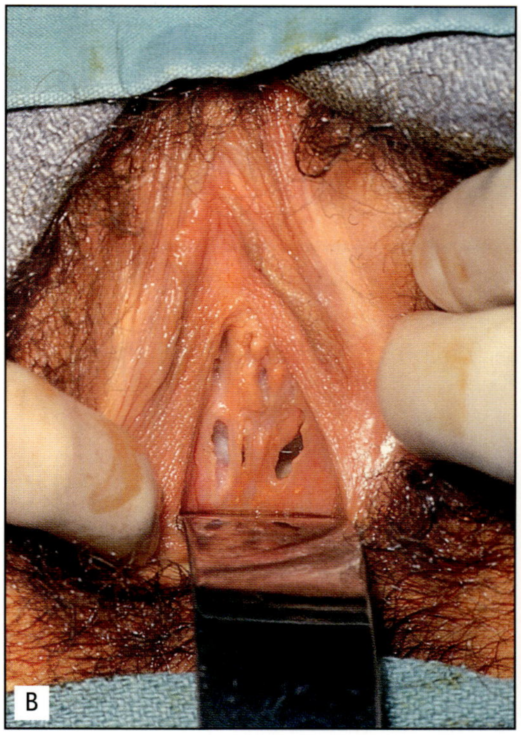

FIGURE 3-6. *(Continued)*
B, Septate hymen. The hymeneal membrane has been perforated sufficiently to allow the flow of menses and other secretions but not sufficiently to allow intercourse. (*Courtesy of* R. H. Kaufman, MD)

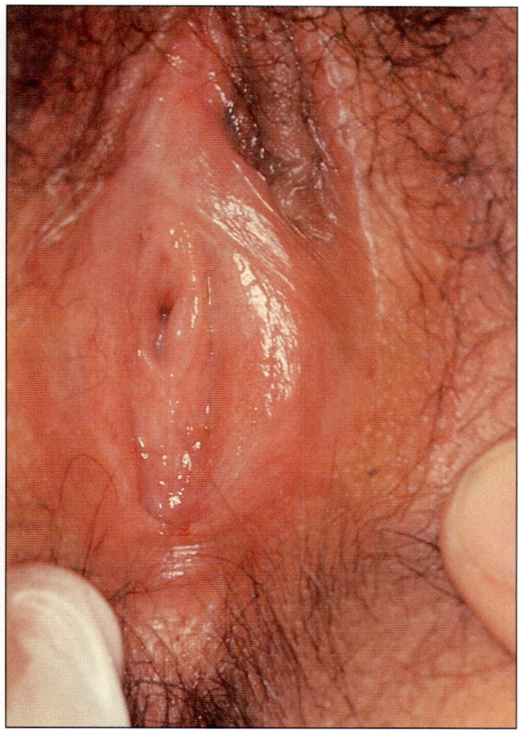

FIGURE 3-7.
Vaginal agenesis. Congenital anomalies relate to the developmental failure that caused them. Congenital absence of the vaginal wall will result if the müllerian ducts fail to form or if the wolffian duct is absent. The latter would deprive the mullerian duct of the template it uses to guide its migration into the pelvis. The urogenital sinus would then form a blind pouch. Because vaginal patency is required to stimulate the metaplastic conversion of columnar to squamous epithelium, the pouch would be lined by mucous-secreting cells. Urologic anomalies are commonly found on the same side as vaginal anomalies (including renal agenesis, pelvic kidney, and ureteric anomalies). Complete vaginal agenesis occurs in 1 in 5000 female births. About 25% of women with vaginal agenesis have a uterus and may have complications associated with retrograde menstruation. In this figure, no introital opening is seen, and there is no bulge at the introitus as might be seen in a woman with an imperforate hymen. (*Courtesy of* R. H. Kaufman, MD.)

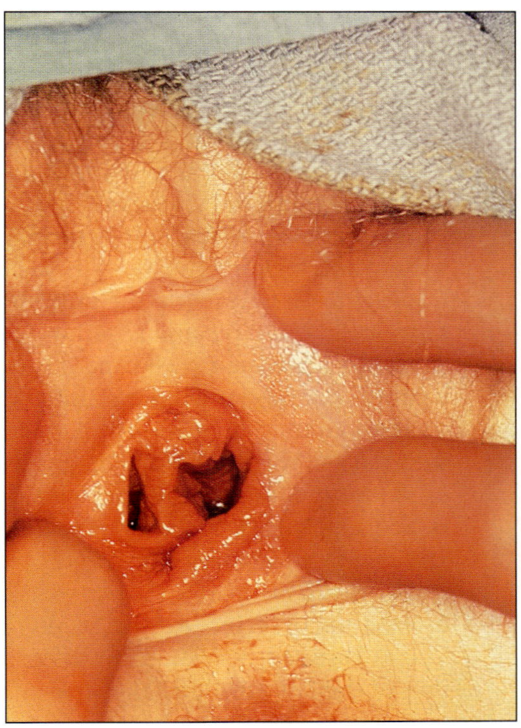

FIGURE 3-8.
Vaginal septum. If the müllerian ducts reach the urogenital sinus but fail to fuse or fuse only partially, a double vagina or a complete or partial longitudinal septum results. A longitudinal vaginal septum seen in the figure is the most common congenital anomaly of the vagina and may also be associated with division of the uterus and cervix. Complete or partial fusion of the müllerian and wolffian ducts may result in a complete or partial transverse vaginal septum at that site. Transverse septa are half as common as longitudinal septa. The inheritance of this anomaly seems to be autosomal recessive. A transverse septum is most commonly found at the junction of the lower and middle third of the vagina. The epithelium of the upper vagina above a complete septum remains columnar and is mucus secreting. (*Courtesy of* R. H. Kaufman, MD.)

VAGINITIS

A. DIFFERENTIAL DIAGNOSIS OF COMMON VAGINAL INFECTIONS

Diagnostic Criteria	Syndrome			
	Normal	**Bacterial Vaginosis**	**Trichomonas Vaginitis**	**Candida Vulvovaginitis**
Vaginal pH	3.8–4.2	>4.5	>4.5	≤4.5 (usually)
Discharge	White, clear, flocculent	Thin, homogeneous, white, gray, adherent, often increased	Yellow-green, frothy, adherent, increased	White, curdy, 'cottage cheese-like', sometimes increased
Amine odor (KOH whiff test)	Absent	Present (fishy)	May be present (fishy)	Absent
Main patient complaints	None	Discharge, bad odor (possibly worse after intercourse), possible itching	Frothy discharge, bad odor, vulvar pruritis, dysuria	Itching/burning, discharge
Microscopic	Lactobacilli, epithelial cells	Clue cells with adherent coccoid bacteria, no WBCs	Trichomonads, WBCs>10/hpf	Budding yeast, hyphae, pseudohyphae (with KOH preparation)

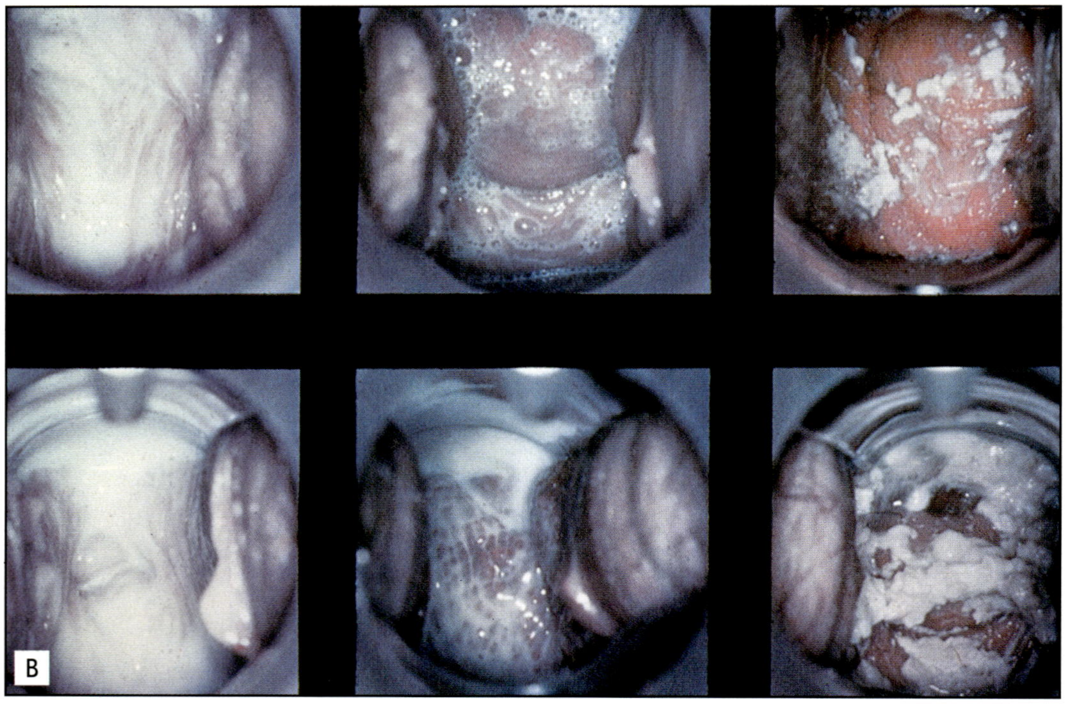

FIGURE 3-9.
Vaginitis. Vaginal infections account for more than 10 million office visits annually. The three most common infections in order of prevalence are bacterial vaginosis, Candida vaginitis, and Trichomonas vaginitis. These three conditions are easily distinguished by the use of a history and pelvic examination, pH determination, microscopic exam, and a whiff test. Bacterial vaginosis and Trichomonas vaginitis are associated with a fishy odor and a high vaginal pH, while with Candida, the odor is absent and the pH is low. Trichomonas and Candida vaginitis cause varying amounts of itching and burning, while with bacterial vaginosis, frequently the only symptoms are a discharge and an odor. The discharge associated with candida vaginitis occasionally has a characteristic "cottage cheese" appearance. **A**, is a summary of the differential diagnosis of the most common vaginal infections. **B**, the appearance of bacterial vaginosis, Trichomonas vaginitis, and Candida vaginitis (*left to right*). (B *courtesy* of the International Society for the Study of Vulvar Disease (ISSVD), from the collection of the late Dr. Herman Gardner.)

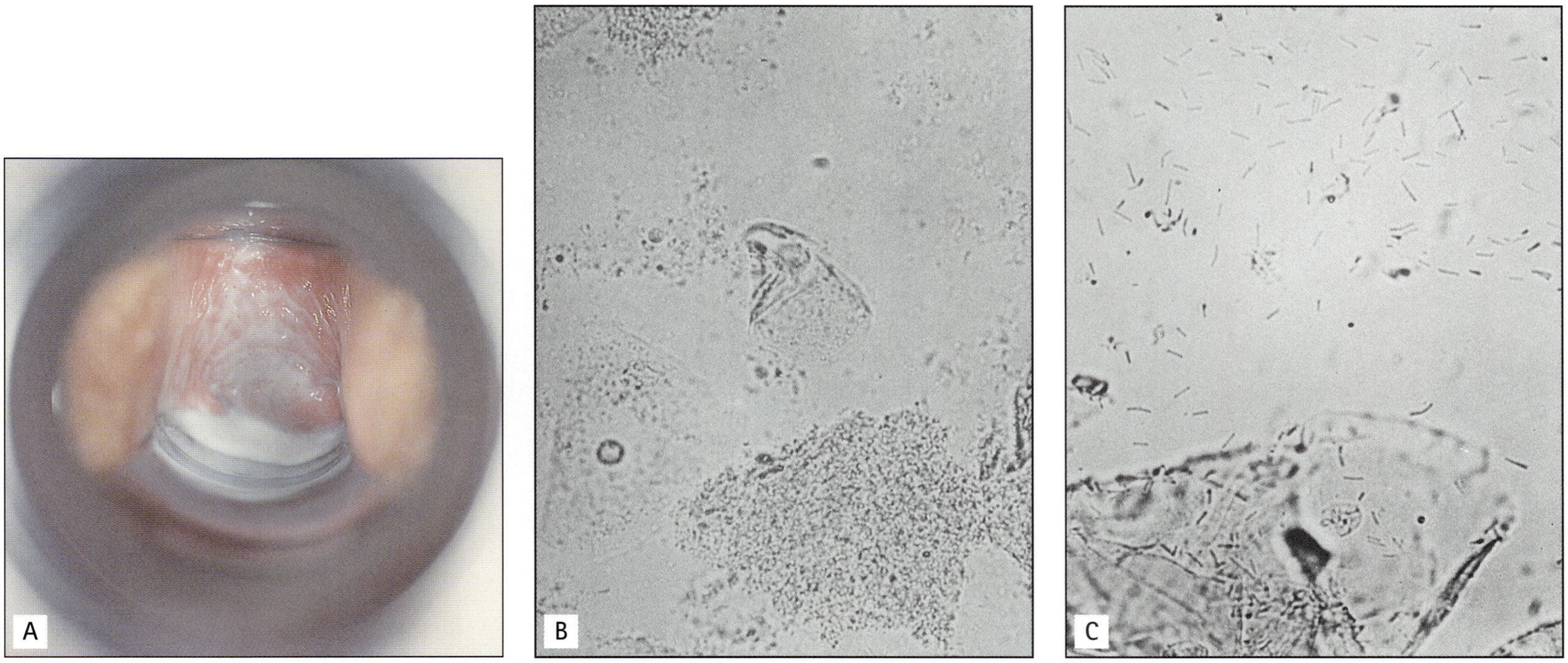

FIGURE 3-10.

Bacterial vaginosis—microscopic features. **A**, Bacterial vaginosis (BV) is the most prevalent vaginal infection and accounts for up to half of all vaginitis complaints. The most common complaint among women with BV is a discharge with an unpleasant or fishy odor which is often exacerbated after menstruation or intercourse. Vaginal irritation and itching are uncommon. The characteristic fishy odor can be elicited by placing two drops of 10% to 20% potassium hydroxide in the discharge. Recently, evidence has been mounting that BV is associated with a variety of significant obstetric and gynecologic conditions including: preterm delivery, premature rupture of membranes, amnionitis, pelvic inflammatory disease, and postoperative infections. Bacterial vaginosis is actually a shift in the vaginal flora from one in which lactobacilli dominate to one with a mixed, predominantly anaerobic flora (*Bacteroides, Peptostreptococcus, Peptococcus, Mobiluncus,* and *Gardnerella*). Concentrations of anaerobic bacteria increase 100- to 1000-fold, and hydrogen peroxide– producing lactobacilli are absent or greatly reduced. The odor associated with BV results when amine byproducts of anaerobic metabolism are exposed to an alkaline pH. On wet mount, the diagnosis of BV can be confirmed by the presence of clue cells (**B**). These are epithelial cells with a heavily stippled surface and borders obscured by the presence of large amounts of adherent bacteria. This is contrasted with a normal epithelial cell with normal lactobacilli flora (**C**). (*B* and *C courtesy of* the International Society for the Study of Vulvar Disease.)

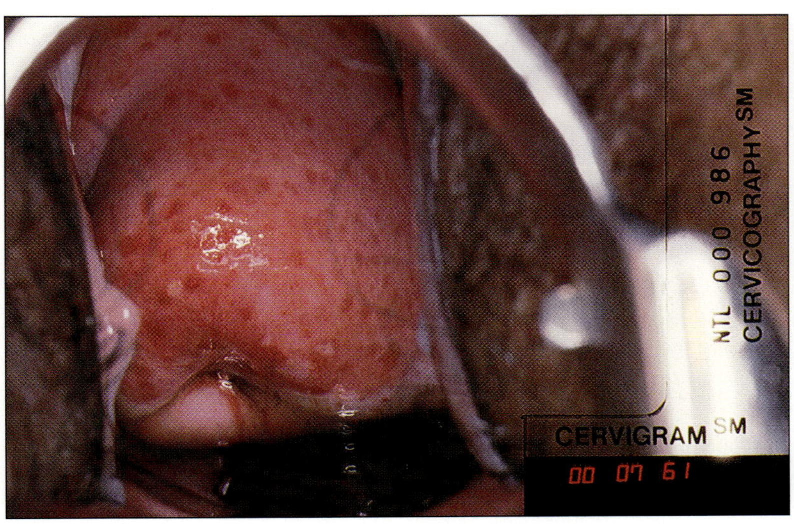

FIGURE 3-11.

Trichomonas vaginitis. Trichomonas vaginitis is a sexually transmitted disease (STD). Consequently, it is more common among women with multiple sexual partners and with a history of other STDs. The male partners of women with *Trichomonas* infection harbor the organism in 15% to 85% of cases, but are usually asymptomatic, so reinfection by an untreated partner is common. Symptoms include severe vulvovaginal itching and burning, dysuria, dyspareunia, a profuse greenish discharge that may be frothy, and a foul or fishy odor. Petechiae, (as seen in the figure) may be seen on the cervix ("strawberry cervix") in 2% to 3% of cases. The vagina is intensely red and swollen with an elevated pH.

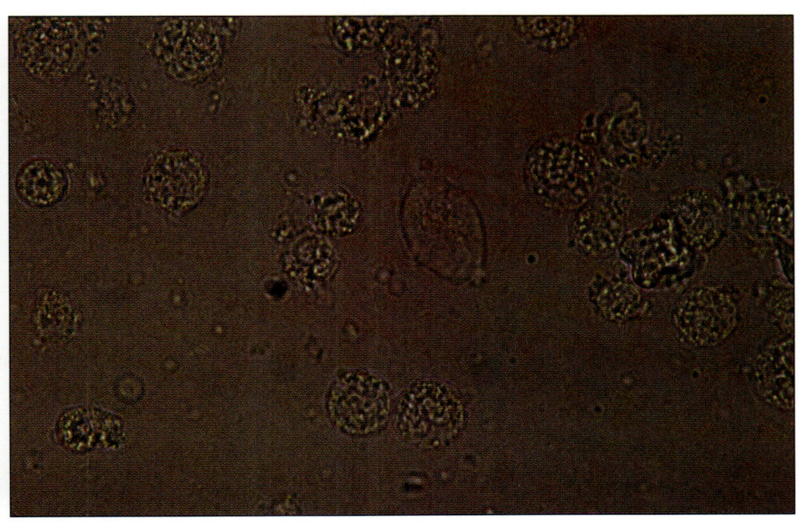

FIGURE 3-12.

Trichomonas vaginitis—microscopic features. Trichomonas vaginitis is caused by a single-celled anaerobic flagellated protozoan called a trichomonad. These motile organisms, which are slightly larger than a polymorphonuclear leukocyte, are easily identified on wet mount. Because of the intense inflammatory response, there are also many white blood cells present. The accompanying microflora is mixed with a marked increase in the number of anaerobes (predominantly *Bacteroides* sp) and a decrease in the number of lactobacilli. (*Courtesy of* D. Ferris, MD.)

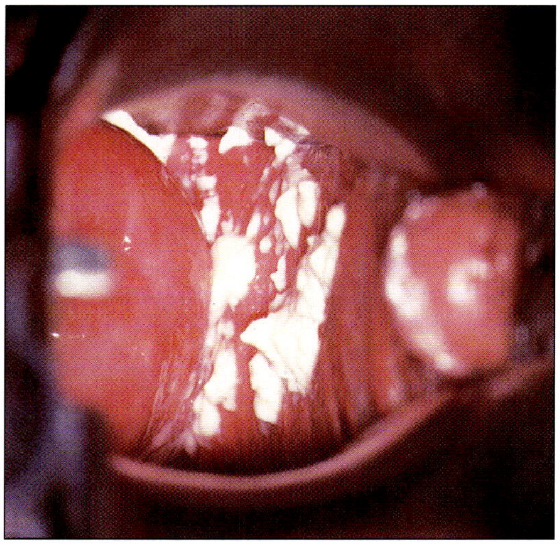

FIGURE 3-13.

Candida vaginitis. Candidal vaginitis accounts for about a third of all vaginal infections. Although *Candida* is part of the normal flora in the vagina, certain conditions may favor the growth of Candida species and result in their overgrowth. Conditions that increase vaginal glycogen (*eg*, pregnancy), increase vaginal glucose (*eg*, pregnancy, diabetes), decrease cellular immunity (*eg*, pregnancy, systemic corticosteroid use, immune deficiency), or reduce the normal bacterial flora (*eg*, broad-spectrum antibiotics) may promote the overgrowth of *Candida* organisms in the vagina. The most common complaints associated with candida vaginitis include a white or yellowish "cottage cheese–like" or "curds and whey" discharge with intense vulvovaginal itching or a sense of vaginal dryness. The discharge is odorless, and the vaginal pH is in the normal range. The appearance of candidal infections may vary. Most have a thick, clumpy, or pasty discharge with an erythematous vaginal epithelium (shown in the figure).

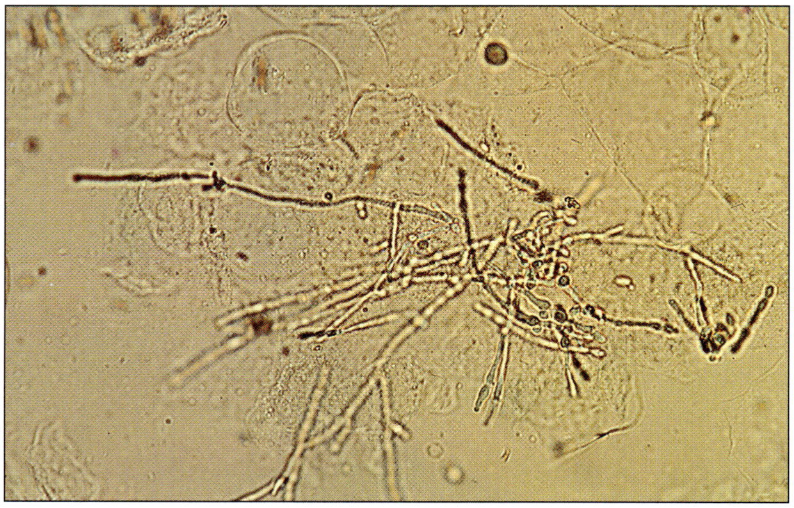

FIGURE 3-14.

Candida vaginitis—microscopic features. The most common *Candida* species is *Candida albicans*. The incidence of *C. glabrata*, *C. tropicalis*, and other less common species of *Candida* varies with the population being studied. The diagnosis of *C. albicans* is made by identifying hyphae and spores on potassium hydroxide (KOH) wet mount as seen in the figure. White blood cells are common. The KOH dissolves cellular elements leaving behind "ghost cells" and making the identification of spores and pseudohypae easier. *C. glabrata* does not have pseudohyphae. The sensitivity of KOH wet mount ranges from 50% to 80%. Culture is still the most sensitive of the diagnostic tests, and typing of the species can provide valuable information in the treatment of resistant cases. (*Courtesy of* D. Ferris, MD.)

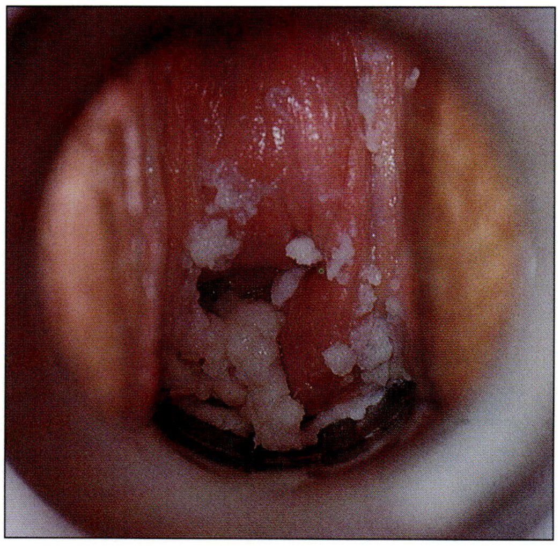

FIGURE 3-15.

Cytolytic vaginosis. (Döderlein's cytolysis). The existence of Döderlein's cytolysis is controversial. Normal vaginal discharge consists of cervical mucus mixed with intact and disintegrated squamous cells and normal flora, predominantly lactobacilli. When this thick white discharge is abundant, the woman may complain of an abnormal discharge with irritation and itching. The clinical picture resembles *Candida* infection and may be confused with it unless the patient is evaluated with a wet smear, a potassium hydroxide (KOH) smear, or a *Candida* culture. Some have associated this clinical presentation with an excess of lactobacilli or abnormal lactobacilli. Treatment with bicarbonate douches, which are mucolytic, may provide symptomatic relief. The figure shows the similarity in appearance between Döderlein's cytolysis and *Candida* vaginitis. Both are associated with a thick, pasty, or clumpy discharge. However, note the complete absence of vaginal erythema in this case of Döderlein's cytolysis. (*Courtesy of* the International Society for the Study of Vulvar Disease.)

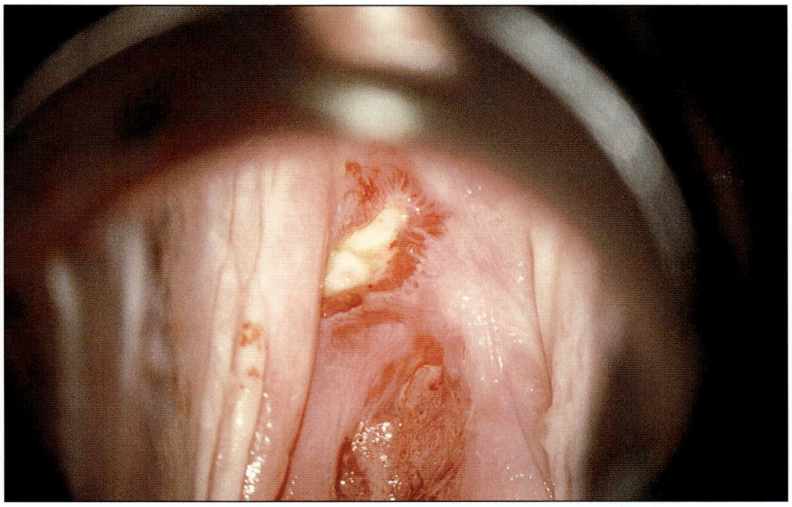

FIGURE 3-16.
Herpetic lesions of the vagina. Herpes simplex virus (HSV) is one of the most common sexually transmitted diseases in the United States. The virus is introduced by direct skin to skin contact. Initial infections ensue in 60% to 70% of seronegative patients approximately 6 days after contact with an infected individual. Lesions progress from papules to vesicles that rupture and produce shallow, painful ulcers that heal slowly without scarring. Untreated primary infections usually resolve in 2 to 3 weeks but may take up to 6 weeks to heal. Recurrent episodes usually present within the same anatomic site and have milder symptoms and a shorter duration. After the initial infection is limited by the individual's humoral and cell-mediated immune systems, the virus remains latent in the nerve ganglion of the infected area. The diagnosis is suspected by clinical observation of a cluster of 1 to 2 mm. vesicles or shallow ulcers in the genital area, and confirmed by culture. Typing of HSV isolates is of limited clinical value since type 1 and type 2 isolates infect both the oral and genital area, however, it may be of some prognostic value, as HSV-1 infection of the vulva and vagina recurs much less often than HSV-2 infection. The figure shows a large vaginal herpetic ulcer anterior to the cervix in a human immunodeficiency virus–positive woman. The ulcer crater is filled with exudate.

HUMAN PAPILLOMAVIRUS, PRENEOPLASTIC VAGINAL DISEASE, AND VAGINAL CANCERS

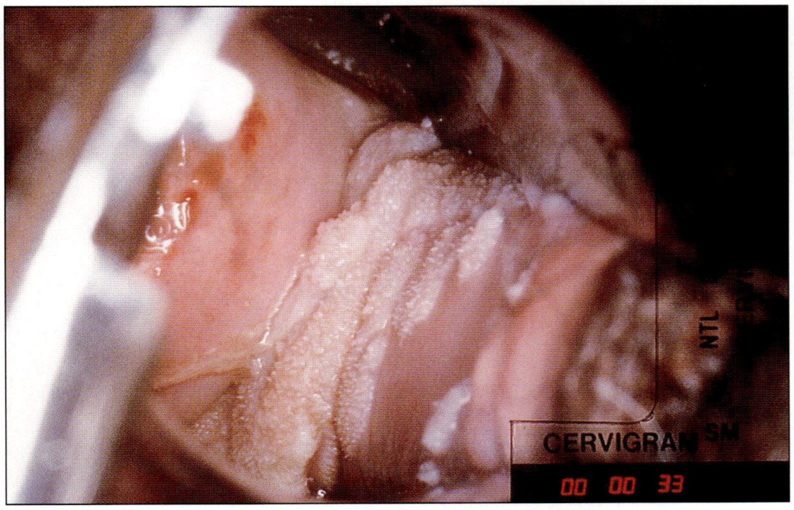

FIGURE 3-17.
Vaginal condyloma. Vaginal and cervical condylomas have a similar appearance. Exophytic vaginal condylomas are usually found in the lower vagina in association with vulvar condylomatas or in the upper vagina associated with cervical condylomas, but they may be found in any part of the vagina. Vaginal condylomas are usually asymptomatic but are an important reservoir of disease that must be identified so that treatment of the associated cervical or vaginal disease is not inadequate. Large, exophytic vaginal condylomata, as pictured in this colpophotograph, are much less common than their subclinical counterparts.

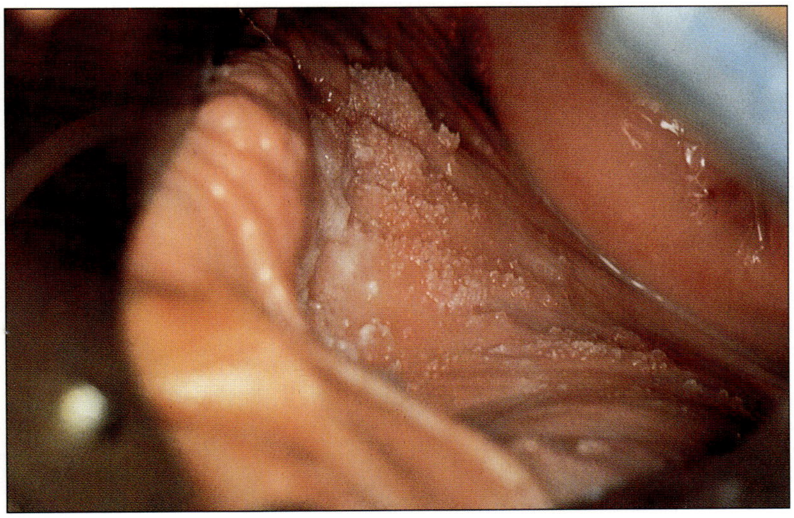

FIGURE 3-18.
Subclinical papillomavirus infection. This infection may exist independently or in conjunction with cervical, vaginal, or vulvar intraepithelial lesions or overt condylomas. Most women with microscopic vaginal condylomas are asymptomatic, and the disease is not evident on routine vaginal inspection. However, at times the vagina may have a sandpaper-like feel on bimanual examination. Exaggerated normal vaginal rugae may be confused with subclinical papillomavirus infection. Most cases of this infection need not be treated, because the hope of complete eradication of the virus is low relative to the morbidity involved in treatment. When treatment is elected, the entire vagina must be treated. This is best accomplished using topical 5-fluorouracil cream.

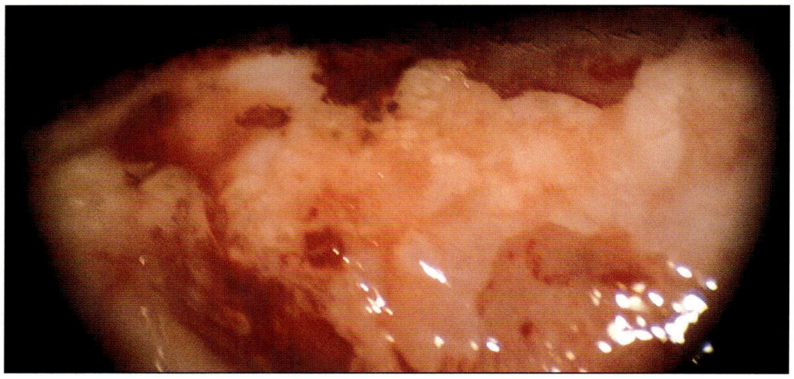

FIGURE 3-19.
Vaginal intraepithelial neoplasia (VaIN). Most cases of VaIN arise in the transformation zone which extends from the cervical squamocolumnar junction and in some women extends onto the vaginal fornices. The etiology and natural history of VaIN is similar to that of cervical intraepithelial neoplasia (CIN). VaIN may occur independently, but most often it coexists with CIN. Failure to eradicate the vaginal extension during therapy of a CIN lesion may result in a persisting abnormality. VaIN is usually asymptomatic. It is usually discovered during colposcopic assessment of a woman with an abnormal Pap smear. VaIN lesions should be suspected in women with a history of CIN or abnormal Pap smears in whom the colposcopic assessment of the cervix is normal, or in women with an abnormal Pap smear after hysterectomy or pelvic irradiation. The colpophotograph shows thick acetowhite epithelium with peeling borders consistent with high-grade VaIN. Biopsy of these lesions is important not only to confirm the diagnosis but also to rule out invasive cancer in the adjacent ulcerated areas.

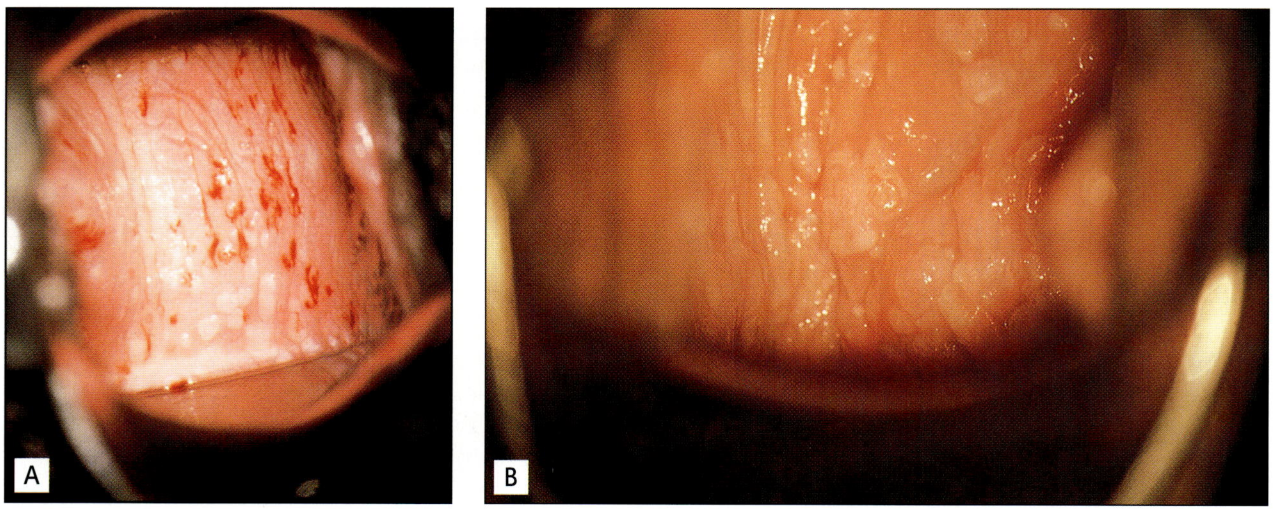

FIGURE 3-20.
Vaginal intraepithelial neoplasia (VaIN)—colposcopic features. Colposcopic inspection of the vagina is considerably more difficult than that of the cervix because of the vaginal rugae. Furthermore, the anterior and posterior walls of the vagina which are ordinarily covered by the vaginal speculum, need to be exposed and examined by rotating or slowly withdrawing the speculum after the vagina has been washed with 3% to 5% acetic acid. The colposcopic appearance of VaIN is similar to that of cervical intraepithelial neoplasia and includes acetowhite epithelium, punctations, and mosaic patterns. Acetowhite lesions may be multifocal and usually have a sharply demarcated border. In cases in which colposcopy is otherwise unrevealing, the vagina may be stained with Lugol's iodine. This allows for more rapid inspection of nonstaining areas that represent potential locations for biopsy. VaIN is difficult to distinguish from more benign lesions. **A**, shows a typical flat vaginal condylomata. **B**, lesions not markedly different proved to be VaIN III on biopsy. (*A, courtesy* of B.A. Krumholz, MD)

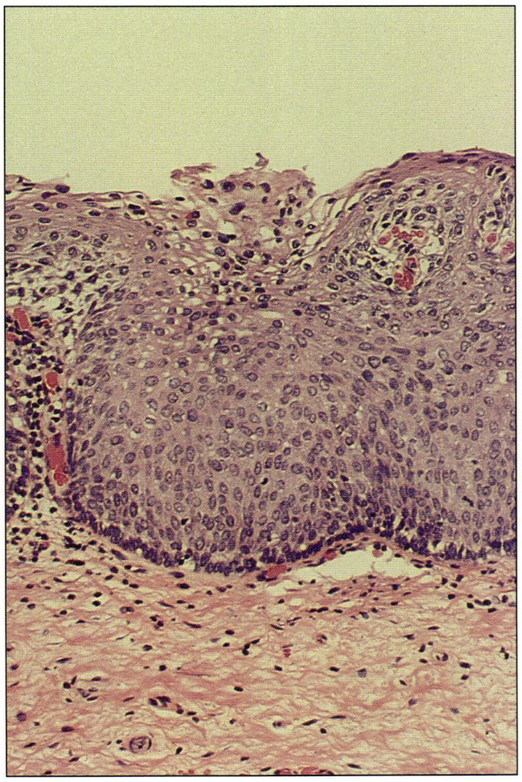

FIGURE 3-21.

Vaginal intraepithelial neoplasia (VaIN)—Microscopic features. The incidence of VaIN is less than 1% of the incidence of cervical disease. The highest incidence is found in women greater than 60 years, with the mean age of VaIN III at 53. The majority of women with VaIN have preexisting or coexisting intraepithelial or invasive lesions of the cervix or vulva. Microscopically, VaIN is almost indistinguishable from cervical intraepithelial neoplasia. Rather than the normal maturation process described earlier, abnormal cells with nuclear enlargement, hyperchromasia, and clumped chromatin are found at progressively higher levels of the epithelium. There is also increased mitotic activity, abnormal mitotic figures, and disordered maturation. The lesions are graded as VaIN I, II, or III based on the degree of maturation, the level at which mitotic activity is found, and the degree of nuclear abnormality. The natural history of VaIN is uncertain, with as many as 5% of lesions progressing to invasive cancer. Suggested therapies have included surgical excision, laser vaporization, topical 5-fluorouracil, and partial or complete vaginectomy. Care must be taken to avoid injury to the bladder and rectum when treating vaginal disease surgically, by laser or electrosurgical loop excision. When using 5-fluorouracil, the vulva must be protected from spillage of the cream which may cause severe vulvar irritation. (*Courtesy of* P. Wasserman, M.D.)

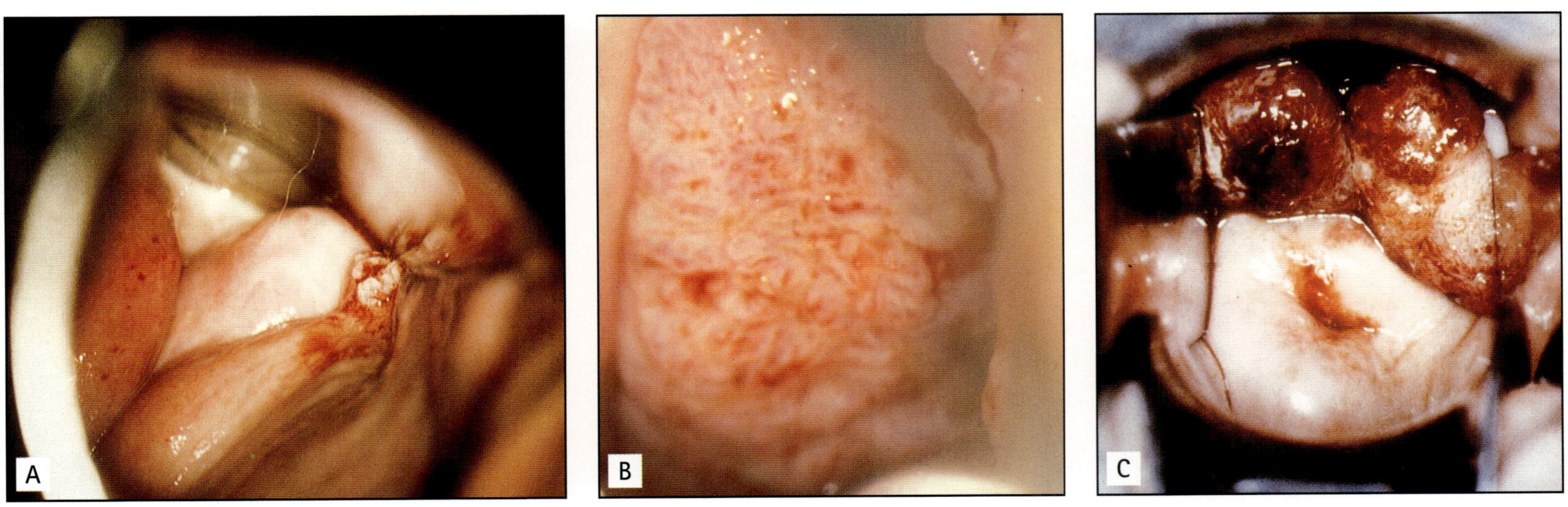

FIGURE 3-22.

Squamous cell carcinoma. Primary squamous cell cancer of the vagina is rare comprising 1% to 2% of all gynecologic malignancies. The vast majority of vaginal cancers are metastatic from the cervix or vulva, so extension from either of these sites must be excluded before confirming the diagnosis as a primary vaginal cancer. The mean age of onset is between 60 and 65 years. It is most commonly found in the posterior wall of the upper vagina and may readily extend to the bladder, rectum, and paravaginal and parametrial tissue. The most common presenting complaint is vaginal bleeding or discharge, or an abnormal Pap smear. **A** to **C**, Various stages of invasive vaginal cancer are shown. In *A*, a small raised cancer can be seen along the right vaginal wall. In *B*, a larger cancer with atypical vessels is seen alongside the cervix. In *C*, a large vaginal tumor invading the entire anterior fornix. (A and C, *courtesy of* B. A. Krumholz, MD.; B, *courtesy of* R. H. Kaufman, MD.)

FIGO STAGING FOR CARCINOMA OF THE VAGINA

Stage 0	Carcinoma *in situ* intraepithelial carcinoma
Stage I	Carcinoma limited to the vaginal wall
Stage II	Carcinoma involves the subvaginal tissue but does not extend to the pelvic wall
Stage III	Carcinoma has extended to the pelvic wall
Stage IV	Carcinoma has extended beyond the true pelvis or has clinically involved the mucosa of the bladder or rectum
Stage IVa	Spread of the growth to adjacent organs and/or direct extension beyond the true pelvis
Stage IVb	Spread to distant organs

FIGURE 3-23.

International Federation of Gynecology and Ostetrics (FIGO) staging system for vaginal cancer. Cancer of the vagina is clinically staged similar to cervical cancer. (*From* Petterson F, ed: *Annual Report on the Results of Treatment in Gynecologic Cancer*, vol 20. Stockhom: International Federation of Gynecology and Obstetrics; 1988; with permission.)

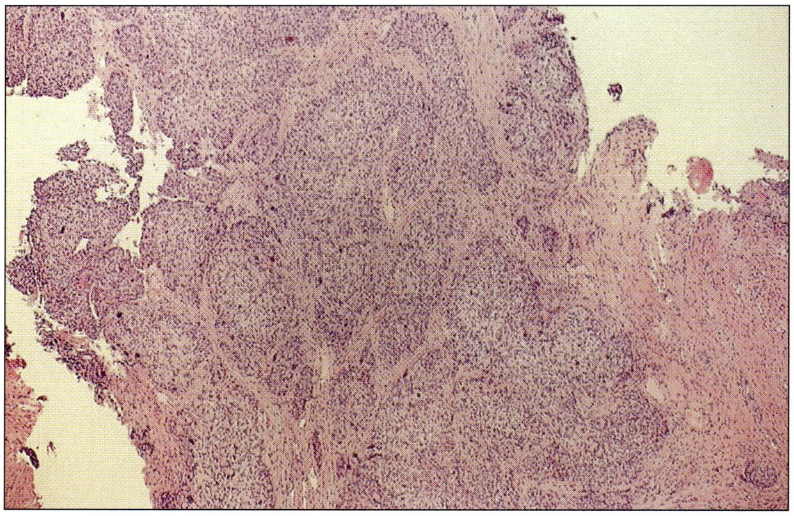

FIGURE 3-24.

Squamous cell vaginal cancer—microscopic features. Primary vaginal squamous cell cancers may be indistinguishable from cancer that extends from the cervix or vulva. Establishing a vaginal origin for the cancer involves excluding a history of cervical or vulvar cancer. Histologically, the well-differentiated tumor may be keratinized with squamous pearls and intracellular bridges. More poorly differentiated lesions may not show keratinization. (*Courtesy of* P. Wasserman, MD.)

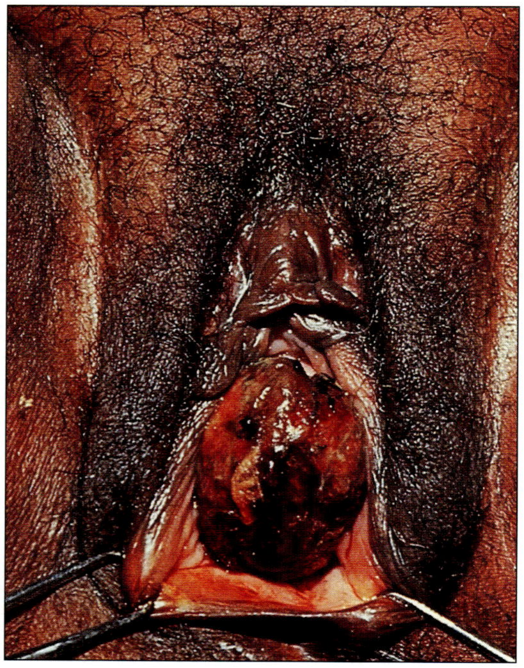

FIGURE 3-25.

Vaginal sarcoma. Vaginal sarcomas are very rare tumors. In general, tumors respond well to local excision if they have few mitotic figures per 10 high-power fields, are well circumscribed, and do not infiltrate at the margins. More aggressive sarcomas, such as the one shown protruding through the introitus, have a poorer prognosis. Fortunately, hematogenous dissemination usually occurs later in the course of the disease. Surgical excision and local radiation are the mainstays of therapy. (*Courtesy of* R. H. Kaufman, MD.)

DIETHYLSTILBESTROL EXPOSURE

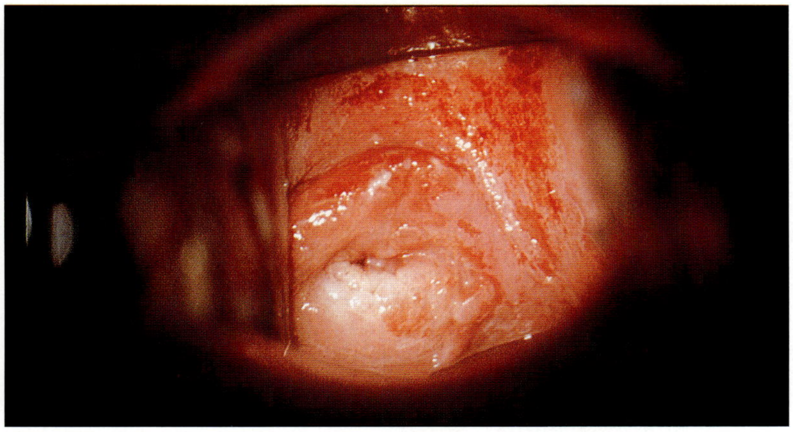

FIGURE 3-26.

Vaginal adenosis. Vaginal adenosis (the presence of mucous secreting glandular epithelium in the vagina) is common among women who were exposed *in utero* to diethylstilbestrol (DES) and uncommon in the rest of the population. The percentage of DES-exposed women with vaginal adenosis ranges from 15% to 20%, and each woman may have varying amounts of adenosis. The anterior wall is most commonly affected followed by the posterior wall. The upper vagina is more commonly affected than the lower vagina and the epithelium is usually of endocervical type. The lower vagina often is involved with tubo- endometrial epithelium. Adenosis eventually regresses spontaneously through the process of squamous metaplasia. Although the rates of regression vary, most adenosis resolves by the time a woman reaches her thirties. In 18% to 33% of DES-exposed women a variety of structural changes of the cervix and vagina occur. The vaginal changes include absent pars vaginalis and apical narrowing of the vagina. DES-exposed women also have an increased risk of clear cell adenocarcinoma of the cervix and vagina (about 1 in 1000 exposed women). Clinically, adenosis is suspected in a woman who was born between 1941 and 1971 and presents with lesions on the vaginal mucosa that are patchy or diffuse, red and stippled, granular or nodular (as in this colpophotograph), and do not stain with iodine. Small cysts or ulcers may also be present. (*Courtesy of* B. A. Krumholz, MD.)

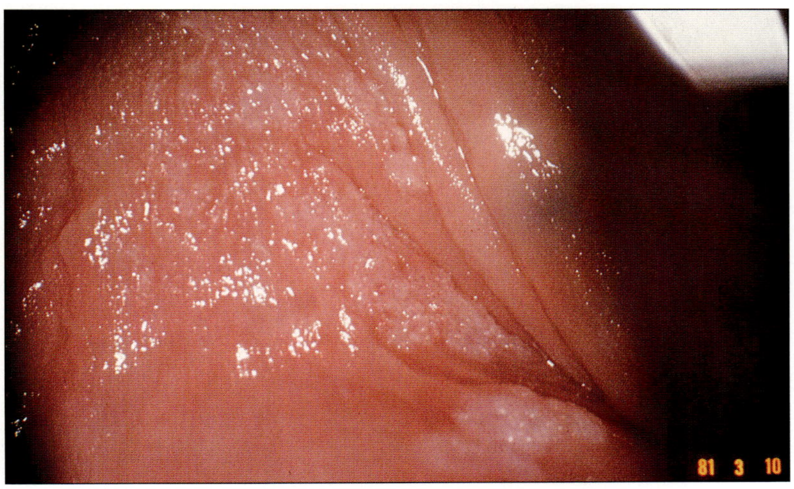

FIGURE 3-27.

Vaginal adenosis—management of the diethylstillbestrol (DES)–exposed woman. Colposcopy of the vagina in a DES-exposed woman is very difficult. Changes of acetowhite epithelium, punctations, and mosaic patterns are common and are significant only when they represent a change. The figure shows patches of vaginal acetowhite epithelium consistent with vaginal adenosis that has undergone squamous metaplasia. Ideally, annual colposcopic follow-up should be performed by the person who is experienced in the evaluation of DES-exposed women. This way, deviation from the normal maturation process can be identified. (*Courtesy of* B. A. Krumholz, MD.)

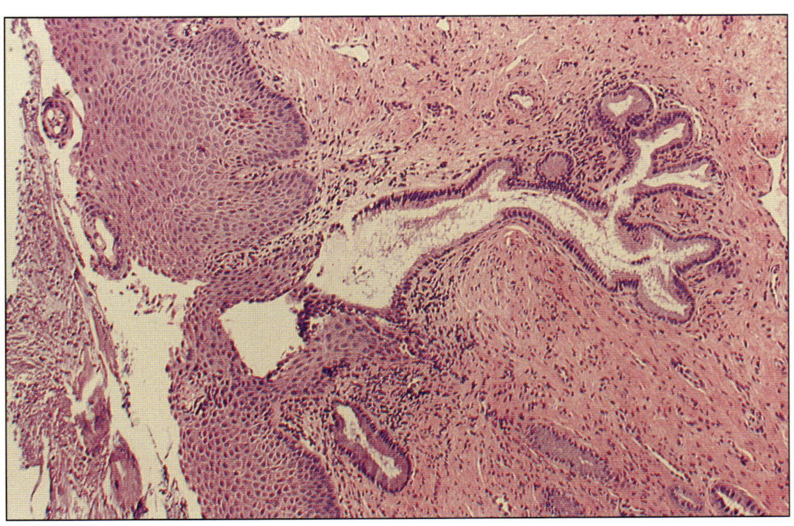

FIGURE 3-28.

Vaginal adenosis—microscopic features. Microscopically, mucinous columnar cells comprise the glandular epithelium in 62% of vaginal adenosis. It is the only type that replaces superficial vaginal epithelium and is the epithelial type most recognized colposcopically. Tubal- and endometrial-type cells, which are found in 21% of adenosis specimens, are found increasingly in adenosis of the lower vagina, and also in the lamina propria. Squamous metaplasia is present to some extent in all biopsies. The figure shows vaginal adenosis in its earlier stages with glandular epithelium evident. (*Courtesy of* P. Wasserman, MD.)

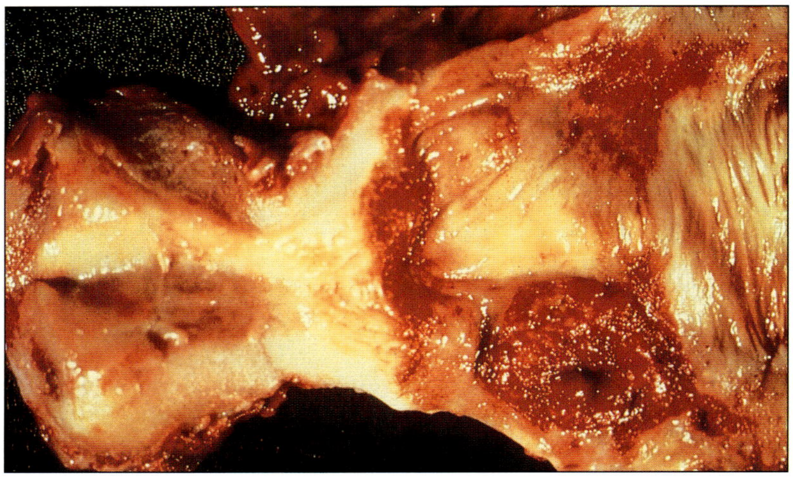

FIGURE 3-29.
Vaginal clear cell adenocarcinoma. Clear cell adenocarcinoma of the vagina is exceedingly rare in women without prenatal exposure to diethylstillbestrol (DES). In non-DES–exposed women, clear cell adenocarcinoma is found after menopause. In DES-exposed women, its incidence begins at age 7, peaks between the ages of 15 and 20, with some cases present until age 40 (or higher). Women at greatest risk were those exposed to DES before the 20th week of gestation. The majority of women with this disease complain of abnormal bleeding and discharge. About one fifth are asymptomatic. The majority of the lesions are vaginal, and about one third are cervical. The lesions are polypoid or flat indurated plaques with ulceration. The diagnosis may be suspected by vaginal cytology but is confirmed by colposcopically directed biopsy. Treatment is by radical hysterectomy and partial vaginectomy with pelvic lymphadenectomy and conservation of the ovaries. As seen in this surgical specimen, the cancer is the granular lesion seen near the vaginal vault. Pelvic irradiation has also been used but is less desirable because it castrates a young woman. (*Courtesy of* R. H. Kaufman, MD.)

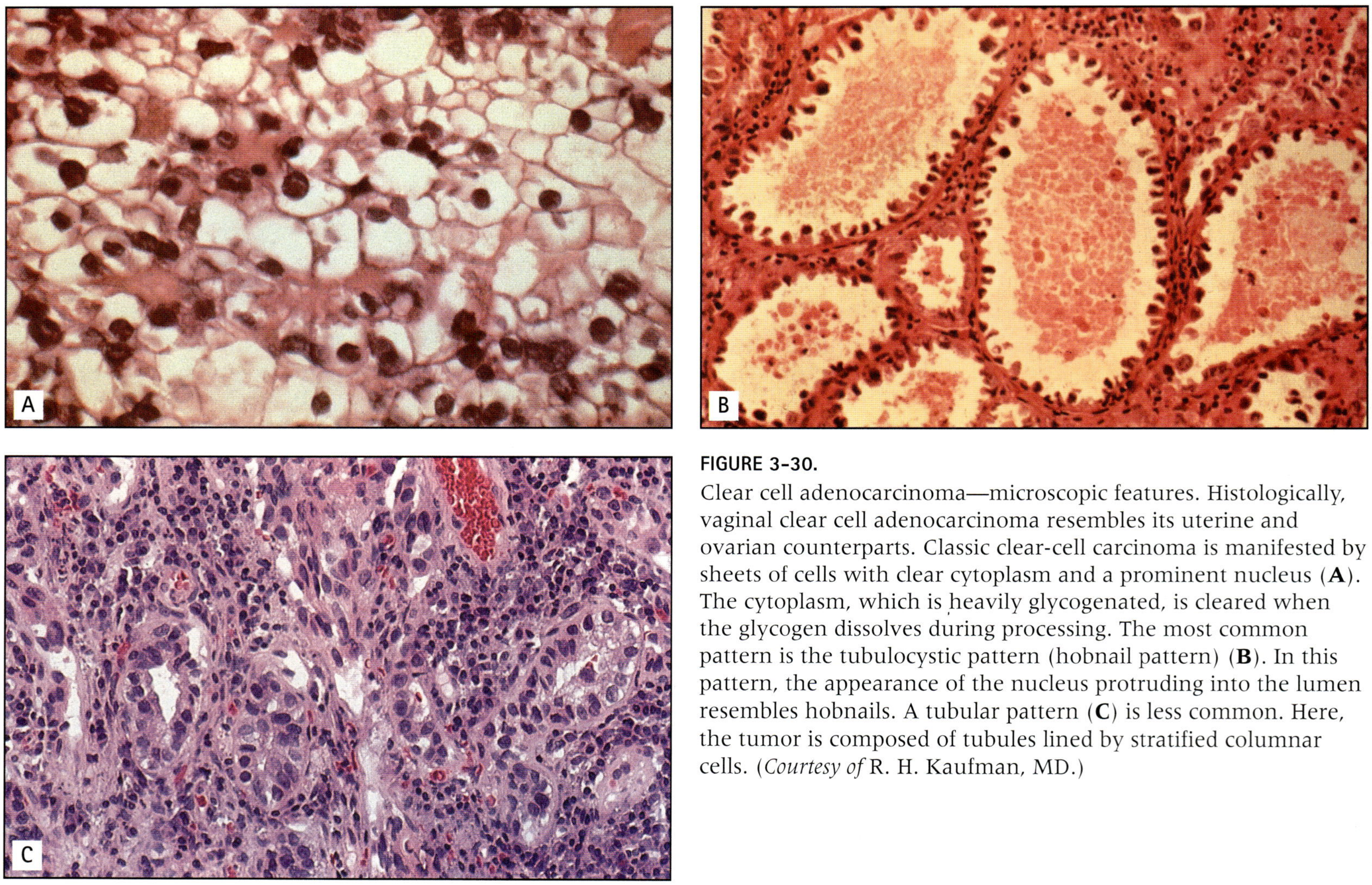

FIGURE 3-30.
Clear cell adenocarcinoma—microscopic features. Histologically, vaginal clear cell adenocarcinoma resembles its uterine and ovarian counterparts. Classic clear-cell carcinoma is manifested by sheets of cells with clear cytoplasm and a prominent nucleus (**A**). The cytoplasm, which is heavily glycogenated, is cleared when the glycogen dissolves during processing. The most common pattern is the tubulocystic pattern (hobnail pattern) (**B**). In this pattern, the appearance of the nucleus protruding into the lumen resembles hobnails. A tubular pattern (**C**) is less common. Here, the tumor is composed of tubules lined by stratified columnar cells. (*Courtesy of* R. H. Kaufman, MD.)

*U*NUSUAL LESIONS

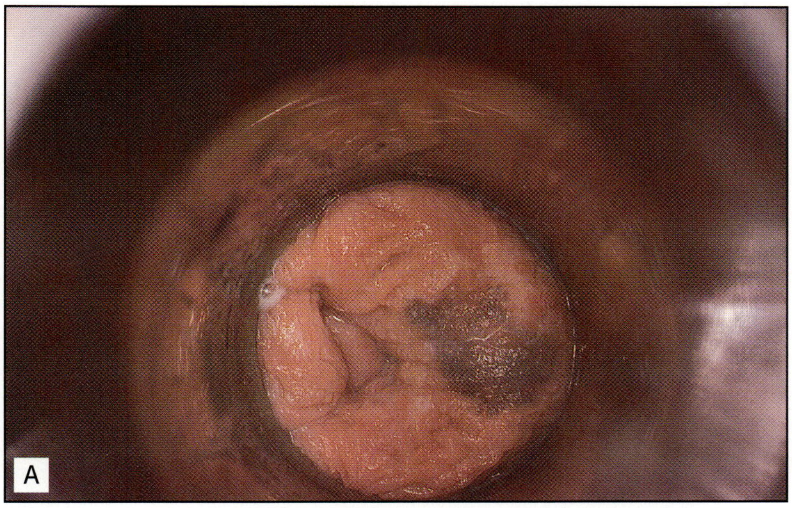

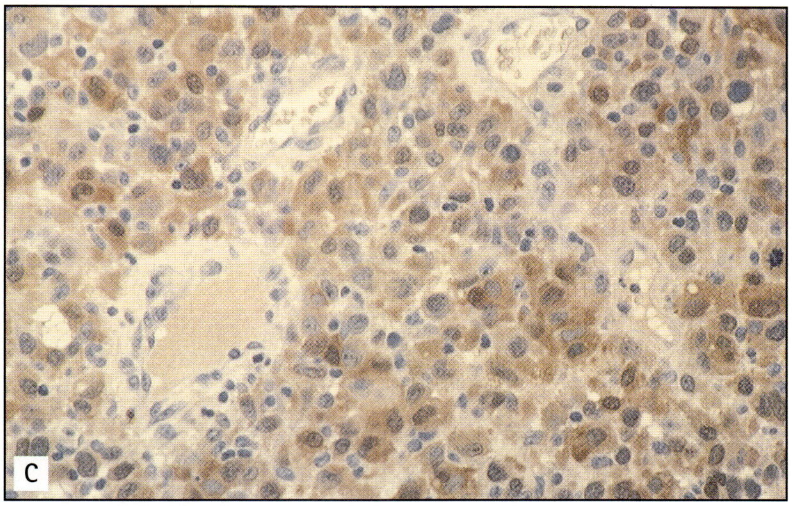

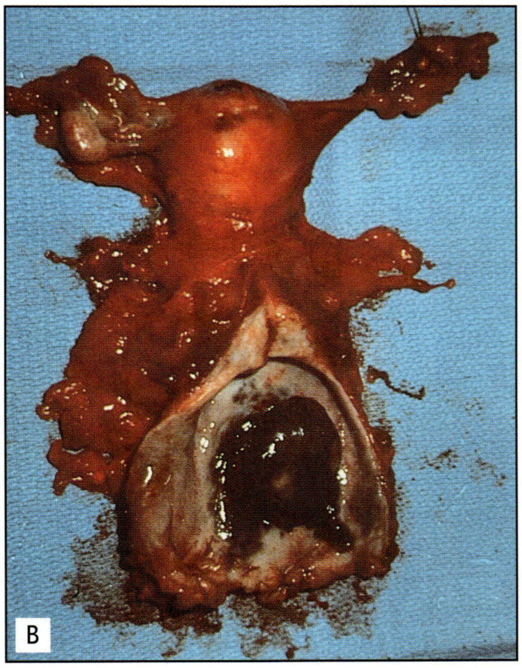

FIGURE 3-31.
Pigmented vaginal lesions. Benign pigmented lesions in the vagina are extremely rare, and so melanoma must be suspected whenever a pigmented lesion is seen. Histologically, the cells may be spindle-shaped, epithelial, or small and may not be pigmented. The prognosis is usually poor. Examples of benign pigmented lesions include lentigo (melanosis) (**A**) and endometriosis (*see* Fig. 3-32). Because these lesions are so rare and the prognosis of melanoma is so poor, the diagnosis must always be confirmed with a biopsy regardless of the benign appearance of the gross lesion. Vaginal malignant melanoma (**B**) is also very rare. It is most commonly found in the anterior vaginal wall in the lower vagina and usually in postmenopausal women. Lesions may be single or multiple, pigmented or nonpigmented. The predominant symptoms are bleeding, discharge, and the feeling of a mass. When vaginal malignant melanoma does occur, it is often metastatic, and a primary focus must be sought. Melanomas can occur in any portion of the vagina but are most frequent in the lower third. The gross and microscopic appearance of melanomas in the vagina, is the same as when they are present in other locations. They show considerable variation in size, color, and growth pattern. **C,** The photomicrograph shows a classic vaginal melanoma with sheets of melanocytes. (A, *courtesy of* the International Society for the Study of Vulvar Disease; B and C, *courtesy of* R. H. Kaufman, MD.)

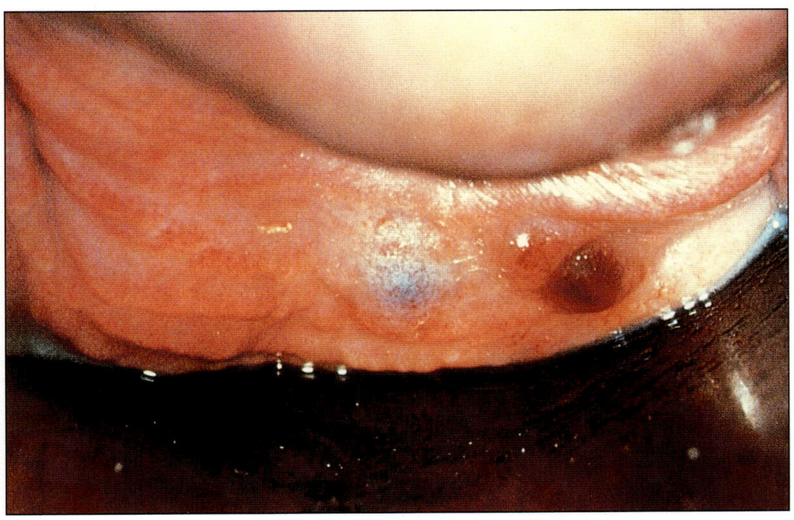

FIGURE 3-32.
Endometriosis. The vagina is a less common site for endometriotic implants. Vaginal endometriosis is almost invariably associated with endometriosis elsewhere in the pelvis. Endometriosis may penetrate the vaginal wall from the cul-de-sac, may develop from peritoneal remnants in the rectovaginal septum, or may implant during an episiotomy repair. The typical appearance is that of blue-domed cysts in the posterior vaginal fornix at the attachment of the uterosacral ligaments and along the rectovaginal septum. Active endometriotic implants that respond to cyclic ovarian stimulation may result in an endometrial cyst. Vaginal endometriosis is often painful and may cause dyspareunia. Surgical excision may be difficult because the condition may be associated with a dense fibrotic reaction. This colpophotograph shows both red- and blue-domed lesions in the posterior vaginal fornix. (*Courtesy of* R. H. Kaufman, MD.)

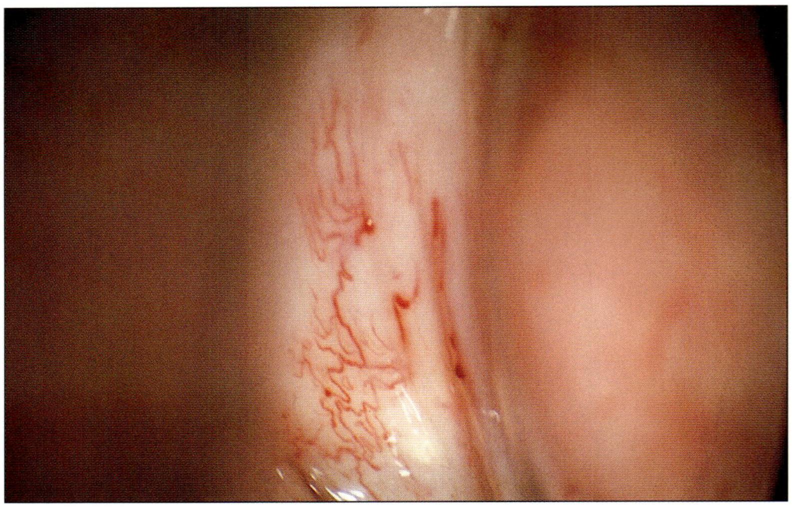

FIGURE 3-33.

Radiation changes. In the treatment of many gynecologic cancers, radiation is used primarily or as an adjunct to treatment along with surgery. After radiation, bizarre vascular patterns may be seen in the vagina on a white background or on a pale atrophic background as represented in this colpophotograph. These vessels may be indistinguishable from those found in malignant disease and must be distinguished from recurrent malignancy by a directed biopsy.

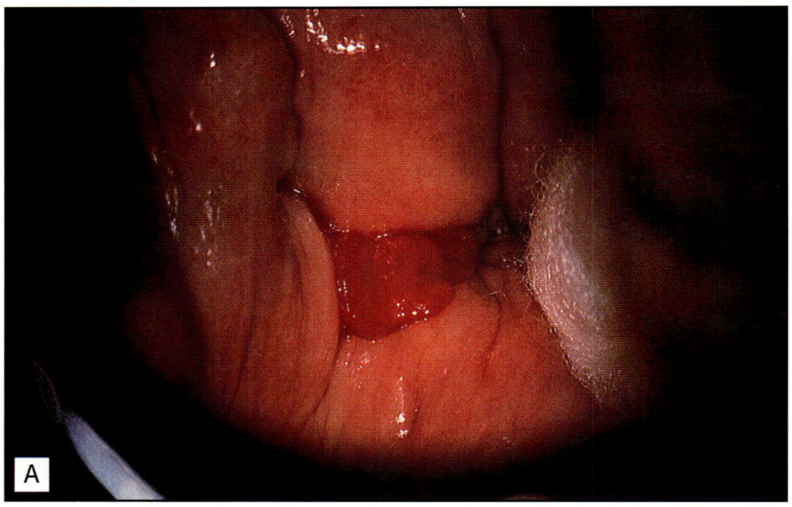

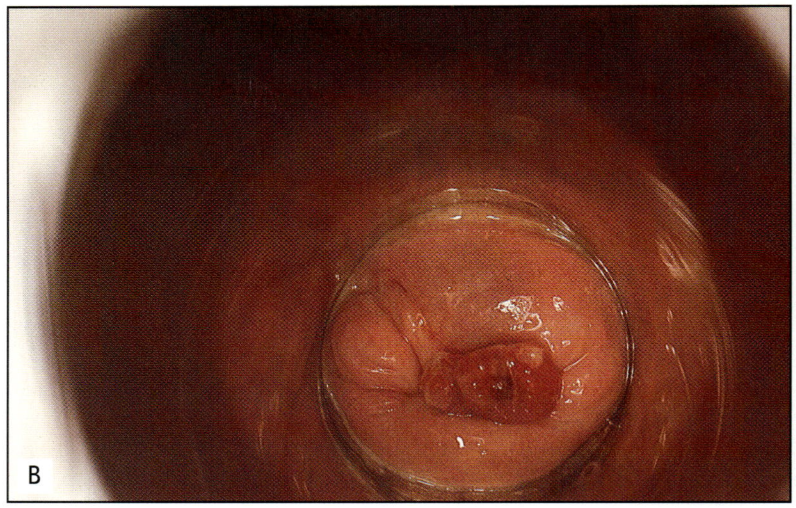

FIGURE 3-34.

Granulation tissue—prolapsed Fallopian tube. Four or more weeks after hysterectomy, some patients are found to have a fleshy lesion at the vaginal vault (**A**). The lesion often bleeds when touched, and the patient may complain of postcoital bleeding. These lesions are easily and painlessly removed in the office by excisional biopsy, and their base should be cauterized with silver nitrate to discourage recurrence. In patients in whom the Fallopian tubes were not removed, consideration must be given to the possibility that this lesion represents prolapse of the Fallopian tube (**B**). These patients complain of persistent and profuse vaginal discharge, lower abdominal pain, and occasionally dyspareunia. Any attempt to remove or biopsy these lesions in the office without anesthesia causes extreme pain, making the diagnosis obvious. (B *courtesy of* the International Society for the Study of Vulvar Disease.)

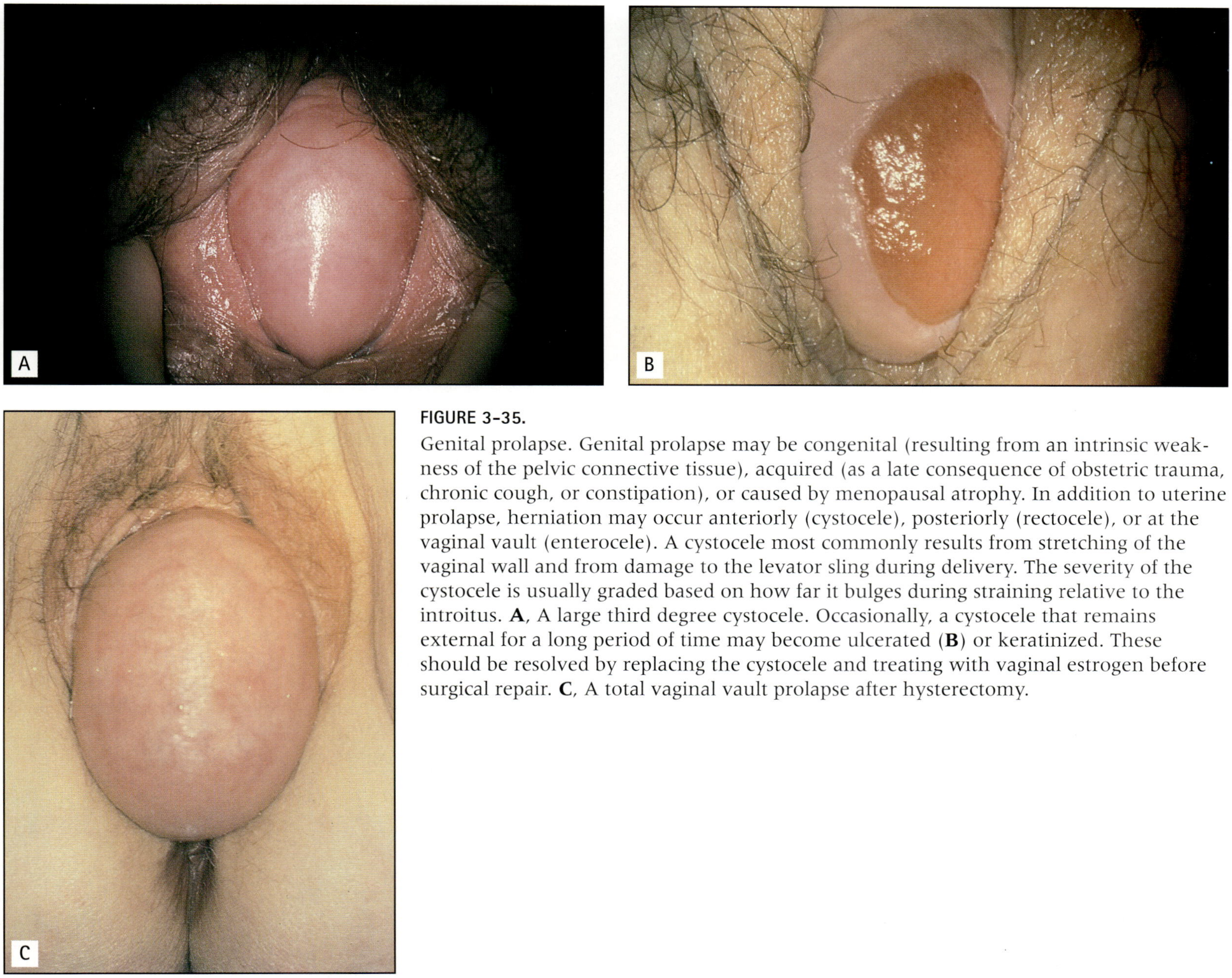

FIGURE 3-35.

Genital prolapse. Genital prolapse may be congenital (resulting from an intrinsic weakness of the pelvic connective tissue), acquired (as a late consequence of obstetric trauma, chronic cough, or constipation), or caused by menopausal atrophy. In addition to uterine prolapse, herniation may occur anteriorly (cystocele), posteriorly (rectocele), or at the vaginal vault (enterocele). A cystocele most commonly results from stretching of the vaginal wall and from damage to the levator sling during delivery. The severity of the cystocele is usually graded based on how far it bulges during straining relative to the introitus. **A**, A large third degree cystocele. Occasionally, a cystocele that remains external for a long period of time may become ulcerated (**B**) or keratinized. These should be resolved by replacing the cystocele and treating with vaginal estrogen before surgical repair. **C**, A total vaginal vault prolapse after hysterectomy.

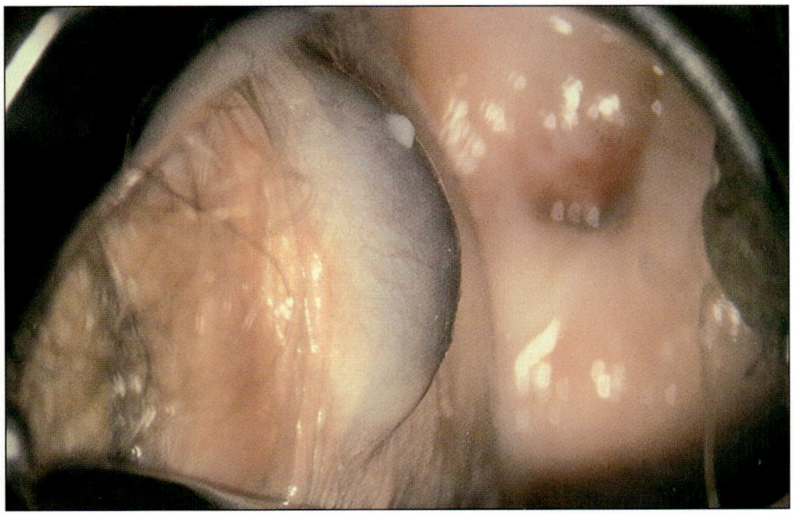

FIGURE 3-36.

Developmental cysts. Developmental cysts found in the vagina are remnants of the müllerian or wolffian duct. Müllerian remnants are lined by epithelium typically found elsewhere in the genital tract; wolffian remnants may contain similar epithelium or low cuboidal epithelium with a prominent basement membrane. Gartner's cysts (wolffian remnants), which may be single or multiple and are seldom very large, classically occur in the anterolateral vaginal wall but may occur anywhere in the vaginal canal. They are usually asymptomatic and do not need treatment unless they become large or symptomatic. Occasionally, they become large enough to be confused with a cystocele and may cause pain, dyspareunia, or even dystocia in labor. Because they may extend into the broad ligament and involve critical structures such as the ureter, surgical management should be undertaken with great caution. Pictured is a large Gartner's duct cyst on the lower lateral vaginal sidewall. (*Courtesy of* R. H. Kaufman, MD.)

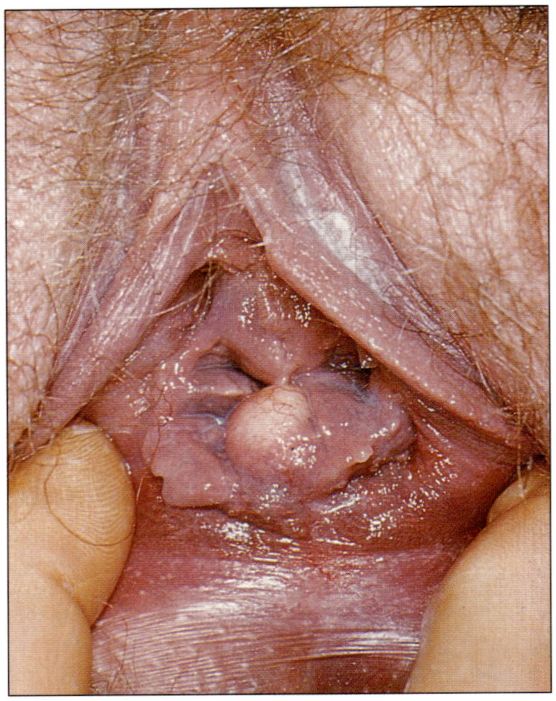

FIGURE 3-37.
Inclusion cysts. The most common vaginal cyst is an inclusion cyst secondary to trauma. These are usually small and asymptomatic and are frequently found at the site of an episiotomy repair, as shown in the figure. They may occur when squamous mucosal epithelium is buried during the repair. When a patient complains, it is usually of dyspareunia or the presence of a lump. Inclusion cysts are easily removed surgically. (*Courtesy of* the International Society for the Study of Vulvar Disease.)

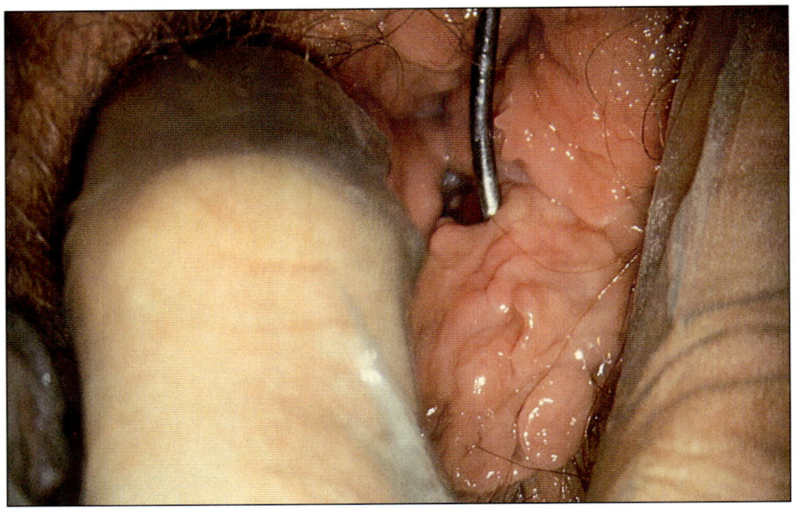

FIGURE 3-38.
Rectovaginal fistula. Rectovaginal fistulas occur most commonly as a result of obstetric trauma. Less common causes include radiation enteritis, tuberculosis, lymphogranuloma venereum, and regional enteritis. Obstetric fistulas are almost always related to an undiagnosed or improperly repaired fourth-degree laceration. The diagnosis is suspected when the patient complains of involuntary loss of feces from the vagina or uncontrolled flatulence. Rectovaginal fistulas can be separated into those close to the introitus, which can be repaired by creating an episioproctotomy followed by a layered closure, or those more distal to the introitus, for which the fistulous tract is excised and the defect is closed in layers. The figure shows a small rectovaginal fistula close to the introitus. By passing a probe through it, its track can be confirmed. (*Courtesy of* R. H. Kaufman, MD.)

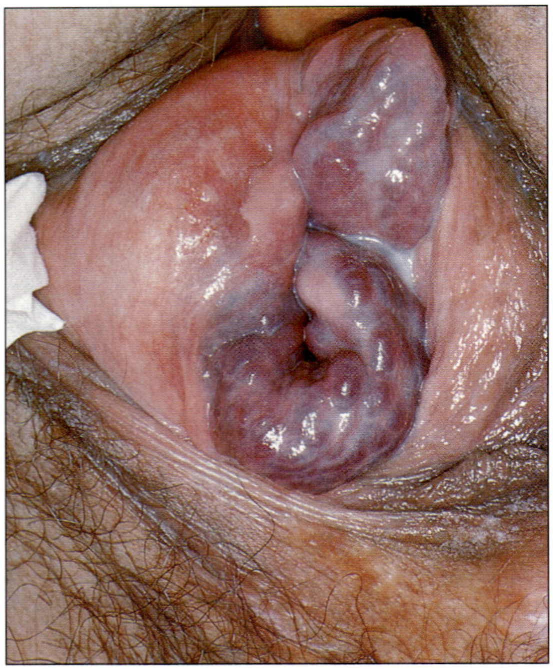

FIGURE 3-39.
Vaginal varicosities. The combination of congenital predisposition, vascular congestion, and relaxation associated with advanced pregnancy and prolonged standing can result in vaginal varicosities. When they are as large as the ones seen in the figure, they are sometimes painful and may on rare occasion rupture spontaneously resulting in profuse hemorrhage. Care must be taken to avoid laceration of these vessels during delivery or via episiotomy repair. (*Courtesy of* R. H. Kaufman, MD.)

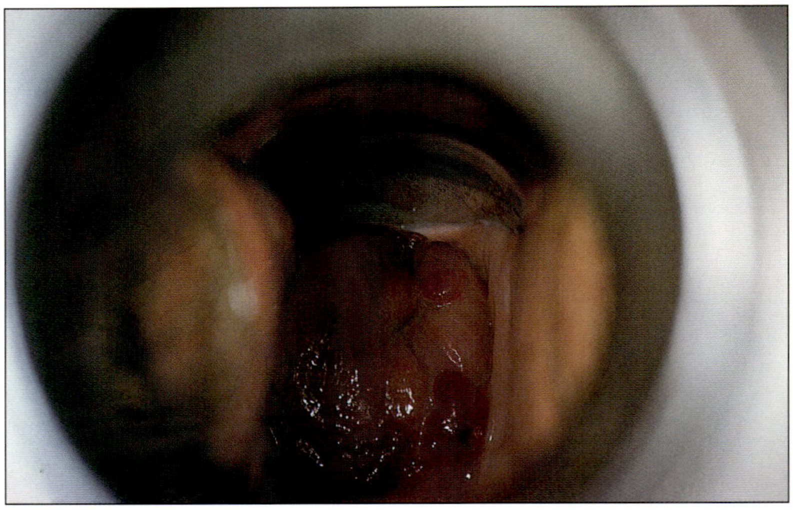

FIGURE 3-40.
Decidual reaction. Decidual reactions may be seen on peritoneal surfaces or mucous membranes during pregnancy. It is usually a response of indigenous stromal cells to high circulating levels of estrogen and progesterone. The decidual foci are visible as small, soft, reddish patches that bleed easily on contact. (*Courtesy of* the International Society for the Study of Vulvar Disease.)

SELECTED BIBLIOGRAPHY

Kaufman RH, Friedrich EG Jr, Gardner HL: *Benign Diseases of the Vulva and Vagina*. Chicago: Year Book Medical Publishers; 1989.

Smith ML, Scott JL Jr: Benign neoplasms of the vagina. In *Gynecology and Obstetrics*, vol 1. Edited by Sciarra JJ. Philadelphia: Harper and Row; 1984.

Woodruff JD, Angtuaco TL, Parmley TH, eds: Vagina. In *Atlas of Gynecologic Pathology*. New York: Raven Press; 1993.

Zaino RJ, Robboy SJ, Bentley R, Kurman RJ. Diseases of the vagina. In *Blaustein's Pathology of the Female Genital Tract*. Edited by Kurman RJ. New York: Springer-Verlag; 1994:131–183.

CHAPTER 4

Pathology of the Uterine Cervix

Jo Ann Benda

The uterine cervix is a relatively easily visualized internal organ that is accessible to pathologic evaluation. Detection of cancerous and precancerous lesions with Pap smear, colposcopy, and biopsy followed by appropriate therapy has led to a significant drop in the incidence of invasive cervical cancer. Infections, anatomic variations, and hormonal responses can also be identified in biopsy specimens. The first section of this chapter illustrates microscopic anatomic variations of the cervix that in some cases could be misinterpreted as a disease process. Variations in hormonal stimuli can also alter the histologic appearance of the cervix. Several of the more common inflammatory processes that may be found in biopsy material are included. The second section of the chapter demonstrates the precancerous lesions of the cervix, including cervical intraepithelial neoplasia of the squamous type and glandular lesions. The histologic effects of some biopsy techniques will be demonstrated, with suggestions for prevention of excess damage to the tissue specimens. The third section describes the invasive cervical cancers in particular, the most common, squamous cell carcinoma. The histologic subtypes of squamous cell carcinoma, adenocarcinoma, and small cell carcinoma are illustrated. The last section illustrates some of the most unusual primary tumors of the cervix as well as metastatic lesions that can be mistaken for primary disease clinically.

MICROSCOPIC ANATOMIC VARIATIONS OF THE CERVIX

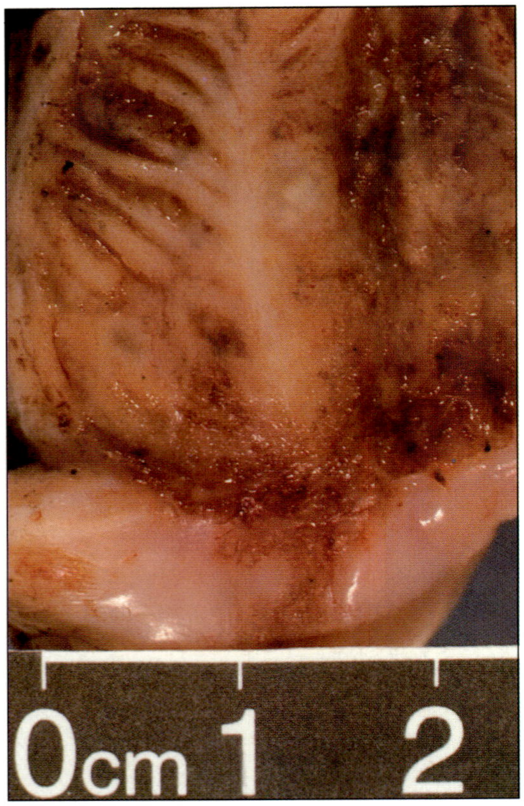

FIGURE 4–1.

Normal cervix. At the bottom of the photograph the smooth, glistening pink squamous mucosa is evident. The endocervix is actually composed of deep, complex folds that grossly resemble the fronds of palm leaves; these are the plicae palmatae. The tissue appears redder than the squamous mucosa because the epithelium is a single layer of columnar cells with the underlying blood vessels closer to the surface. When the columnar epithelium is present on the ectocervix, it is sometimes called "erosion," because of the red color, when in fact it is eversion of the normal endocervical mucosa. A true ulcer or erosion should be differentiated from this normal phenomenon. The two epithelial cell types meet at the squamocolumnar junction.

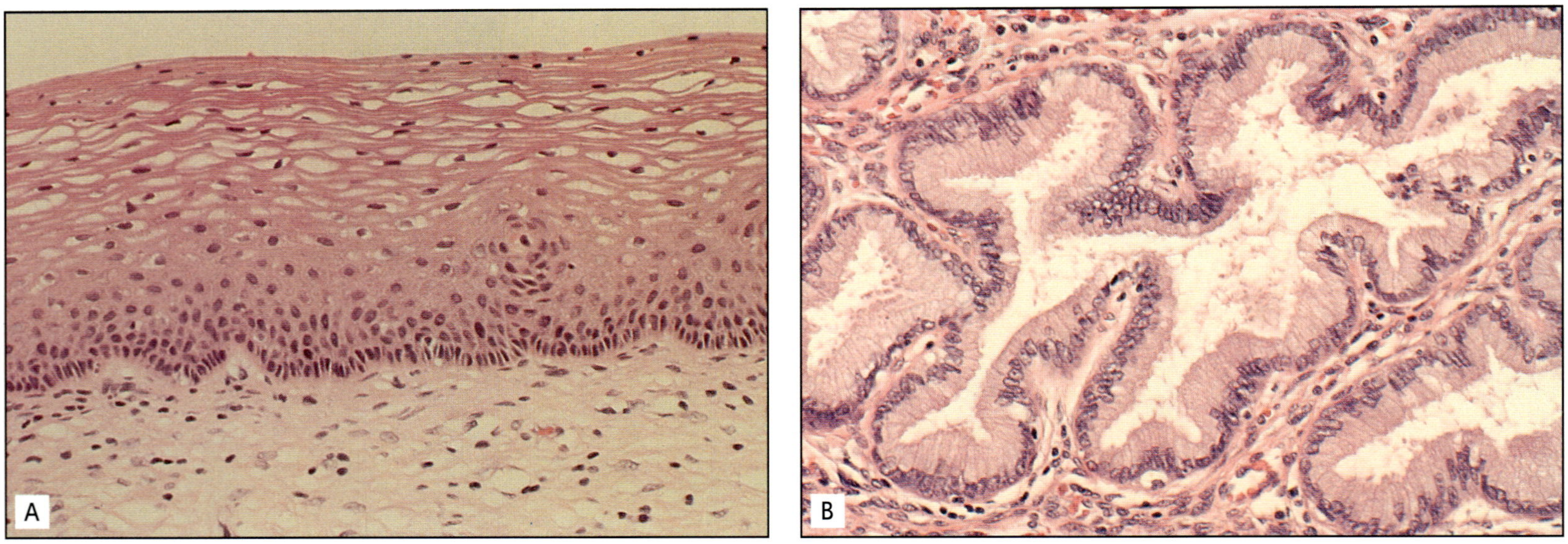

FIGURE 4–2.

Normal squamous and glandular epithelium of the cervix. **A**, Normal squamous epithelium of the ectocervix, characterized by a single layer of well demarcated basal cells, transition to a horizontal orientation of cells in the midportion of the epithelium, accumulation of cytoplasm in the upper layers with a decreasing nuclear to cytoplasmic ratio, small pyknotic nuclei at the surface, and no granular cell or keratin layers. Mitotic activity is confined to the basal layer. **B**, Normal columnar epithelium of the endocervix, characterized by tall columnar cells with small basal nuclei, intracytoplasmic mucin globules, and minimal mitotic activity. The amount of mucin present is dependent to some degree on the hormonal status of the patient.

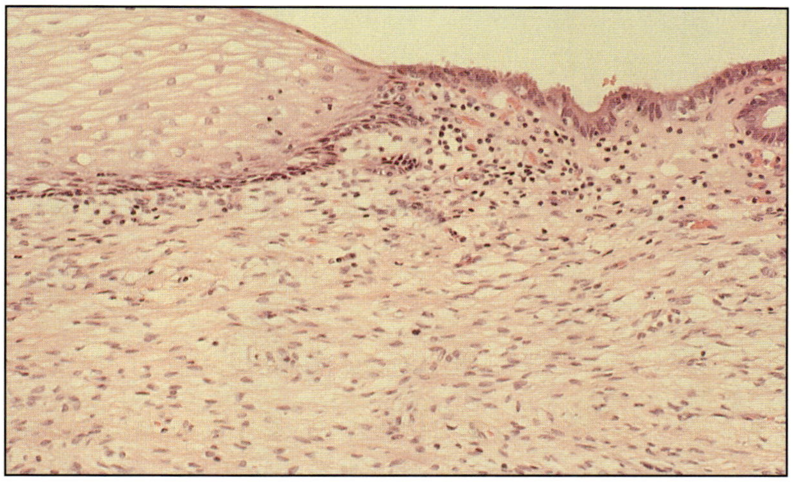

FIGURE 4-3.

Squamocolumnar junction. The squamocolumnar junction is the site where the glandular cells meet the squamous cells. During the reproductive years the squamocolumnar junction is usually visible with the naked eye and with colposcopic examination. Most squamous intraepithelial neoplastic lesions begin at this junction. As they spread out onto the ectocervix, the squamous lesions are visible by colposcopic examination. Newer information suggests that preneoplastic glandular lesions also begin at the squamocolumnar junction. However, they are not easily visualized by colposcopic examination. Theoretically, squamous lesions are visible after the application of acetic acid because the hypertonic solution temporarily dehydrates the cytoplasm and the nuclear material compacts. Because there are an increased number of cells and cells with more nuclear material, the epithelium appears more opaque, or white. The glandular lesions are not highlighted by acetic acid, and because they grow into the clefts of the endocervix are not so amenable to visualization.

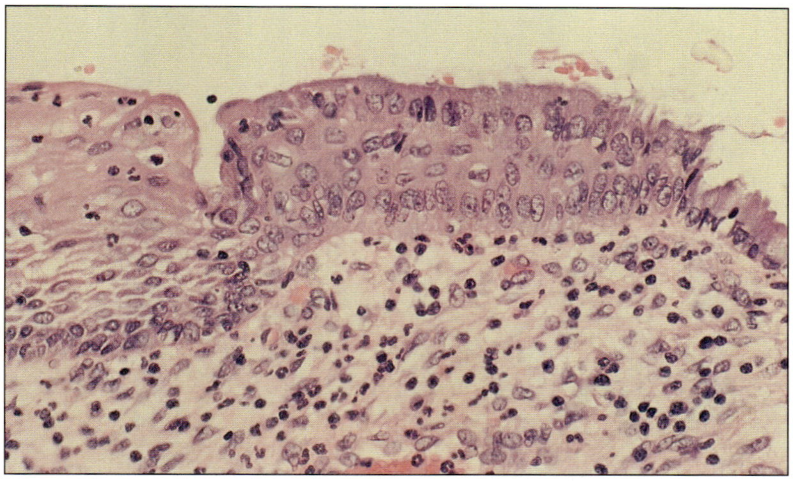

FIGURE 4-4.

Squamous metaplasia. Squamous metaplasia occurs at the squamocolumnar junction during the reproductive years when the endocervical glandular epithelium is exposed to the acidic vaginal environment. The basilar or subcolumnar reserve cells attempt to reepithelialize the surface with the more resilient squamous cells by gradual transformation. The cells of the lower part of the epithelium begin to accumulate cytoplasm and lose their columnar appearance, whereas the columnar surface cells appear to be lifted and replaced. Relative to mature squamous cells, the metaplastic cells have a larger, more vesicular nucleus that may contain a nucleolus. This normal process must be carefully excluded from diagnoses of dysplasia or intraepithelial neoplasia.

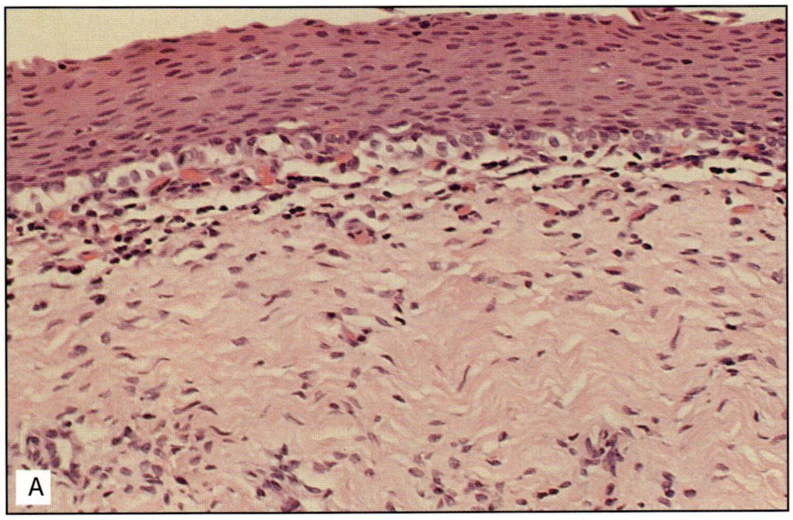

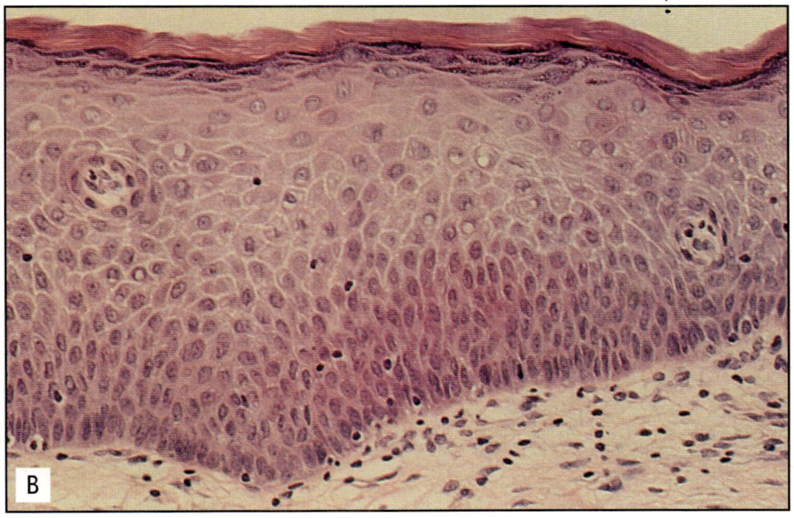

FIGURE 4-5.

Atrophy and keratinization. Although these two processes do not necessarily occur together, they are both commonly seen in postmenopausal women. **A**, Atrophy, the result of lack of estrogen, is demonstrated. The normal superficial cells of a mature squamous epithelium do not develop resulting in an epithelium composed of intermediate and basilar cells with relatively high nuclear to cytoplasmic ratios. These cells could inadvertently be interpreted as the basilar cells of a preneoplastic lesion. Therefore, the hormonal status of the patient should be included with cytology or biopsy requests for clinical-pathologic correlation of the interpretation. **B**, Keratinization of the type seen here, with a normal underlying squamous epithelium, is most often a result of trauma, usually owing to severe cervical-uterine prolapse.

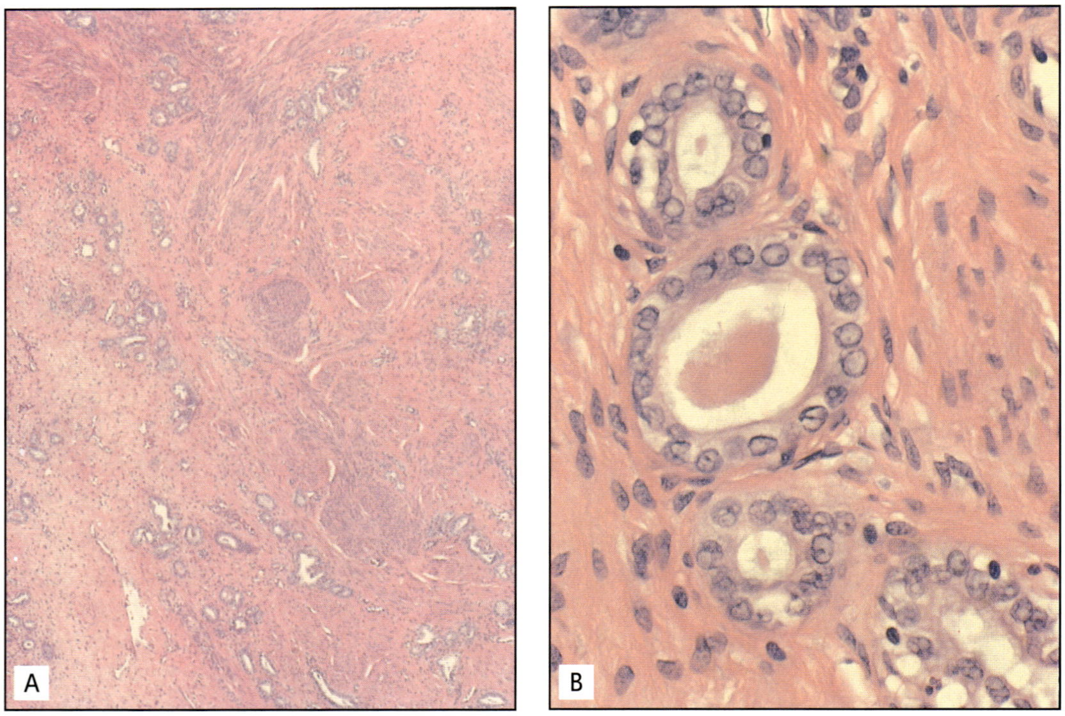

FIGURE 4-6.

Mesonephric remnants. These structures are embryonic remnants derived from mesonephric (wolffian) ducts that persist in about 20% of normal cervices and are usually found at the 3 and 9 o'clock positions (lateral cervix) [1]. At low power (**A**), the glandular structures are fairly diffuse throughout the stroma and are generally deep to the normal endocervical glands. In some cases a long tubular structure runs through the middle of the small glands. At higher power (**B**), the mesonephric remnants are distinguished from cervical glands by the lack of intracellular mucin, low columnar or cuboidal appearance, and the frequent presence of eosinophilic proteinaceous material in the lumens. They must be distinguished from endocervical adenocarcinoma, which is done by noting the lack of nuclear atypia and hyperchromasia, absence of mitoses, and the location in the cervix.

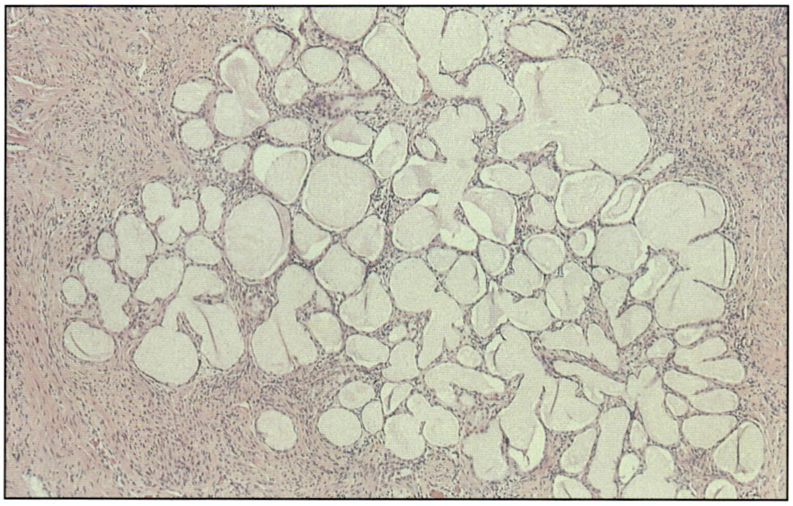

FIGURE 4-7.

Tunnel clusters. Tunnel clusters are aggregates of dilated microcystic endocervical glands that form distinct lobules. The process can become quite florid, but is generally confined to the part of the cervix that normally contains endocervical glands. The major problem with tunnel clusters is misinterpreting them as adenocarcinoma, particularly of the very well differentiated type (minimal deviation) [2]. Location in the inner third of the cervix wall, absence of any atypia or mitoses, and rounded configuration are helpful in distinguishing them from adenocarcinoma. Immunohistochemical studies for carcinoembryonic antigen may also be useful.

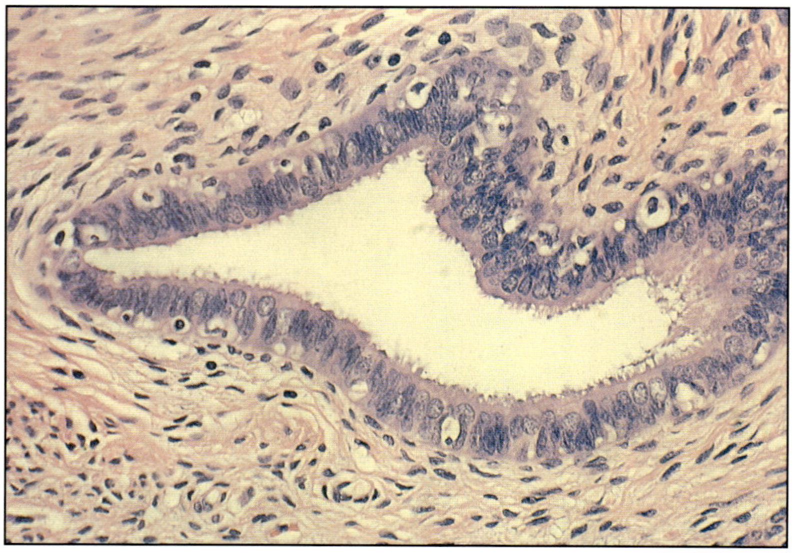

FIGURE 4-8.

Ciliated metaplasia. The upper endocervix is a frequent site of this finding in which the usual mucin-producing endocervical cells are replaced by columnar cells with cilia on the luminal border. In one study 70% of benign uteri and 89% of uteri removed for cervical carcinoma showed this finding [3]. The percentage of cervices in which this was found was dependent on the number of sections taken and whether sampling of the upper third of the cervical canal was done. This may well be considered a variation of normal at the uterocervical junction. The major problem is misinterpreting this as a neoplastic glandular process in Pap smears, particularly since the introduction of the cytobrush, which samples from higher in the endocervical canal.

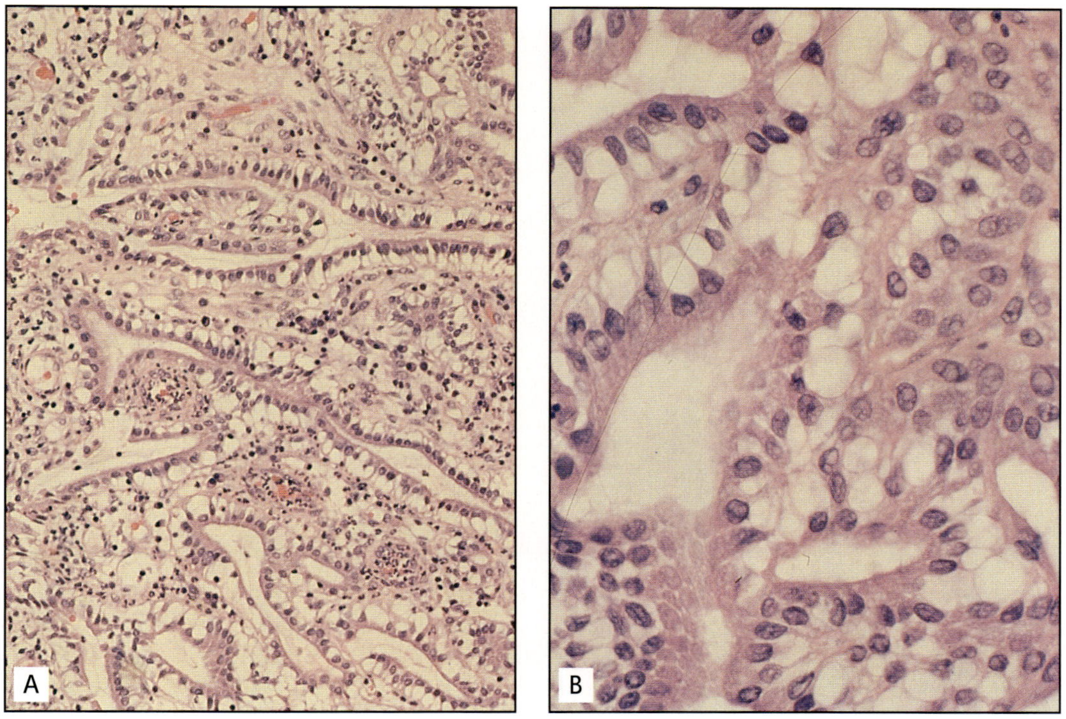

FIGURE 4-9.

Microglandular hyperplasia. This non-neoplastic variation of normal endocervix has been thought to develop under the influence of hormonal stimulation as it is most frequently seen in patients who are pregnant, taking oral contraceptives, or on other forms of hormone therapy. Some recent data would suggest this may be a mistaken impression [4]. **A**, The glands become tightly packed and may have a gland-within-gland pattern. **B**, Vacuolation at the base of the cells is common. Squamous metaplasia or basilar hyperplasia commonly accompany the process. This process may cause the cervix to be somewhat friable, thus symptoms may include vaginal spotting or postcoital bleeding.

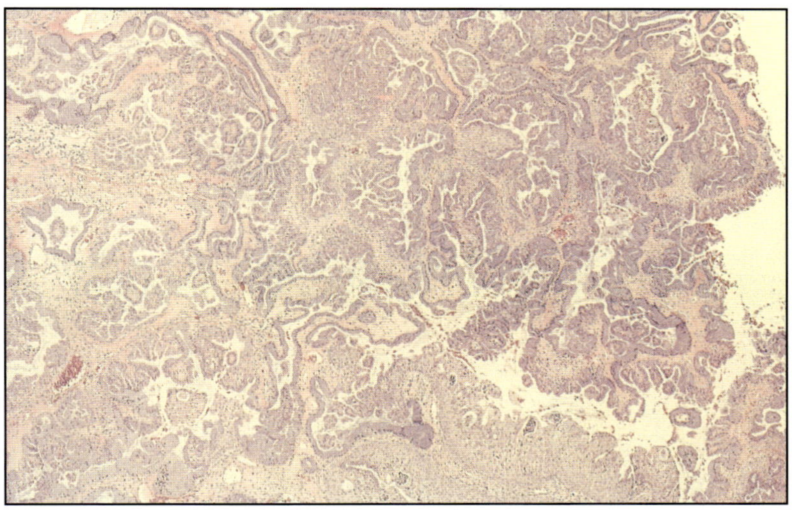

FIGURE 4-10.

Atypical polypoid microglandular hyperplasia. In this photomicrograph the microglandular hyperplasia is so florid it is difficult to identify the stromal component. These cases can be particularly troublesome to distinguish from adenocarcinoma [5]. The bland cells and presence of more typical microglandular hyperplasia nearby can be of assistance. Information about the hormonal status of the patient is most useful in alerting the pathologist to consider this unusual benign condition.

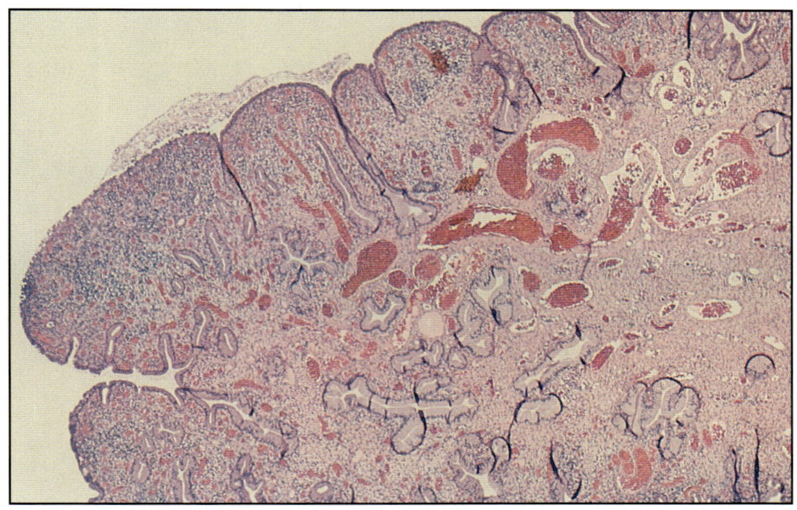

FIGURE 4-11.

Endocervical polyp. Endocervical polyps are more often an exaggeration of the normal folds of the endocervix than true neoplastic polyps. Inflammation and edema make the folds protrude from the cervix. The polypoid structure in the photomicrograph has a surface of normal endocervical glandular epithelium, increased thick-walled vessels within the stroma, and an inflammatory infiltrate below the surface. Because they are easily traumatized, endocervical polyps may cause the worrisome symptoms of intermenstrual or postcoital bleeding. Generally they are easily removed at a clinic visit.

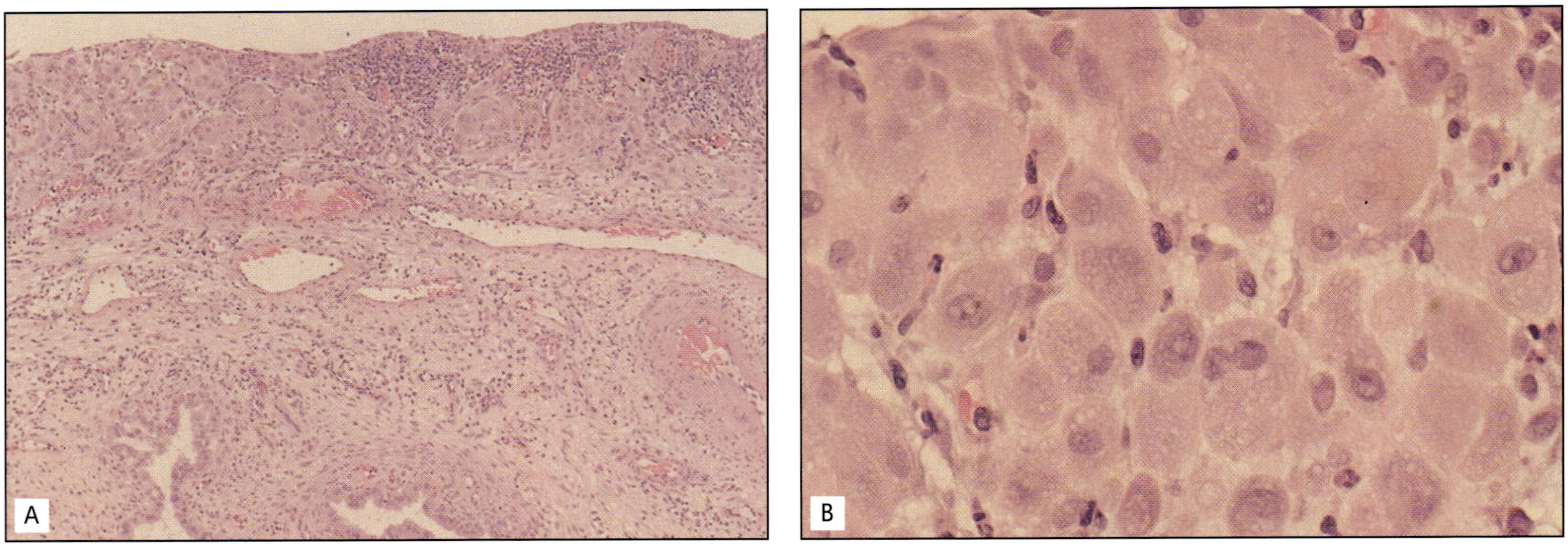

FIGURE 4-12.

Decidualization of the cervical stroma. Decidualization of the cervical stroma occurs during pregnancy. **A**, Photomicrograph shows the decidua just below the epithelium. It can also occur around blood vessels. **B**, Large nuclei with large nucleoli and the abundant cytoplasm of typical decidua are seen. The biggest pitfall with decidua is misinterpreting it as squamous cells invading the stroma, particularly if a patient who is pregnant is biopsied for an abnormal pap smear (or has an intraepithelial lesion). This is yet another instance in which the clinical information may be of great significance in alerting the pathologist to a diagnosis found only in specific clinical circumstances.

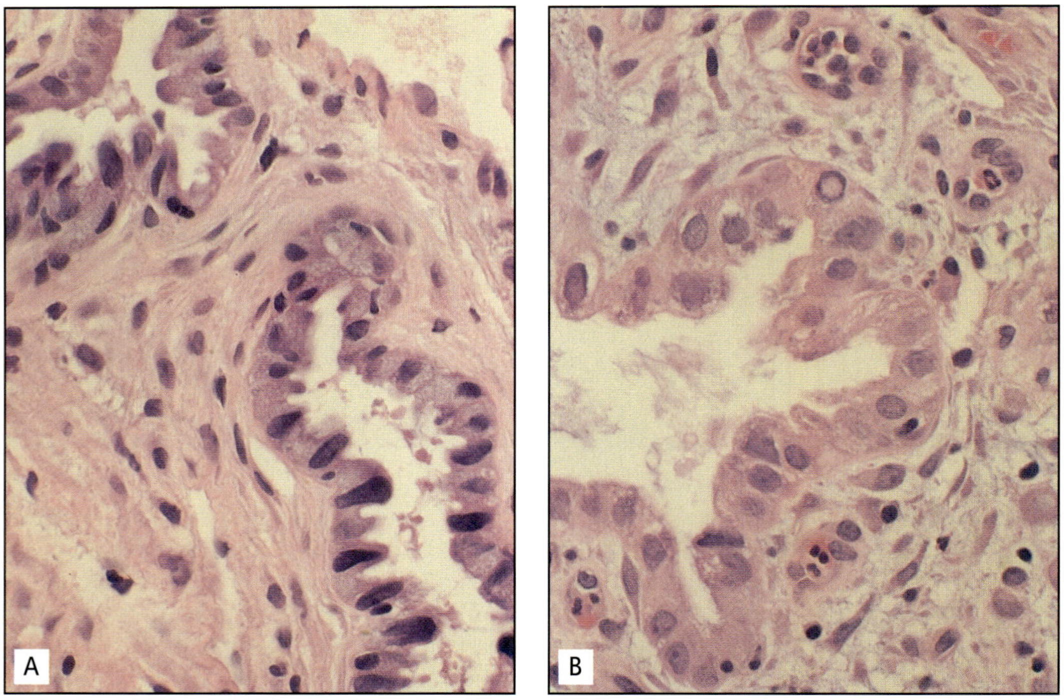

FIGURE 4-13.

Arias-Stella reaction of cervical epithelium. Although Arias-Stella reaction of the endometrium is fairly well-recognized, the same process in the endocervical glands is much less often identified. The process in which the glandular cells show marked cytologic atypia is the result of the hormonal milieu of pregnancy. The nuclei come away from the basement membrane and protrude into the glandular lumen. Nuclei are hyperchromatic and bizarre, mitotic figures are not seen, and mucin depletion is evident. The cells have some similarities to the hobnail cells of clear cell carcinoma. The clinical information of a current pregnancy episode and the lack of mitoses or invasion are useful in preventing identification of this lesion as adenocarcinoma. **A** and **B** demonstrate the variation that can occur within this process.

INFLAMMATORY LESIONS OF THE CERVIX

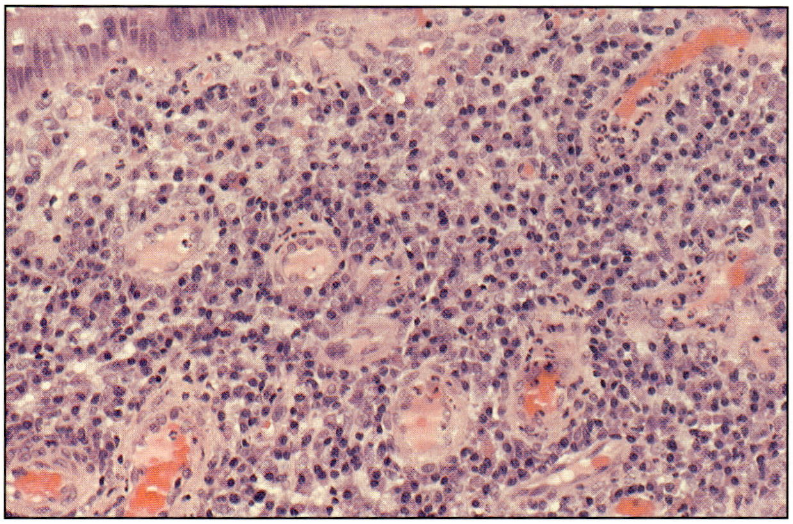

FIGURE 4-14.
Cervicitis. Infiltration of the cervical stroma by mixtures of acute and chronic inflammatory cells is quite common. Many times cervicitis is not reported as a separate diagnosis because it is so common. In this particular case, the infiltrate is almost purely plasma cells, and endothelial hyperplasia is also present. In this circumstance it is prudent to screen the patient for syphilis.

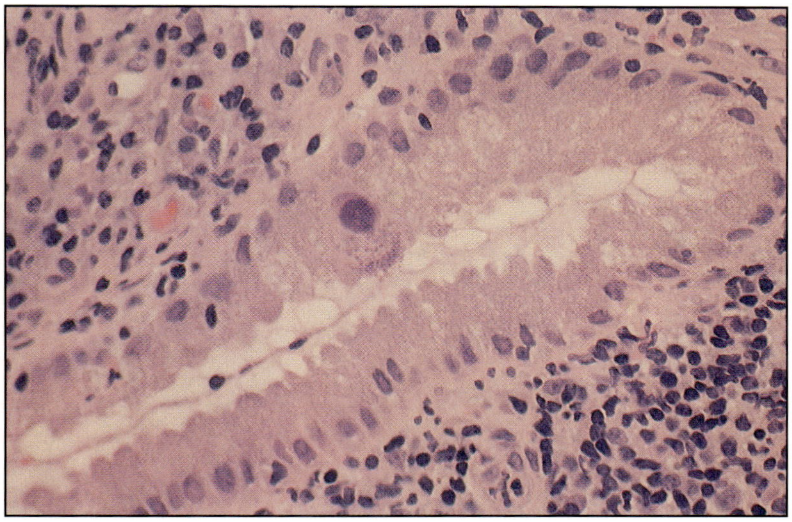

FIGURE 4-15.
Cytomegalovirus (CMV) infection. Acute primary infection with cytomegalovirus produces typical cytoplasmic and nuclear viral inclusions in some patients. The nucleus becomes markedly enlarged with a large intranuclear inclusion, and the cytoplasm shows granular red or blue (in this case) inclusions. In this patient, the biopsy was performed for an abnormal Pap smear and the cytomegalovirus was incidental. Although for most patients this would not be a particularly worrisome finding and probably is self-limiting, this patient was in the second trimester of pregnancy and the fetus could have become infected. If the cells are suspicious for CMV but not classic, an immunohistochemical study on paraffin-embedded, formalin-fixed tissue to identify CMV is currently available.

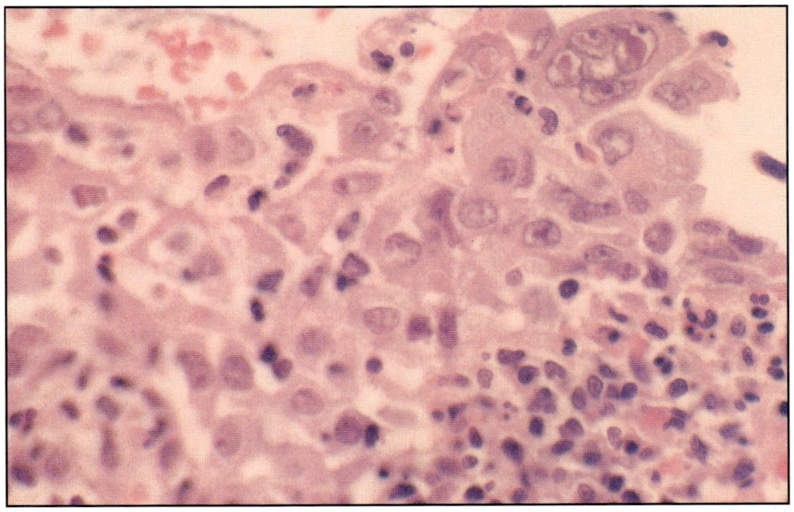

FIGURE 4-16.
Herpes simplex virus infection. In the upper right-hand corner of the photomicrograph the typical multinucleated epithelial giant cell with large, ground-glass nuclear inclusions of herpes simplex virus infection is evident. Individual cells with nuclear inclusions, and a marked inflammatory response are also present. This biopsy was performed for an abnormal Pap smear and this was an incidental finding. Biopsy of herpetic infections is not the usual means of diagnosis; culture is the preferred method. If the patient is known to have genital herpes, this would be useful to include in the clinical information. If the cells are suspicious for herpes but not diagnostic, immunohistochemical studies on paraffin-embedded, formalin-fixed tissue can be used to identify herpes simplex virus types 1 and 2 are currently available.

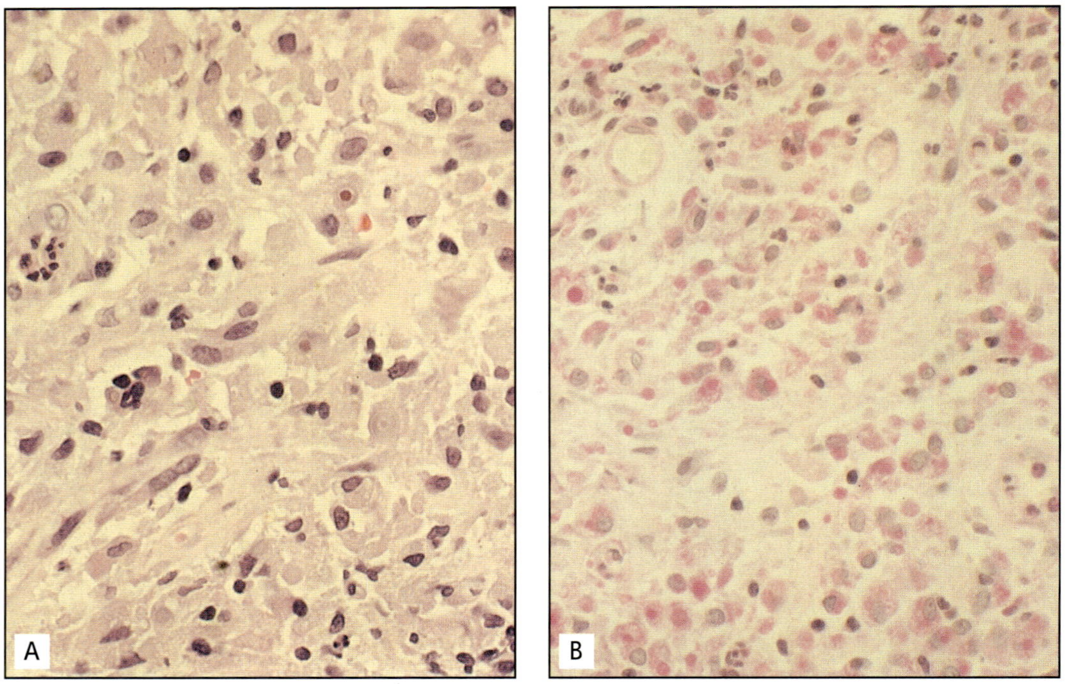

FIGURE 4-17.

Malakoplakia. Malakoplakia is grossly characterized by yellow, raised mucosal plaques microscopically composed of sheets of macrophages. This process is thought to be due to abnormally functioning macrophages that are distended with debris of bacterial origin. Laminated, mineralized concretions known as Michaelis-Gutmann bodies are typical and visible in the hematoxylin and eosin stain (**A**). The granularity of the macrophage cytoplasm is more evident on the periodic acid–Schiff stain (**B**). Malakoplakia is uncommon in the cervix, and most often seen in the urinary bladder.

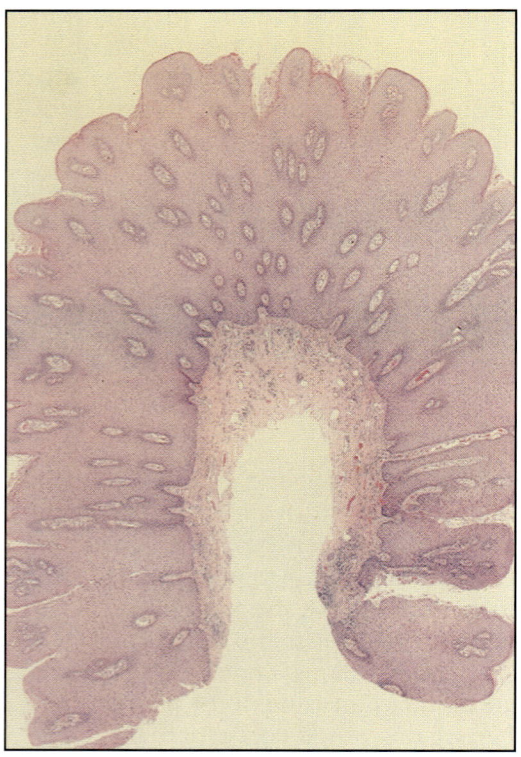

FIGURE 4-18.

Condyloma. Condylomas of the cervix are caused by infection with one of the human papillomaviruses (HPV). The typical gross appearance looks like any wart. Microscopically, there are papillomatous undulations of the surface with abnormal keratinization. Many condylomas are associated with dysplastic lesions.

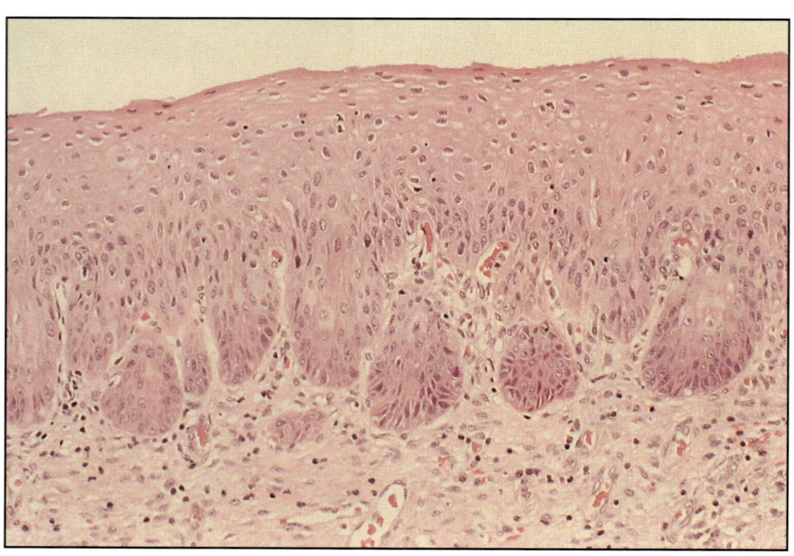

FIGURE 4-19.

Inverting growth pattern. This growth pattern was described many years ago with the caveat not to mistake this benign lobulation of the basal layer for carcinoma [6]. This "inverting pattern" in my experience is frequently associated with condylomas or adjacent to dysplastic lesions. The basal layer has an irregular growth pattern with apparent downgrowth rather than the epithelium being thrown up into folds in the typical condylomatous pattern.

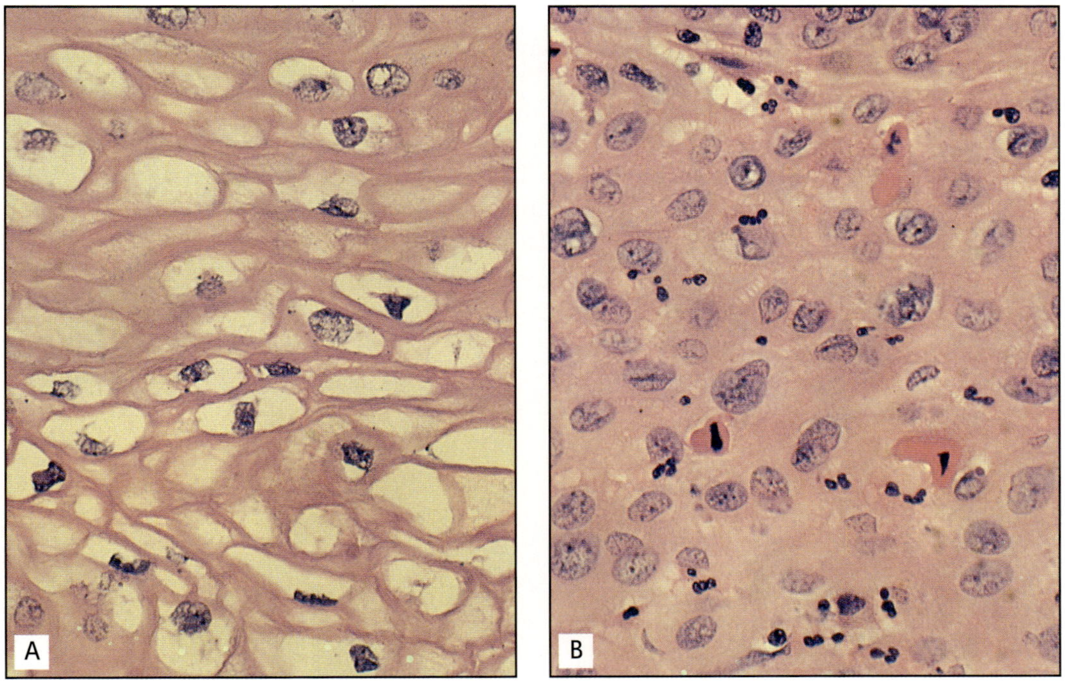

FIGURE 4-20.

Koilocytosis and dyskeratosis associated with condyloma. On higher power examination, typical cellular findings associated with condyloma are koilocytes (**A**) and dyskeratotic cells (**B**). Koilocytes have a cleared out center that looks as though the cytoplasm is pushed to the cell margin, apparently thickened cell membrane (probably owing to the cytoplasm adjacent to the cell membrane), and hyperchromatic nuclei. Classic koilocytes were described with "box-car" shaped (rectangular) nuclei, although the crinkled, "raisinoid" appearance is also fairly typical. The dyskeratotic cells are hypereosinophilic and scattered throughout the epithelium rather than collecting at the surface. Some of these cells may be dying and shrinking rather than producing keratin.

Precancerous Lesions of the Cervix

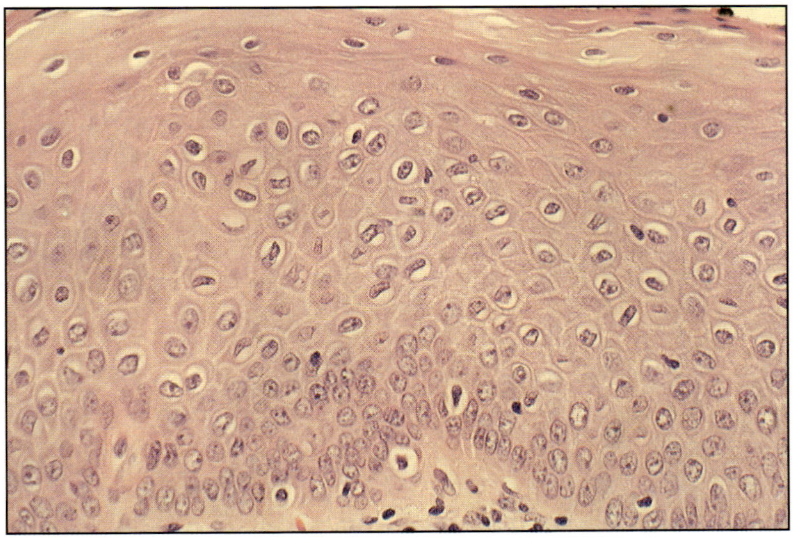

FIGURE 4-21.

Mild dysplasia, or cervical intraepithelial neoplasia grade I (CIN I). All dysplasia or cervical intraepithelial neoplasia (CIN) is defined by two general findings: 1) there must be nuclear atypia in the cells throughout the entire thickness of the epithelium; and 2) the population of basaloid type cells is increased, with more than a single layer present. The nuclear changes include hyperchromasia; clumpy irregular chromatin; irregular nuclear membranes; and increased nuclear to cytoplasmic ratio. In mild dysplasia, the basaloid population occupies no more than the lower one third of the epithelium. Mitoses are generally increased, above the basal layer, and may be atypical with tripolar or dispersed forms. Koilocytosis is common.

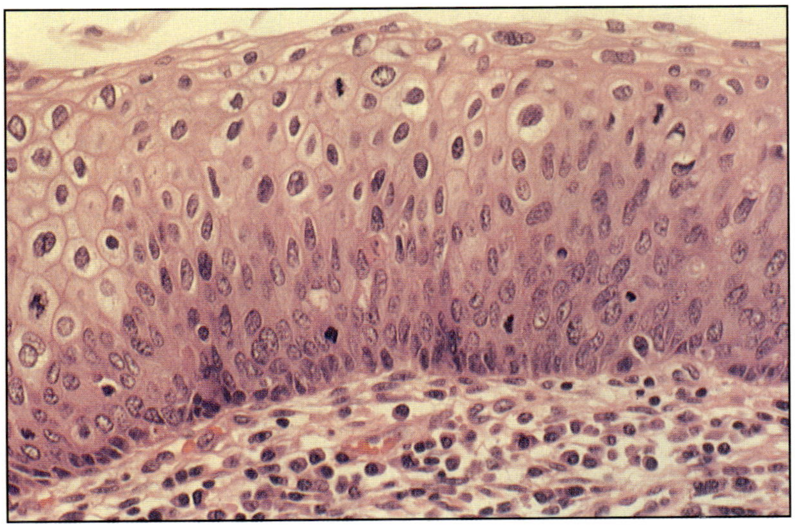

FIGURE 4-22.

Moderate dysplasia, or cervical intraepithelial neoplasia grade II (CIN II). The same basic principles apply to moderate dysplasia (CIN 2) as to any dysplasia–full thickness nuclear atypia and an increase in basaloid cells. However, the degree of nuclear atypia is generally more pronounced as the degree of dysplasia becomes greater. The basaloid population occupies at least one third, but no more than two thirds, the thickness of the epithelium. Mitoses are common, frequently atypical, and may be spread throughout the epithelium. Koilocytes are still quite common, although as the degree of dysplasia becomes greater this finding often disappears.

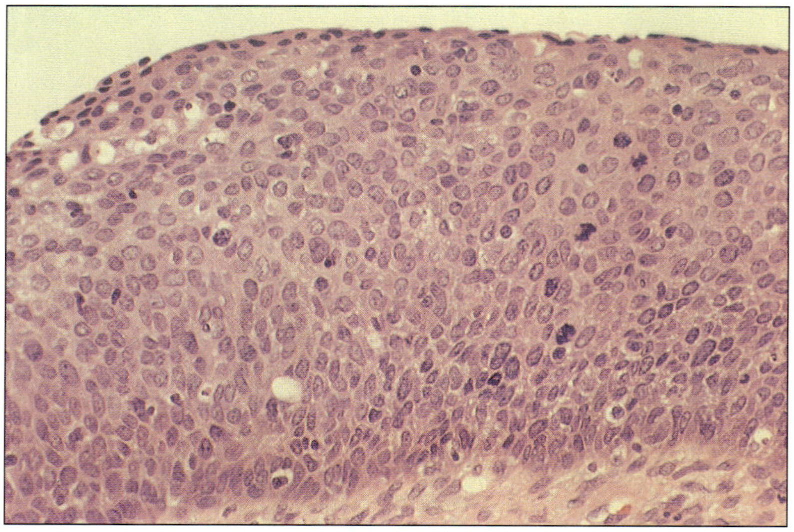

FIGURE 4-23.

Severe dysplasia/carcinoma *in situ* (CIS), or cervical intraepithelial neoplasia grade III (CIN III). The population of cells is entirely basaloid throughout the entire thickness of the epithelium in CIS, whereas a thin layer of slightly more mature cells may be present in severe dysplasia. Mitoses are common and often atypical. Koilocytosis is very uncommon within the lesion, although it may be present in adjacent areas. Any of the dysplastic or CIN processes may involve endocervical glands without evidence of invasion.

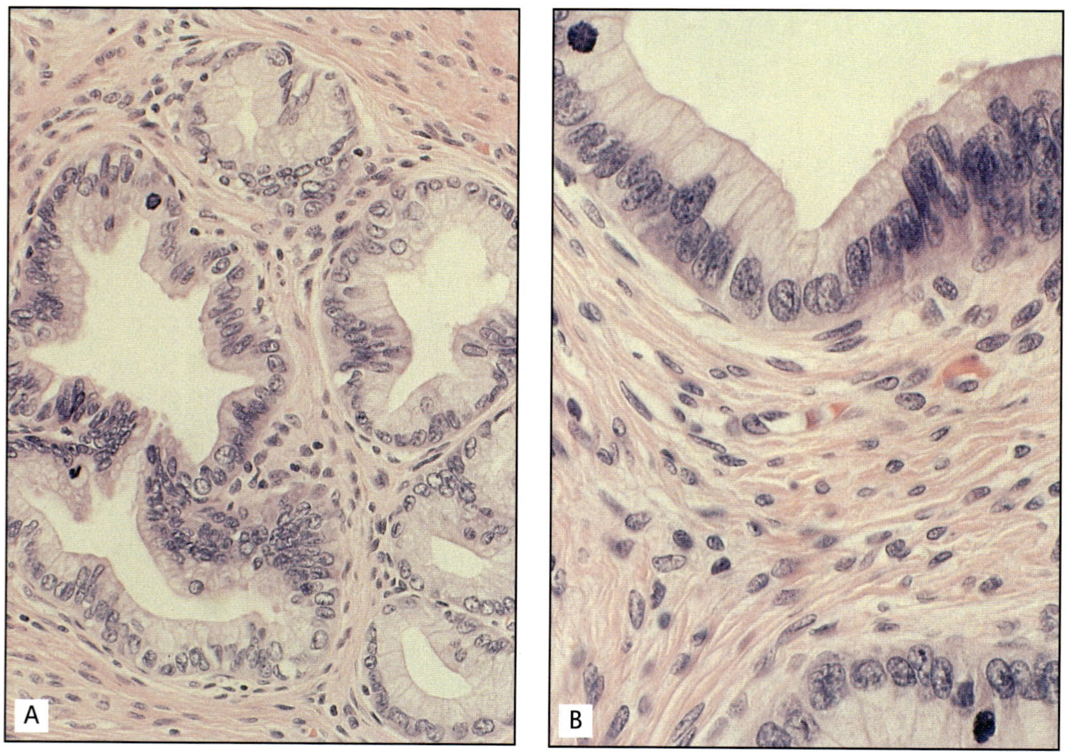

FIGURE 4-24.

Endocervical dysplasia. **A**, The endocervical glands in this photomicrograph are lined by cells containing hyperchromatic nuclei with irregular chromatin that are becoming stratified. **B**, Excess mitotic figures are present. Endocervical dysplasia is not well defined or described; nor is the relationship of endocervical dysplasia to the development of invasive carcinoma well defined. Extrapolations from the behavior of squamous dysplasia have been made, suggesting the lesion shown would have some risk of progression without intervention. Currently, there is no way to evaluate and follow endocervical lesions without removing them, and therefore no good correlations of histologic findings with behavior are available [7].

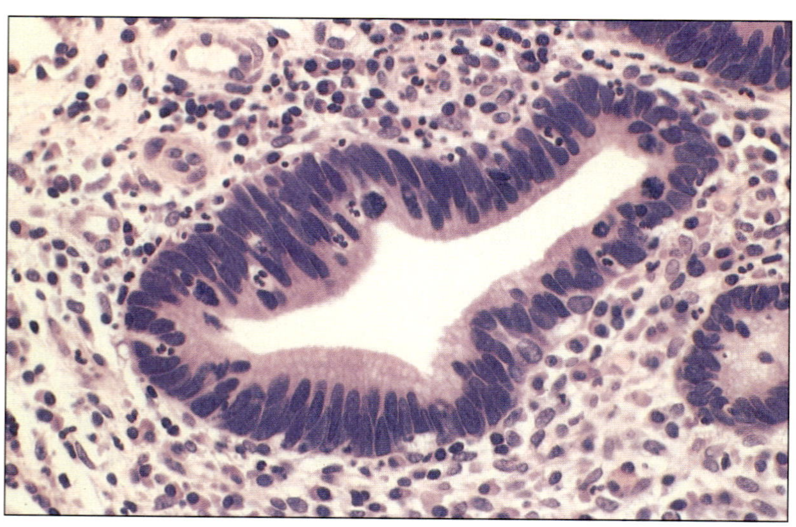

FIGURE 4-25.

Adenocarcinoma *in situ* (ACIS). The endocervical glands in are lined by cells with very hyperchromatic nuclei and mucin depletion. Mitotic figures are significantly increased and frequently atypical. Pseudostratification of cells is present. The cells usually resemble endocervical- or endometrial-type cells, but intestinal-type cells have also been reported. The lesion in the photomicrograph shows no invasion but has spread along the endocervical clefts. It can be difficult to determine the extent of ACIS because it can spread in any direction through the maze of endocervical glandular clefts [8]. Diagnostic procedures that use electrocautery are strongly discouraged in the evaluation of any glandular lesion because the effects of cautery will alter or obscure the cytologic detail of the cells, especially at the margins. Large loop procedures are often too shallow to examine adequately the deep endocervical glands.

PATHOLOGIC ARTIFACTS

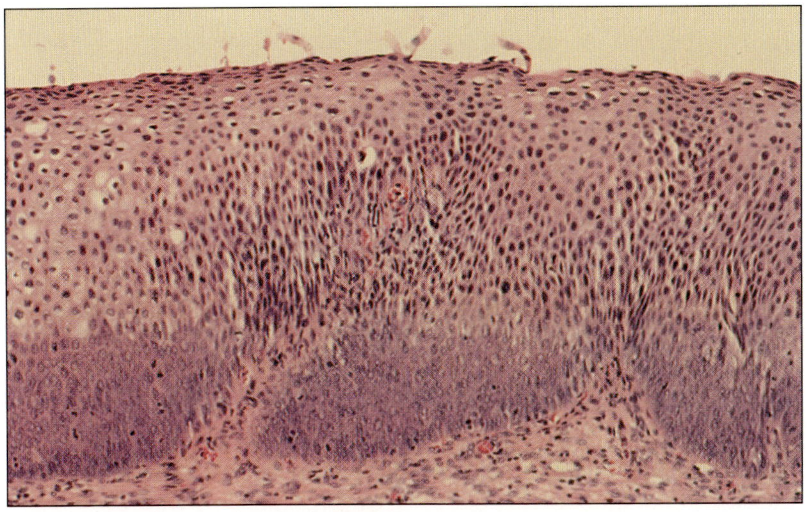

FIGURE 4-26.

Artifact from strong iodine solution (Lugol's solution) applied to the cervix prior to biopsy. A line of demarcation about one third of the way through the epithelium in this biopsy specimen suggests a change in cellular differentiation. However, the change is caused by strong iodine solution (Lugol's) rather than a change in cellular differentiation [9]. This artifact can make determining the degree of dysplasia difficult, particularly in patients who also have atrophic changes. The artifact can be lessened by using a more dilute solution of iodine (Schiller's solution) or using only acetic acid for diagnostic procedures. If an iodine solution is used, it should be noted on the pathology consultation form to alert the pathologist so that the line of demarcation caused by the iodine is not misinterpreted as a change in cellular differentiation, perhaps resulting in an inaccurate assessment of the degree of dysplasia.

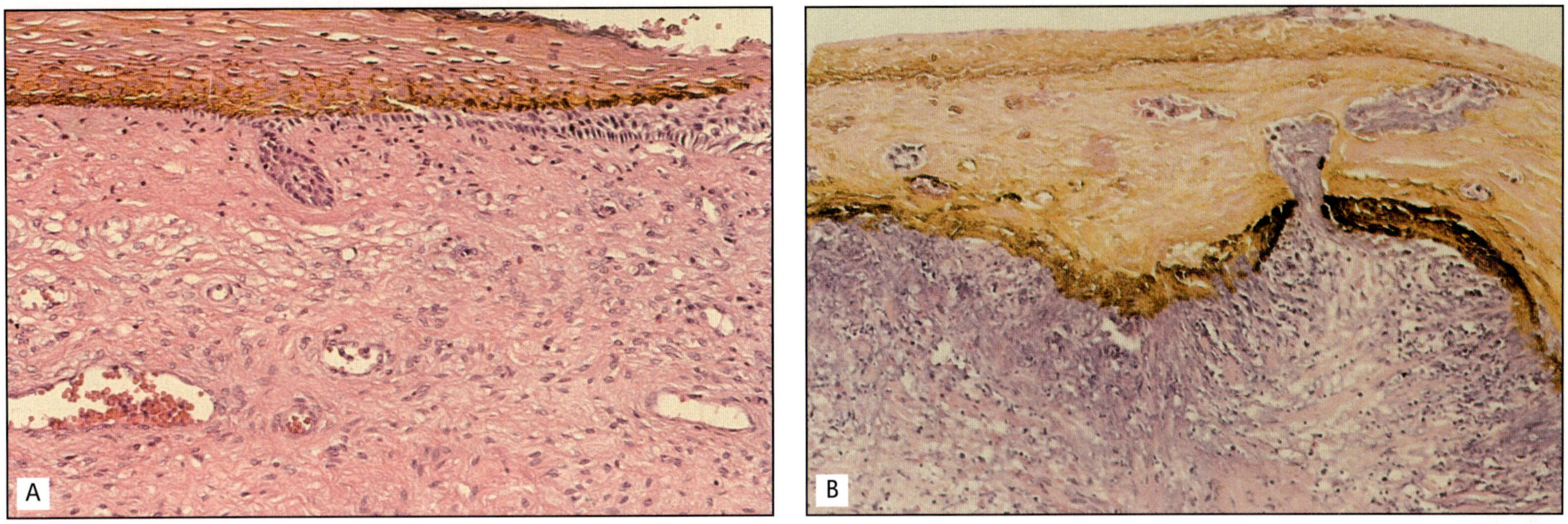

FIGURE 4-27.

Artifacts from Monsel's solution applied to the cervix before biopsy. **A**, The photomicrograph shows the granules from Monsel's solution applied to "another site" just before this biopsy was taken. Complete loss of epithelium (**B**) is seen when Monsel's was applied for colposcopic examination and biopsy the day before a cone biopsy. Monsel's solution (ferric subsulfate) is used to stop bleeding from biopsy sites, but it is also a caustic solution that can damage mucosa, and should be avoided until all biopsies are taken [10].

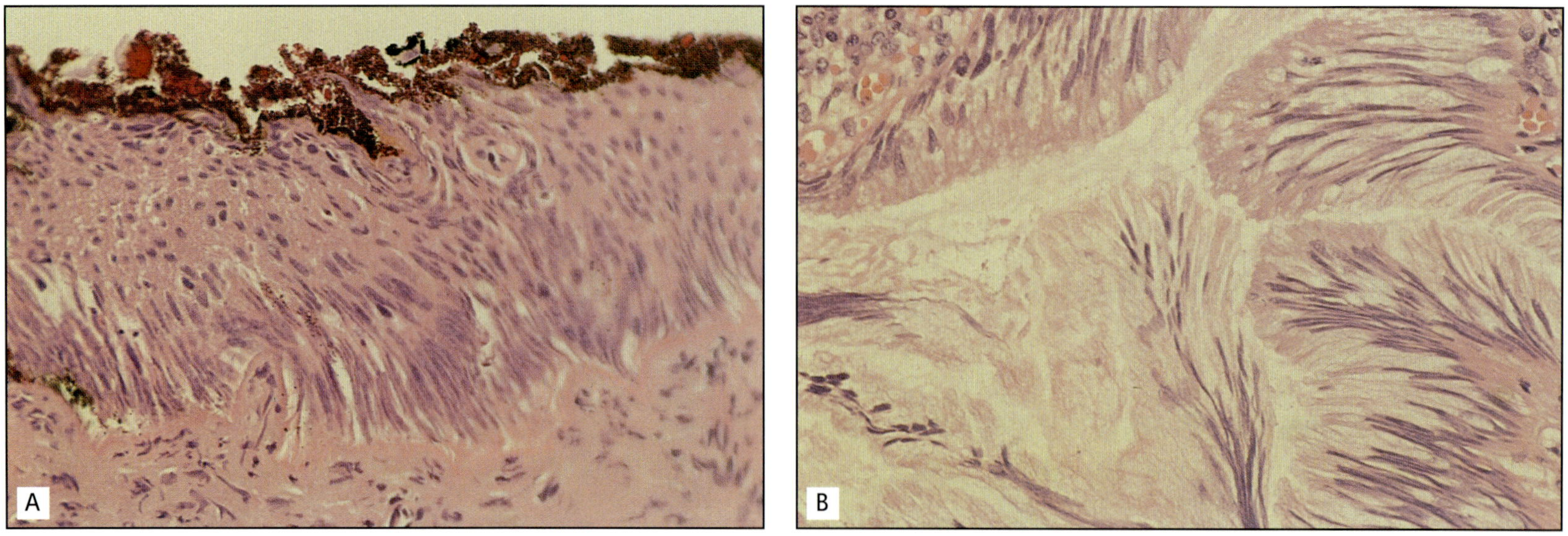

FIGURE 4-28.

Artifact from thermal injury to the cervix (electrocautery artifact). The typical alterations of thermal injury are demonstrated in squamous (**A**) and endocervical (**B**) epithelium. The cauterized cells are long and narrow with hyperchromatic and stretched nuclei ("taffy pulled") [11]. The nuclear features become inevaluable. Thermal artifacts are quite common since the introduction of large loop excisions of the cervix (loop electrosurgical excision procedure [LEEP] and large loop excision of the transformation zone [LLETZ]), often making the edges of the tissue specimens inevaluable. This artifact can make differentiating benign processes from malignant ones difficult, such as mesonephric remnants from well-differentiated adenocarcinoma. If thermal injury affects all of the mucosa, the entire specimen is inevaluable, a frequent problem when a second specimen is obtained from an endocervical canal that has been cauterized from all sides. Immunohistochemical studies also do not work on tissue that has suffered thermal injury. As noted above, procedures using cautery are strongly discouraged for evaluation of glandular lesions of the cervix.

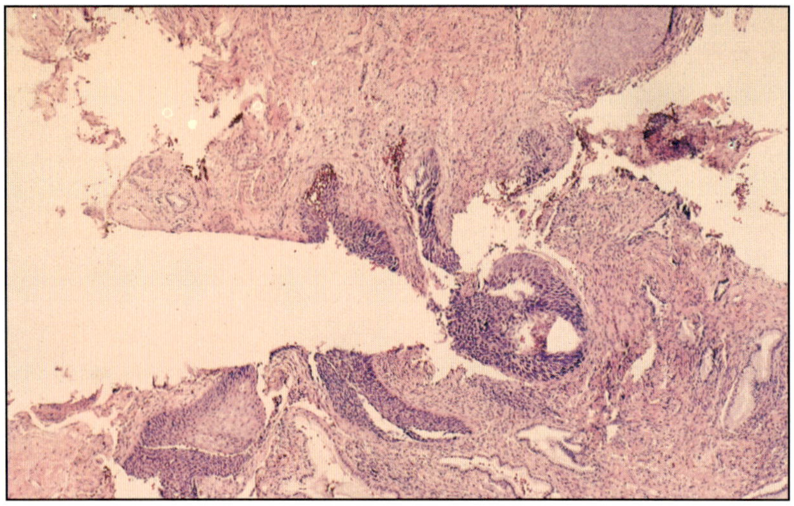

FIGURE 4-29.

Artifact from surgical instrumentation at the time of conization. A pointed instrument, possibly a stenaculum, was used to grasp this cone biopsy. The instrument disrupted an area of carcinoma *in situ*. The carcinoma cells were artificially implanted into the stroma. Because the cells did not appear to incite a desmoplastic response, the lesion was considered noninvasive. When doing a cone biopsy, whether cold knife, laser, or loop, the operator should avoid placing instruments on or through the epithelium of the specimen being removed to prevent disruption of the epithelium. Clamps or sutures can be placed into the stroma or into the part of the cervix not being removed. Similarly, aggressive rubbing of the cervix while applying acetic acid or other solutions during a diagnostic procedure can disrupt or remove fragile dysplastic epithelium.

INVASIVE CERVICAL CANCERS

FIGO STAGING OF CERVICAL CANCER	
Stage I	*The carcinoma is strictly confined to the cervix*
Stage IA	Invasive cancer identified only microscopically. All gross lesions even with superficial invasion are stage IB cancers. Invasion is limited to measured stromal invasion with maximum depth of 5.0 mm and no wider than 7.0 mm
Stage IA1	Measured invasion of stroma no greater than 3.0 mm in depth and no wider than 7.0 mm
Stage IA2	Measured invasion of stroma greater than 3 mm in depth and no greater than 5 mm and no wider than 7 mm
Stage IB	*Clinical lesions confined to the cervix or preclinical lesions greater than stage IA*
Stage IB1	Clinical lesions no greater than 4.0 cm in size
Stage IB2	Clinical lesions greater than 4.0 cm in size
Stage II	*Extension beyond the cervix but not to the pelvic wall. Involves vagina, but nmot the lower third*
Stage IIA	Involves vagina, but not lower third. No obvious extension to parametria
Stage IIB	Involves vagina, but not lower third. Obvious parametrial involovement
Stage III	*Extension to pelvic wall. On rectal examination, no cancer-free space between tumor and pelvic wall. Involves lower third of vagina*
Stage IIIA	No extension to pelvic side wall, with involvement of lower third of vagina
Stage IIIB	Extension to pelvic side wall
Stage IV	*Extension beyond true pelvis or involvement of bladder or rectal mucosa. Bullous edema does not permit a case to be assigned to stage IV*

FIGURE 4-30.

International Federation of Gynecology and Obstetrics (FIGO) staging of cervical cancer. Cervical cancer is the third most common gynecologic malignancy in the United States. There is a close association between human papillomavirus infection and the development of cervical cancer. The most common histologic type of cervical cancer is squamous cell carcinoma, accounting for approximately 80% of all cervical cancers. Adenocarcinomas represent approximately 15% to 20% of cervical cancers. (*From* FIGO [12].)

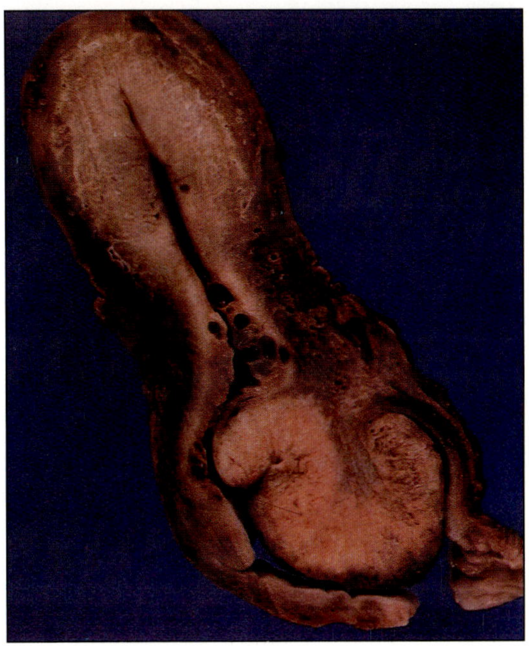

FIGURE 4-31.

Exophytic carcinoma of the cervix. An exophytic carcinoma of the cervix is shown from a hysterectomy specimen cut in the sagittal plane. The upper vaginal canal is distended by the tumor mass. If a visible lesion is seen on the cervix, it should be biopsied. Pap smear alone may not detect cancer cells, even in such an obvious lesion, because necrosis, blood, and cellular debris can obscure the abnormal cells, or the cancer may be growing entirely beneath normal tissues. Therapy should be planned after biopsy confirmation of cancer.

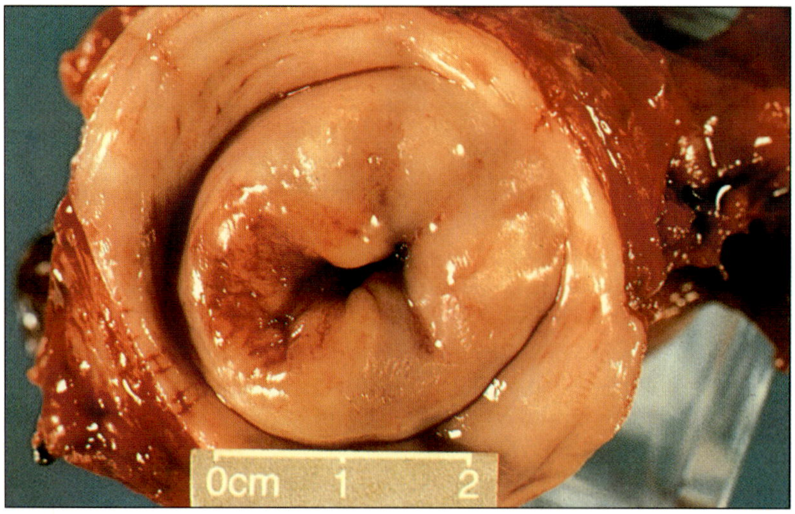

FIGURE 4–32.
Endophytic carcinoma of the cervix. An ulcerated carcinoma is located between 8 and 10 o'clock (right lateral) on the cervix. Cellular debris, necrosis, and blood may obscure abnormal cells on a Pap smear in this ulcerated cancer. Biopsy would also be indicated in this case to confirm invasive cancer.

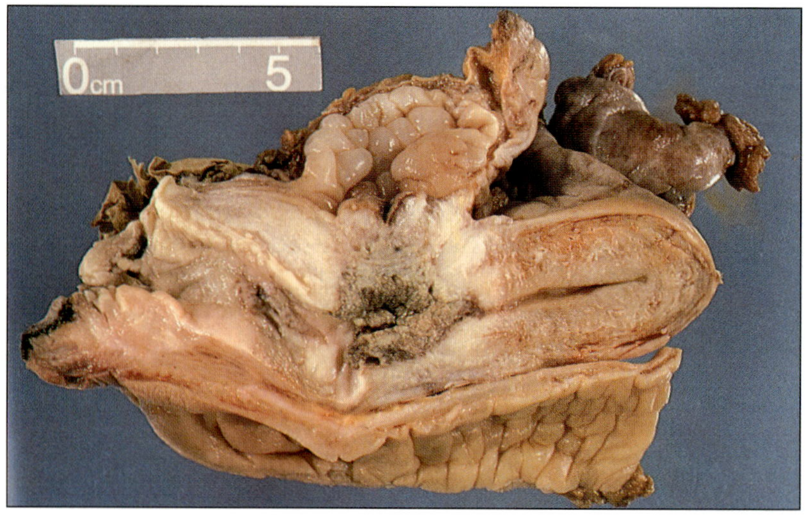

FIGURE 4–33.
Pelvic exenteration in recurrent carcinoma of the cervix. This saggital section of a pelvic exenteration shows a large recurrent mass that has obliterated the cervix and extended into the bladder anteriorly. The rectum posteriorly is not invaded by tumor, but the rectovaginal septum is sufficiently involved to warrant removal of the rectum.

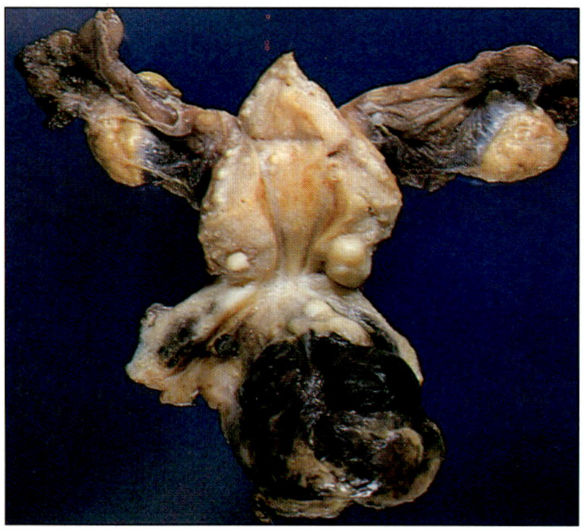

FIGURE 4–34.
Primary malignant melanoma of the cervix. The large, black exophytic lesion represents malignant melanoma. Melanoma is a rare primary cancer of the uterine cervix. (*Courtesy of* Richard Zaino, MD.)

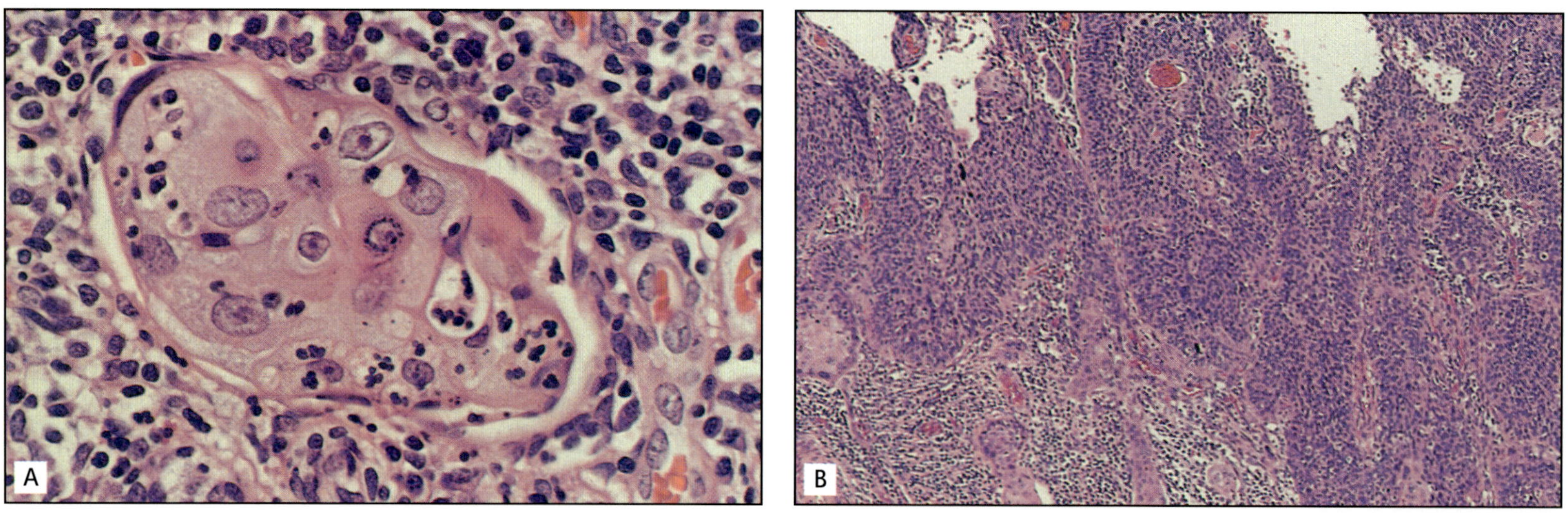

FIGURE 4–35.
"Microinvasive" squamous carcinoma of the cervix. The invading cells have acquired cytoplasm and incited a marked inflammatory response (**A**), likely a host response attempting to hold the cancer in check. Carcinoma *in situ* and small fingers of tumor invading the stroma are present (**B**). In these early carcinomas, there have been many definitions attached to the term "microinvasive." Many gynecologic pathologists have stopped using the term and report the presence of invasion with the measured depth and width of the invasive cancer. This is a more precise method of reporting, and allows for accurate International Federation of Gynecology and Obstetrics (FIGO) staging.

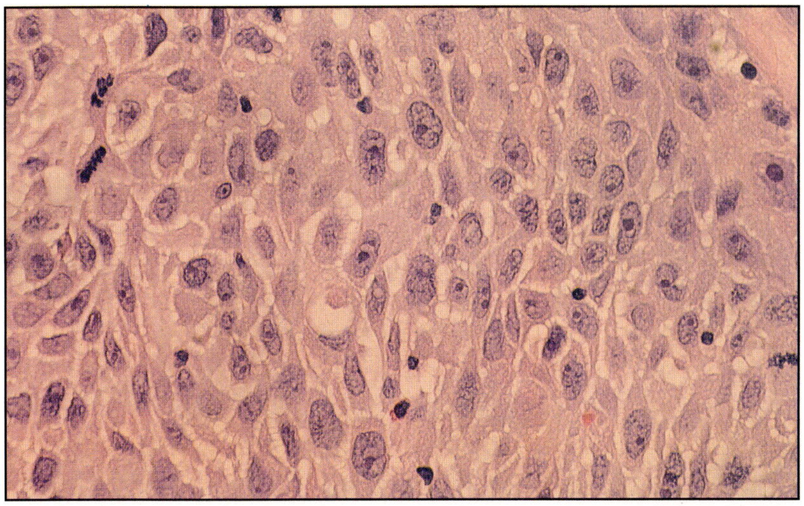

FIGURE 4-36.

Large cell non-keratinizing squamous carcinoma. Cells with abundant cytoplasm and intercellular bridges are typical for large cell squamous carcinomas. Individual cell keratinization may be present in some nonkeratinizing cancers. In cervical squamous carcinomas, intercellular bridges are frequently difficult to identify and cell borders are ill-defined. Some large cell carcinomas have intracytoplasmic mucin, and are more precisely considered adenosquamous carcinoma or poorly differentiated adenocarcinoma. Some data suggest that such cancers behave differently from pure squamous cancers [13]; however, therapy at present is the same for all large cell carcinomas, so special stains for intracellular mucins in large cell carcinomas are not widely done.

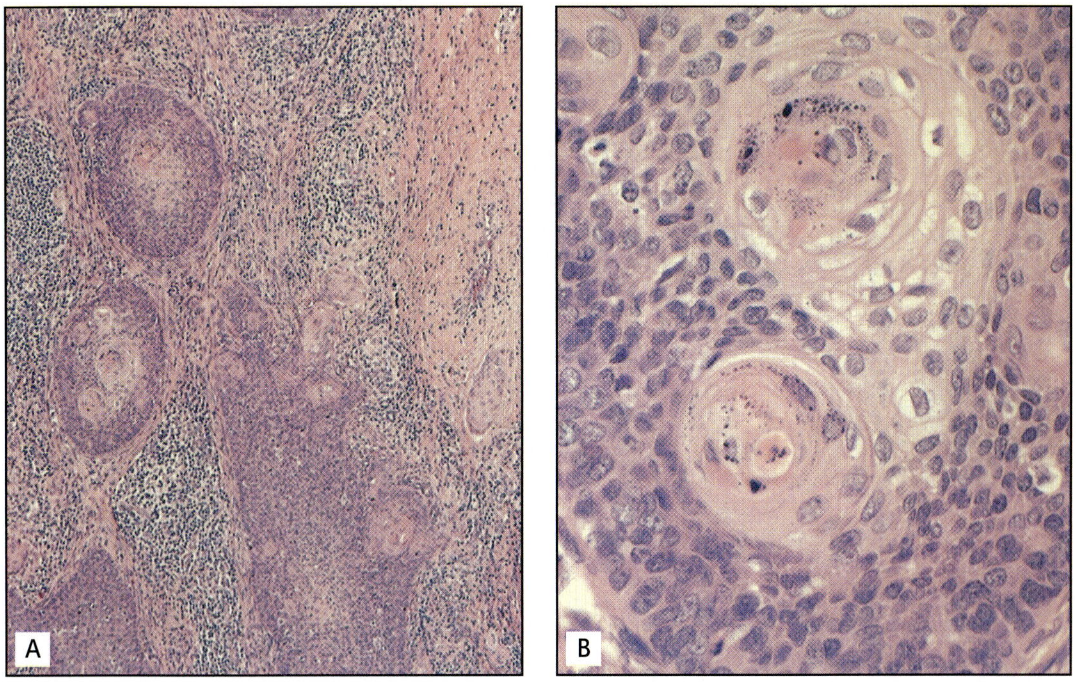

FIGURE 4-37.

Large cell keratinizing squamous carcinoma. **A,** These carcinomas also contain large cells with abundant cytoplasm, but are separated from the nonkeratinizing type by the identification of keratin pearl formation. Individual cell keratinization is not sufficient for the designation of keratinizing type. **B**, A higher power photomicrograph shows the swirling growth pattern of the keratin pearl. With mucin stains, some of these tumors also prove to be poorly differentiated adenosquamous carcinomas.

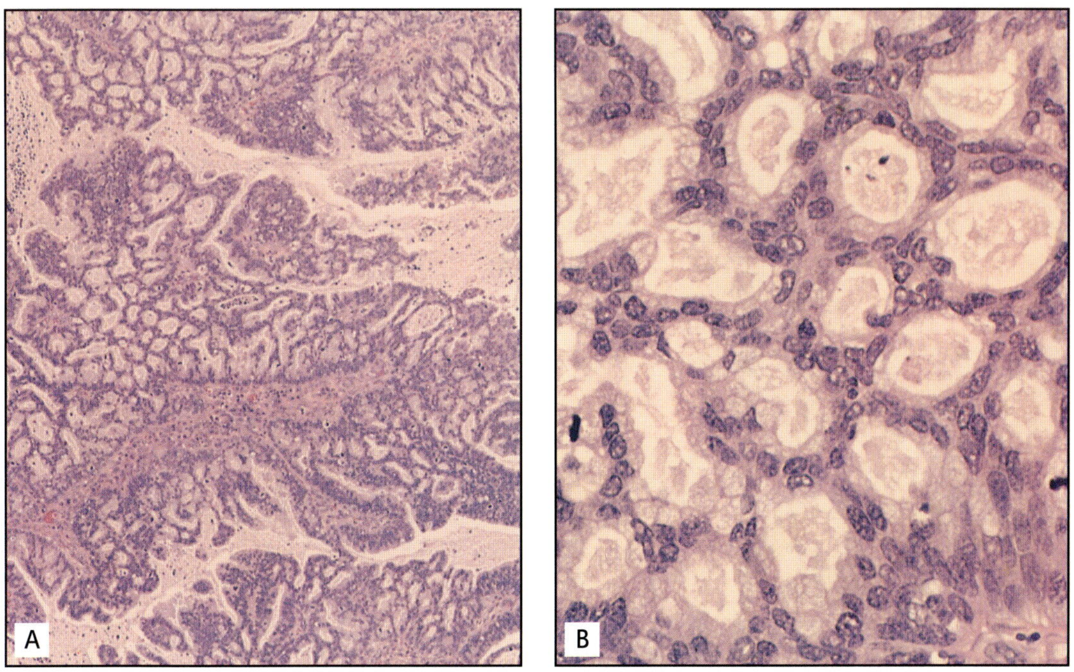

FIGURE 4-38.

Adenocarcinoma—endocervical type. **A**, Thin stromal stalks with excess growth of glandular cells showing intracellular mucin production are present in this tumor. The mucin producing cells also invade the stroma. The purely glandular invasive carcinomas are divided into types by the resemblance of the cells to normal structures and by growth pattern. Because normal endocervical glands contain intracellular mucins, this example is designated endocervical type. **B**, Pure adenocarcinoma as a group have a poorer 5-year survival rate than squamous carcinomas, and have a propensity for earlier metastasis to distant sites such as lung. There has been a relative increase in the number of adenocarcinomas, mostly owing to the decrease in squamous cell carcinoma over the last 30 years, but the incidence of the disease found in population-based data has not increased [14].

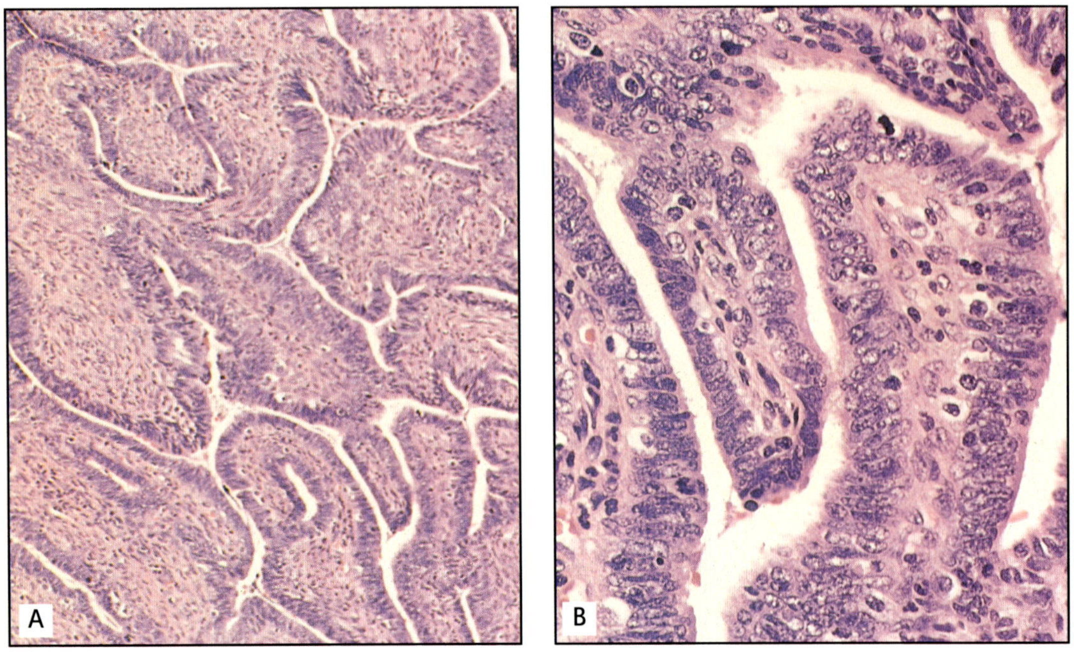

FIGURE 4-39.
Adenocarcinoma—endometrioid type. **A**, This tumor grows at the surface as papillary structures with thick, fibrous stromal cores and invades the cervix in deep clefts. **B**, The cells resemble endometrial cells, and contain no intracytoplasmic mucins. When any carcinoma of the endocervix is of the endometrioid type, extension of endometrial adenocarcinoma from the corpus must be excluded.

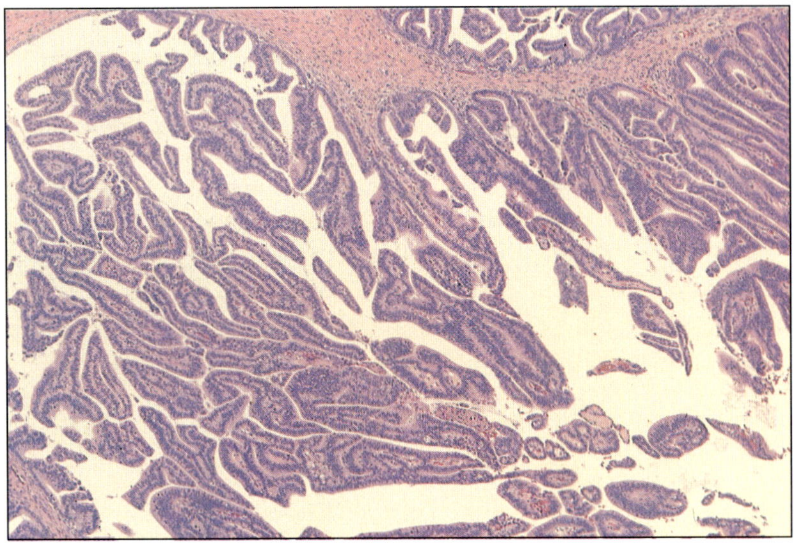

FIGURE 4-40.
Adenocarcinoma, villoglandular type. The villoglandular type of adenocarcinoma is typified by thin fibrovascular cores and a broad invasive front. The cytologic features of the cells are endometrioid type. When a cervix carcinoma is all villoglandular type, it appears to have a better prognosis, even if there is deep invasion and marked destruction of cervical stroma. Diagnosis of invasion with biopsy may be difficult as only the tips of the villiform structures may be sampled. Typical features of invasion may not be evident on a small biopsy. Cone biopsy may be necessary to evaluate invasion because depth of the villoglandular growth into the cervical wall may be the only evidence of stromal destruction.

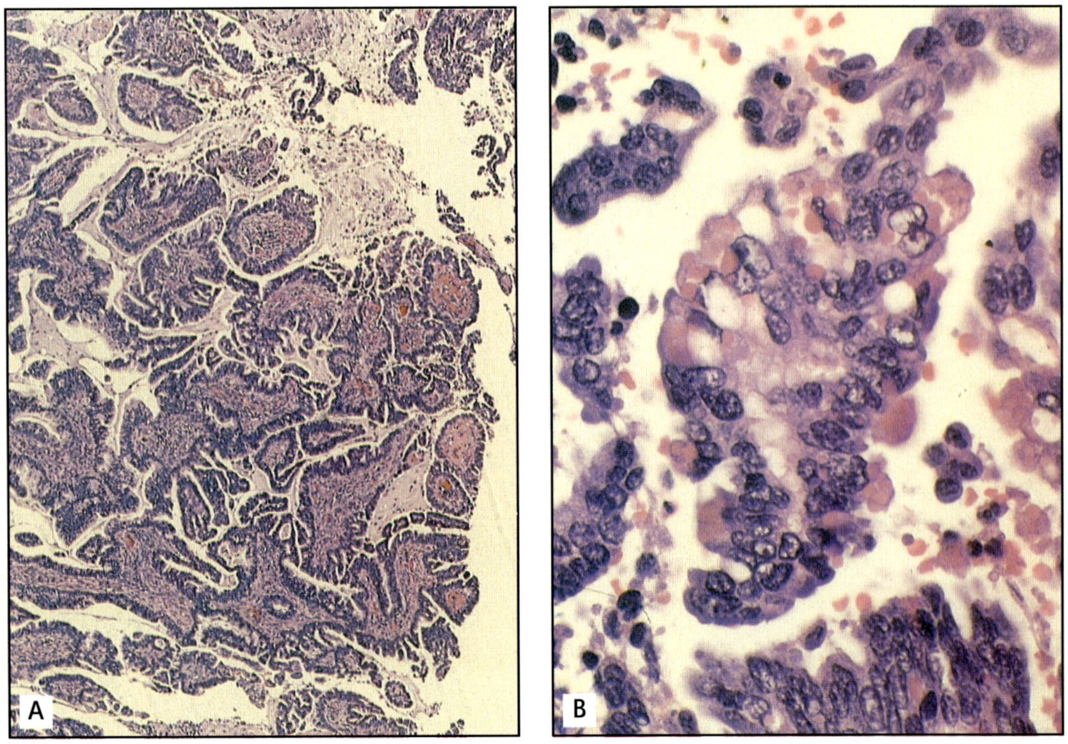

FIGURE 4-41.
Adenocarcinoma—serous type. **A**, Serous carcinoma is typified by tumor cells growing on thin fibrovascular cores. **B**, The cells also grow in small tufts from the surface of the papillary structures, and small clusters of cells appear to float in the open spaces between the supporting structures. The cells are cytologically very atypical, with pleomorphic and hyperchromatic nuclei. Although large numbers of cases have not been reported, serous cancers of the cervix appear to be more aggressive than other adenocarcinomas, similar to serous cancers of the corpus.

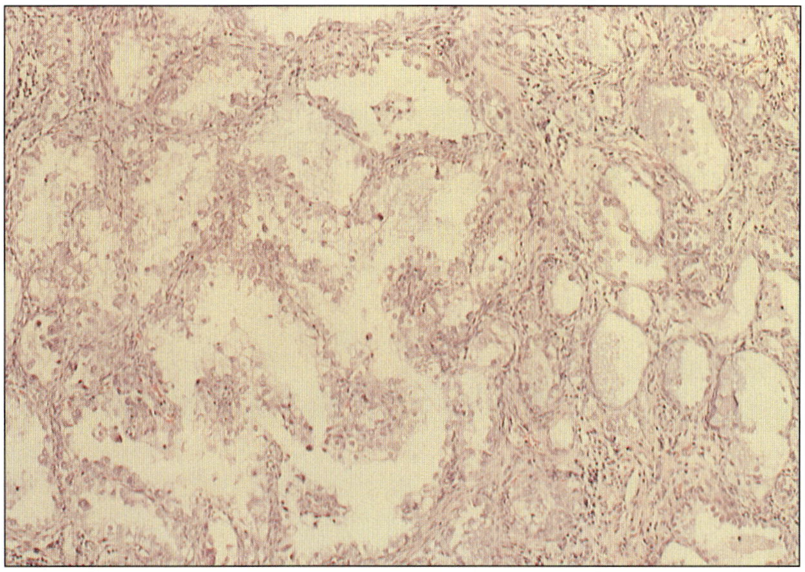

FIGURE 4-42.

Adenocarcinoma—clear cell type. Clear cell carcinoma is typified by cells with abundant, clear cytoplasm. The cells may grow on papillary tufts, in tubular patterns, or as solid nests. The differential considerations include Arias-Stella reaction and florid microglandular hyperplasia. Good clinical information can assist the pathologist in assessing these possibilities. Clear cell carcinoma, although not a common type, has been shown to be associated with prenatal diethylstilbestrol exposure, similar to clear cell carcinoma of the vagina.

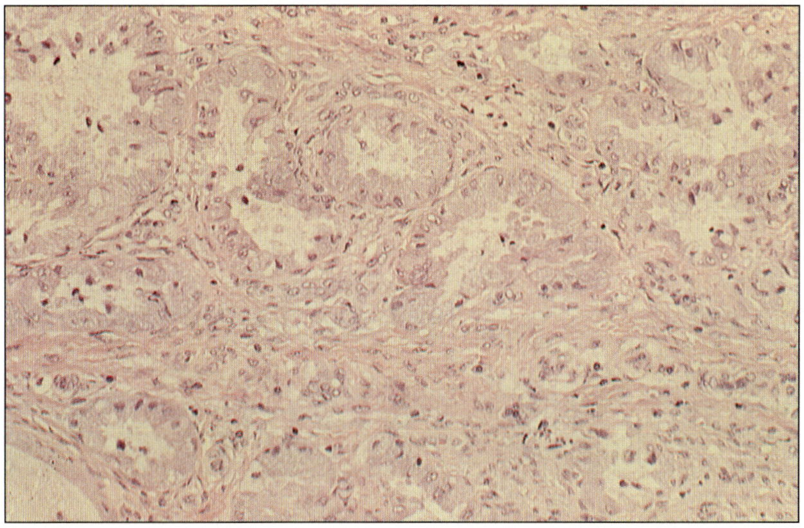

FIGURE 4-43.

Adenocarcinoma—very well differentiated type. The cytologic atypia in this lesion is so minimal it is difficult to separate from normal. However, the pattern of glandular growth is far more complex and deeper into the cervical stroma than the normal glands. Positive carcinoembryonic antigen immunohistochemical staining of formalin-fixed, paraffin-embedded tissue has been helpful in identifying some of these well-differentiated carcinomas, as normal endocervix does not exhibit this marker.

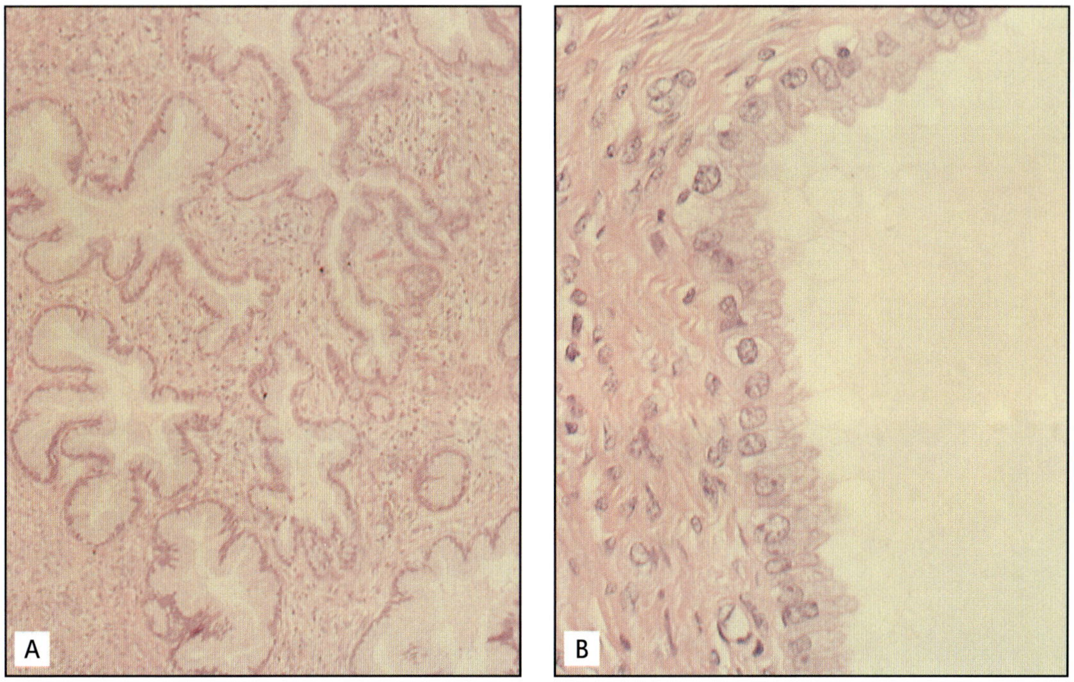

FIGURE 4-44.

Adenocarcinoma—minimal deviation type. This pattern of endocervical carcinoma is difficult to identify. The major finding is minimally abnormal glands that extend deeply into the cervical stroma. Some other features include glands with markedly irregular contours (**A**), described as claw shaped, and glands with pointed ends. The cells themselves are cytologically very similar to normal endocervix (**B**). This tumor type is likely to be diagnosed only on deep cone biopsy or hysterectomy. It has been associated with the Peutz-Jeghers syndrome.

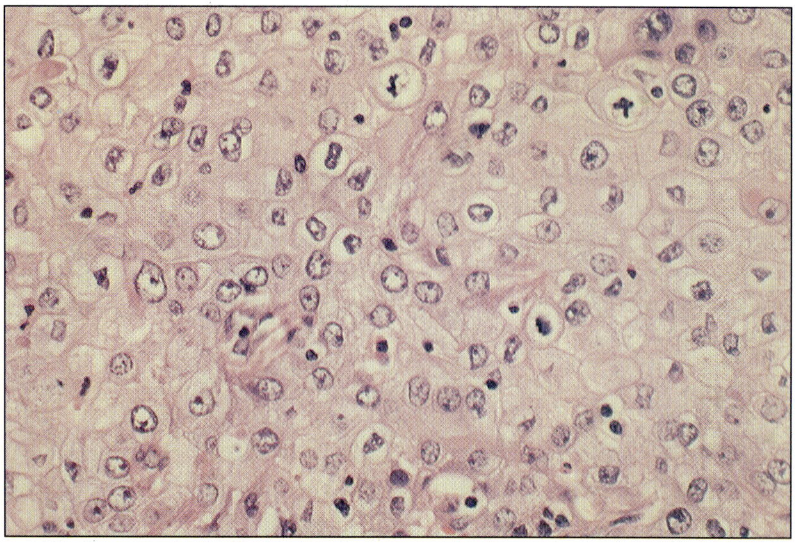

FIGURE 4-45.

Glassy cell carcinoma. This carcinoma is characterized by cells with abundant, ground glass cytoplasm and a distinct cytoplasmic membrane. The nucleus contains a large nucleolus and the chromatin is distributed along the nuclear membrane. This cancer type has been associated with glandular, squamous, and adenosquamous differentiation in electron microscropy studies. Glassy cell carcinoma is most difficult to separate from large cell nonkeratinizing squamous carcinoma, which generally does not have the distinct cell borders or large nucleoli. Glassy cell carcinoma is reported to have a poorer prognosis than typical cervical carcinomas.

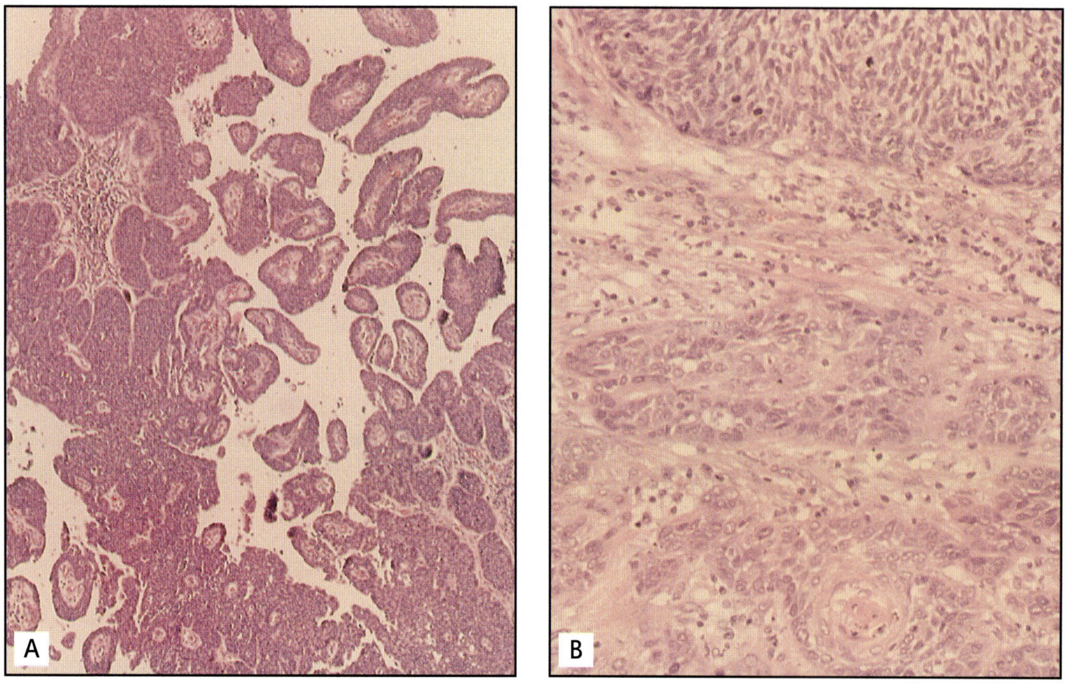

FIGURE 4-46.

Papillary squamous (transitional) cell carcinoma. Papillary structures lined by a primitive basaloid cell population are typical of this cancer (**A**). The invasive component may be a basaloid population identical to the papillary component, or a usual type large cell nonkeratinizing squamous carcinoma, as in this case (**B**). Some cancers in this group have an atypical epithelium with squamous differentiation lining the papillary structures. The behavior is determined by the invasive component.

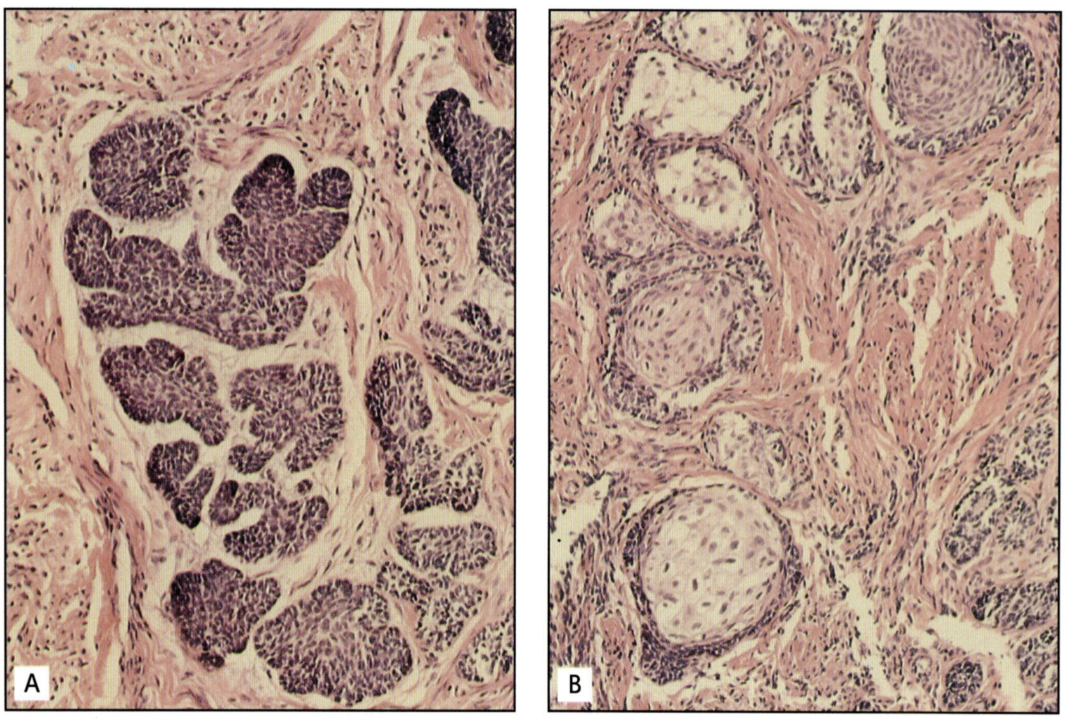

FIGURE 4-47.

Adenoid basal cell carcinoma. This carcinoma most resembles a basal cell carcinoma of the skin with squamous differentiation. **A**, There is a purely basaloid population with a minimal stromal response. **B**, squamous differentiation is evident. This tumor is uncommon, and seen in an older patient population. It may be found in a simple hysterectomy specimen in which surgery was done for a squamous intraepithelial lesion. Few of these lesions have metastasized, so additional therapy beyond hysterectomy is not currently recommended.

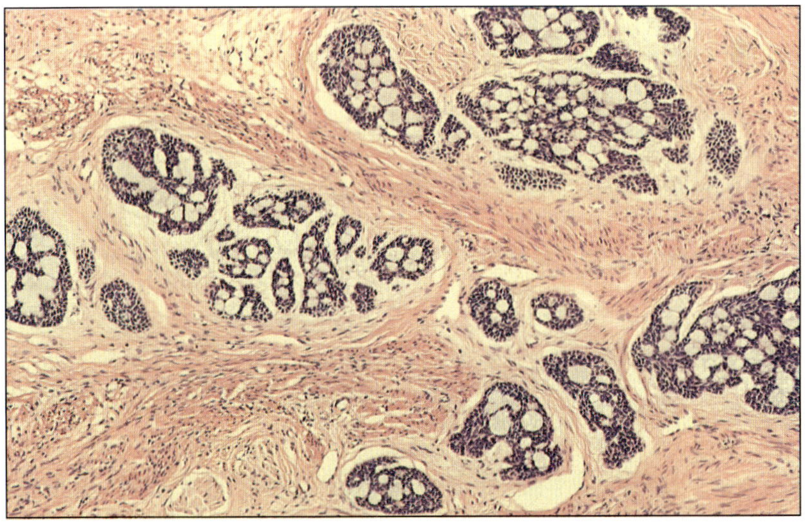

FIGURE 4-48.

Adenoid cystic carcinoma. Adenoid cystic carcinoma is a very uncommon histologic type found in the cervix. The histology is typical of adenoid cystic carcinomas in other sites. It is found in an older patient population, and may be difficult to separate from adenoid basal cell carcinoma. However, it is important to do so, as adenoid cystic carcinoma has a poor prognosis as opposed to the good prognosis of adenoid basal cell carcinoma. (*Courtesy of* Richard Feddersen, MD.)

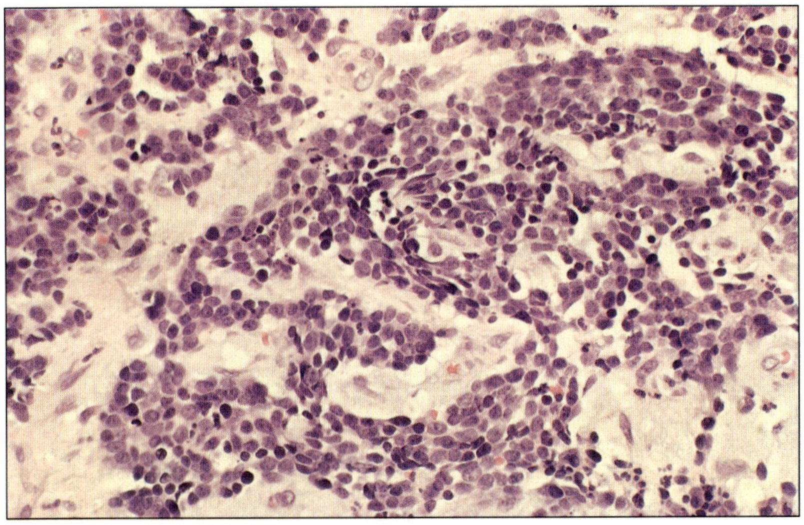

FIGURE 4-49.

Small cell carcinoma. Small cell carcinoma is composed of cells with little cytoplasm and hyperchromatic oval to spindled nuclei. Mitoses are frequent. Cellular distortion owing to traction or compression from the biopsy process is common. Although formerly classified as a subset of squamous cell carcinoma, small cell carcinomas are now known to exhibit squamous, glandular, or neuroendocrine differentiation. Neuroendocrine differentiation has been suggested to impart a worse prognosis than the other types of small cell carcinoma; however, the group as a whole has a very poor prognosis. This histologic type has been studied extensively because of its distinctively poor outcome, and many studies suggest combined-modality therapy is necessary.

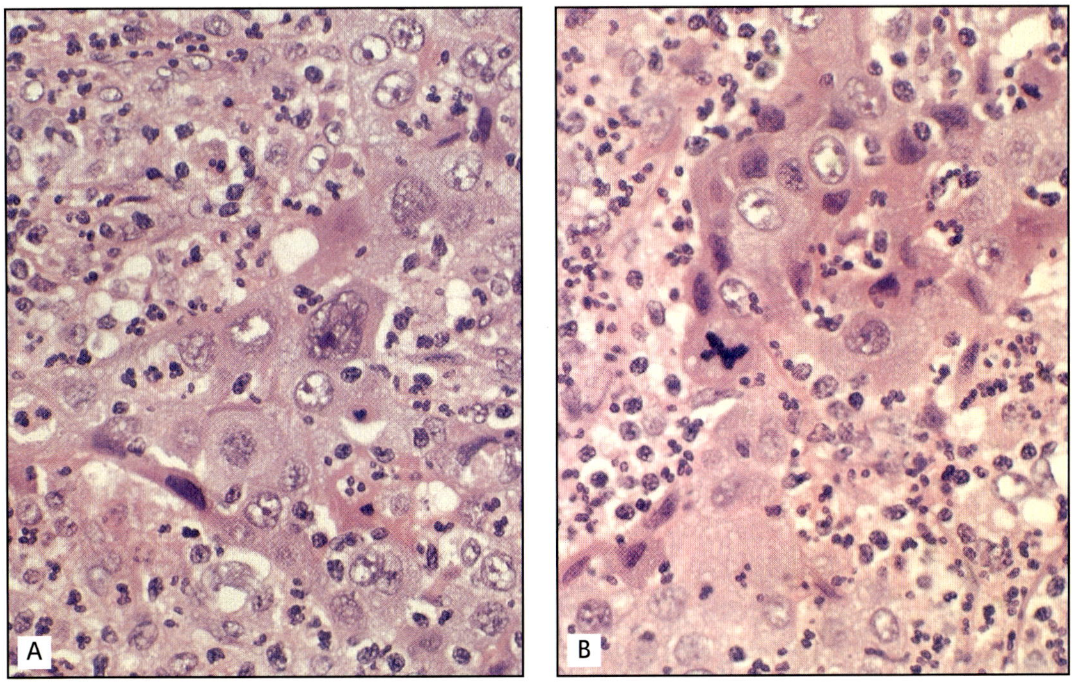

FIGURE 4-50.

Undifferentiated carcinoma. Some carcinomas of the cervix are so pleomorphic they are best regarded as undifferentiated because they show no features of glandular or squamous differentiation. The growth pattern is almost syncytial without demarcation of cell borders (**A**). Markedly abnormal mitoses are seen (**B**). In studies grading cervical squamous carcinomas, it has been shown that most are Broder grade 3 or 4, and that grade of differentiation is of little or no value in predicting behavior.

UNUSUAL PRIMARY TUMORS OF THE CERVIX

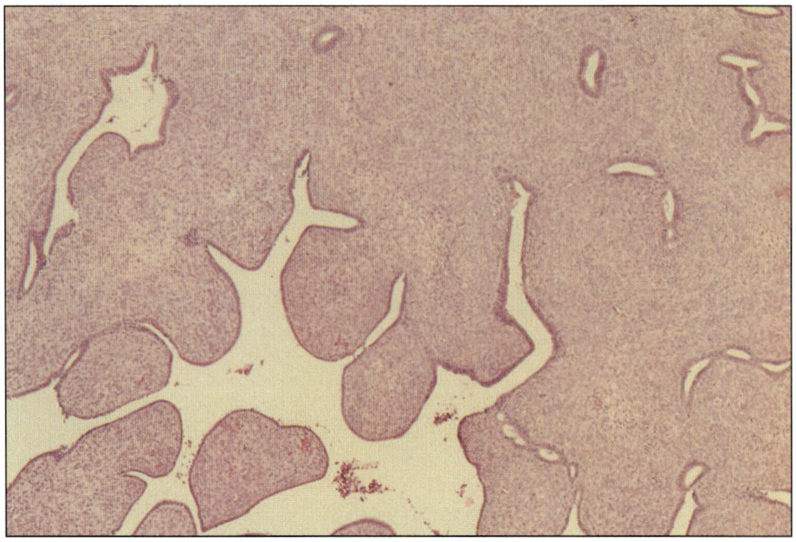

FIGURE 4-51.

Adenofibroma. Adenofibroma is characterized by the lobulated appearance of the surface, both grossly and microscopically. Broad stromal cores are lined by endocervical-type cells or nonspecific cuboidal cells. The main differential consideration is adenosarcoma. This particular case has a somewhat more cellular stroma than usual, but shows no atypical features or excess mitoses. Complete removal of the lesion is sufficient therapy.

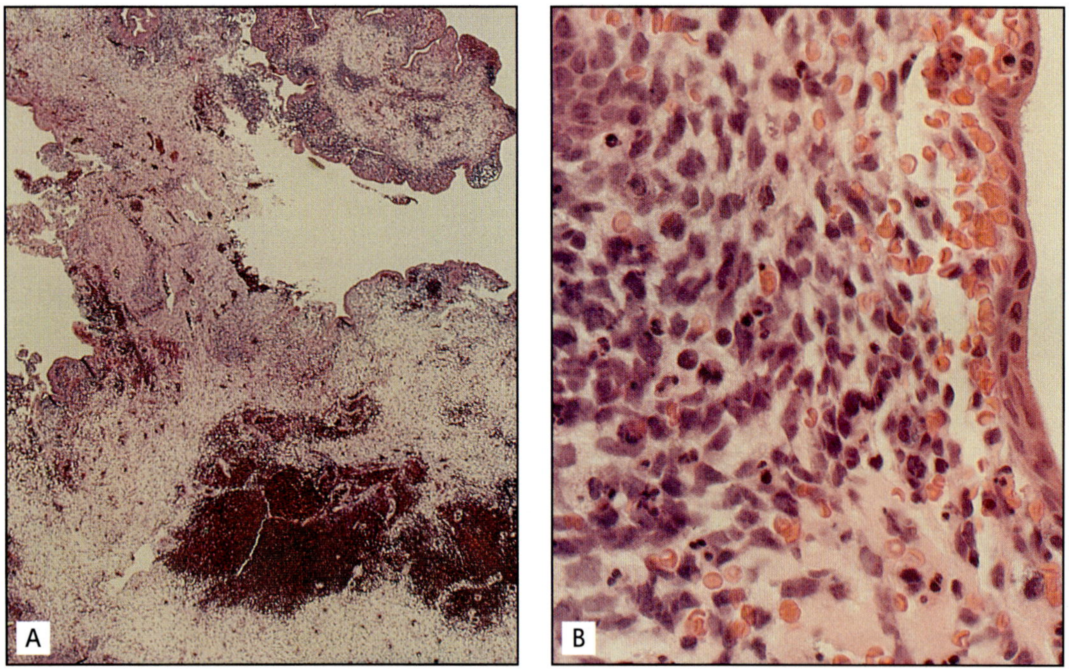

FIGURE 4-52.

Adenosarcoma—müllerian type. In this lesion the stroma is malignant and the epithelium benign in appearance. Broad papillary fronds are present that protrude into clefts and spaces within the stroma. It is common for the most hypercellular areas to be just beneath the epithelium (**A**). The cells are atypical with many mitotic figures. As with most müllerian sarcomas, the malignant cells are capable of many different sarcomatous variations. In this case they resemble endometrial stromal sarcoma (**B**). There is increasing evidence that some of these lesions can be cured with complete excision. Radical therapy may not be required, particularly if the tumor grows on a stalk that can be completely removed by a procedure such as conization and margins can be demonstrated to be negative for tumor.

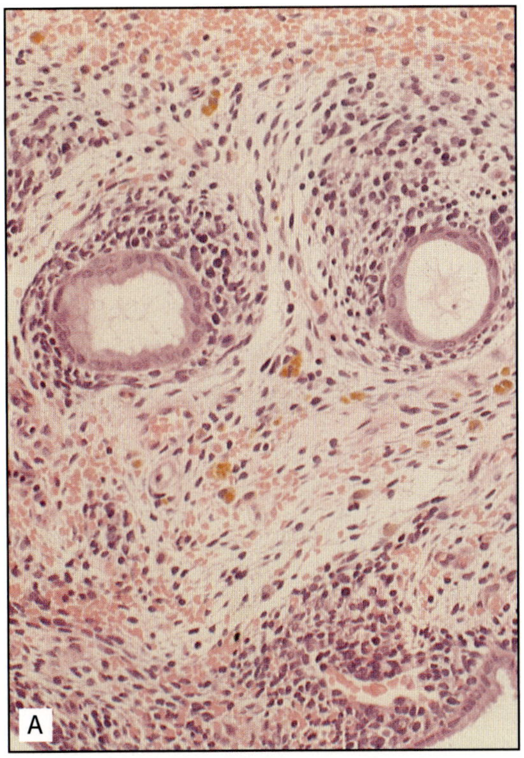

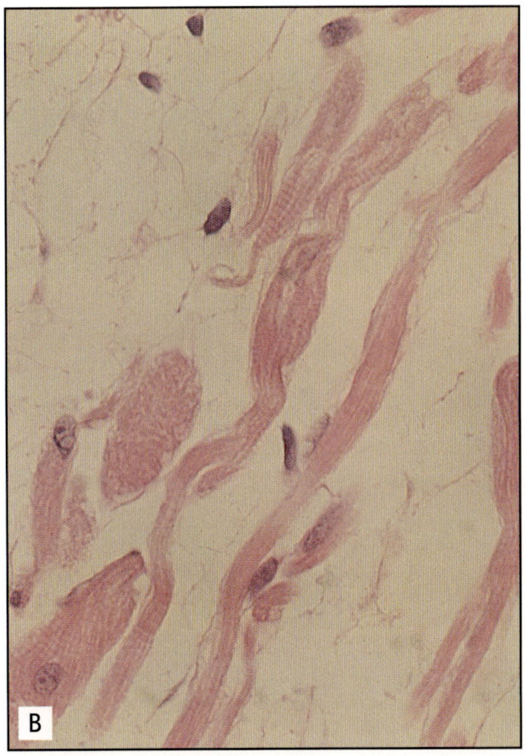

FIGURE 4–53.

Embryonal rhabdomyosarcoma. This tumor is commonly called sarcoma botryoides (from the Greek, "resembling a bunch of grapes") because of its clinical appearance of edematous clusters of polypoid tumor. **A**, In the low-power photomicrograph, the condensation of tumor cells adjacent to the entrapped epithelial cells (cambium layer) is evident. **B**, At high power, skeletal muscle differentiation with striations is evident. This tumor is less aggressive than the same histologic type arising in the vagina of younger patients. A multimodality therapeutic regimen is generally recommended.

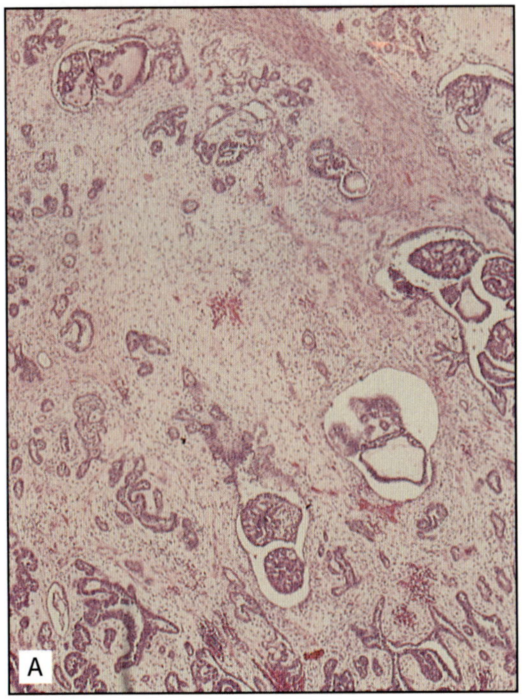

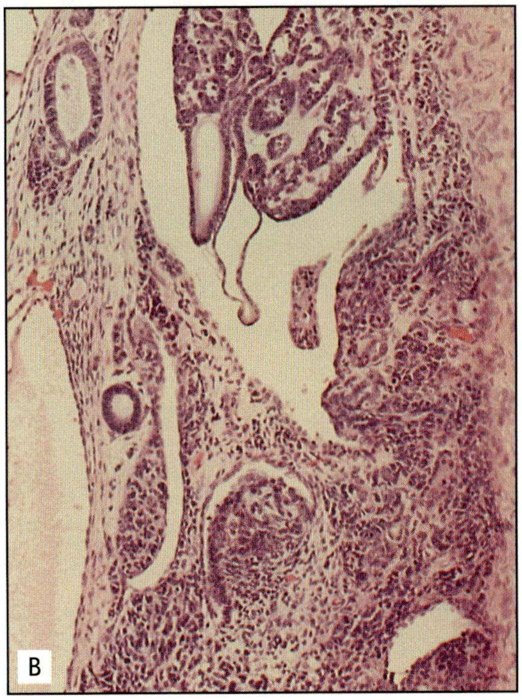

FIGURE 4–54.

Carcinosarcoma (malignant mixed müllerian tumor). In carcinosarcoma, both the glandular and stromal elements appear malignant. The epithelial and stromal components resemble endometrial carcinoma (**A**) and endometrial stromal sarcoma (**B**). These tumors are more rare in the cervix than the corpus, so a corpus primary tumor must be excluded.

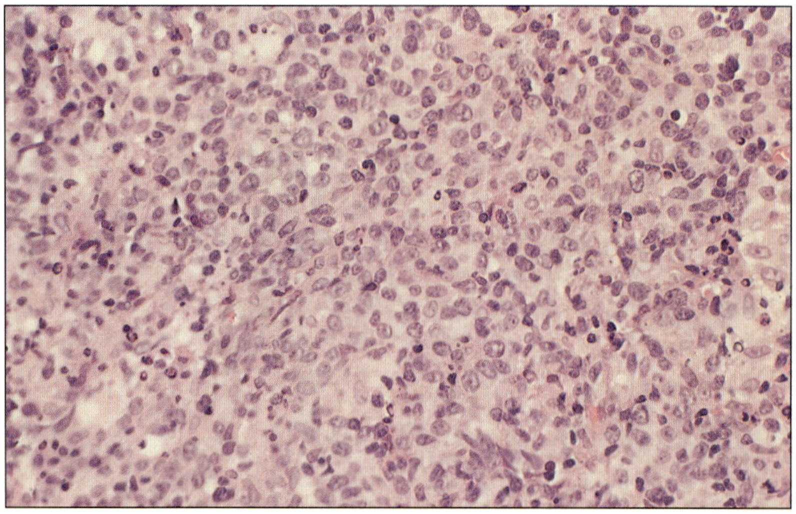

FIGURE 4-55.

Lymphoma. Lymphoma rarely presents as a primary tumor of the cervix; however, in this case the patient presented with vaginal bleeding and a cervical mass. The typical finding on examination is an expanded cervix that may be multinodular, but without the hard, localized mass typical of carcinoma. If lymphoma is suspected, additional material for immunohistochemical, flow cytometry, and molecular studies on fresh or frozen tissue may be needed. Communication between pathologist and gynecologist is imperative in such cases.

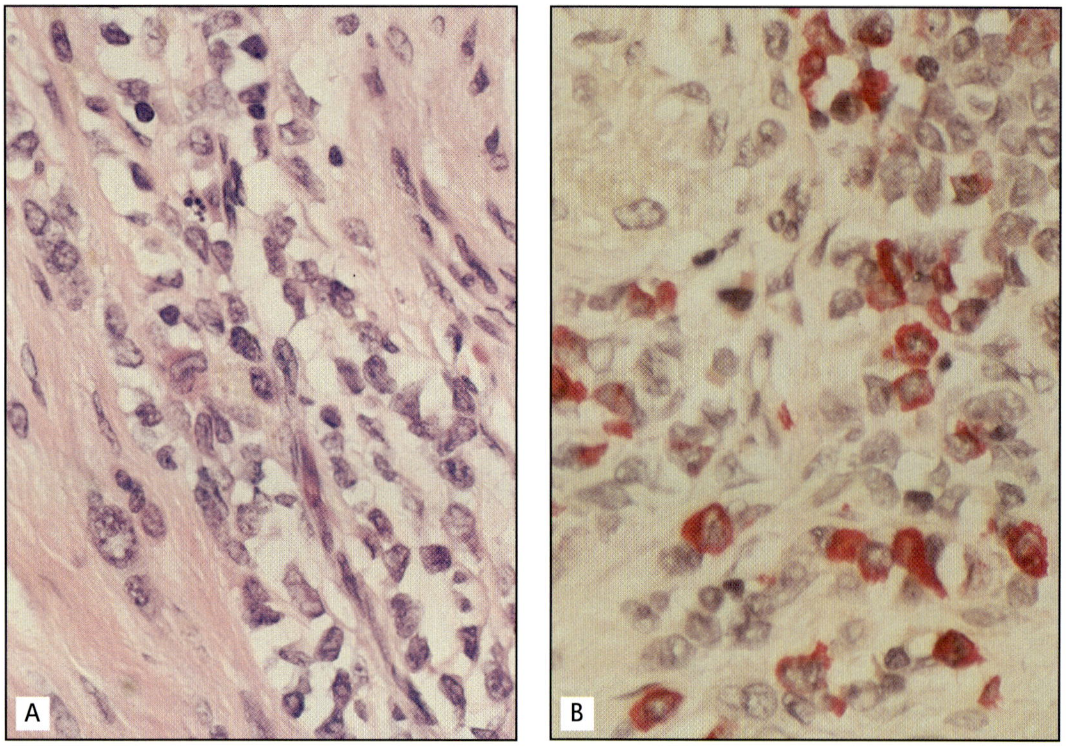

FIGURE 4-56.

Granulocytic sarcoma. This rare condition of the cervix is most likely to be associated with a diagnosis of myelogenous leukemia. In this case the atypical cells clustered around blood vessels. Following the diagnosis on cervical biopsy, the bone marrow was found to be involved. **A**, Some large cells with red granular cytoplasm can be seen, which appear to be eosinophilic myelocytes. **B**, A Leder (chloracetate esterase) stain highlights (*in red*) the granules typical of myeloid differentiation.

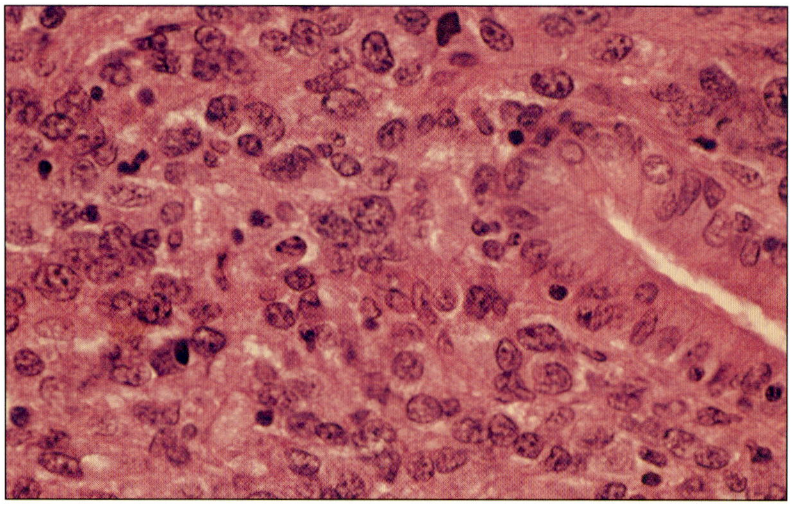

FIGURE 4-57.

Melanoma. Melanoma is an extremely rare primary tumor of the cervix. However, as the great histologic masquerader, it could be mistaken for other large cell tumors of the cervix if it is not clearly pigmented. Noting the presence of pigmentation observed at the time of examination would be most helpful to the pathologist in considering melanoma as a part of the differential diagnosis (*see also* Fig. 4-34) (*Courtesy of* Richard Zaino, MD.)

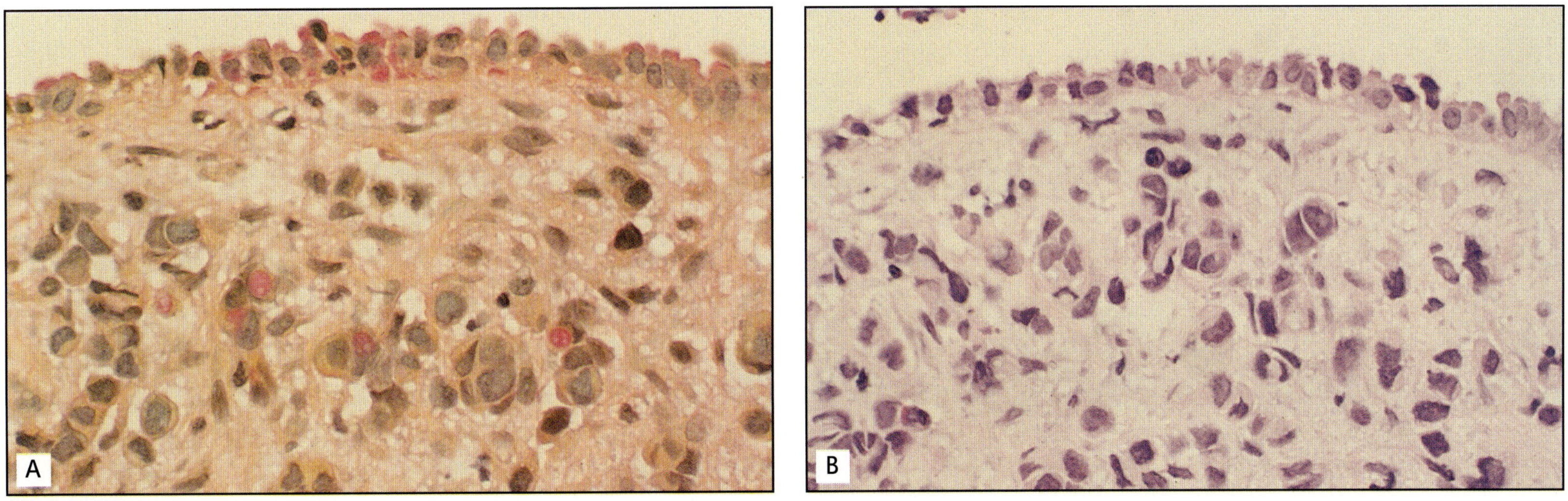

FIGURE 4-58.

Metastatic breast carcinoma. The most common tumor metastatic to the cervix is an endometrial primary, with ovary the second most common. Of tumors not originating in the genital tract, breast is one of the most frequent. **A**, Neoplastic cells have infiltrated the stroma of the cervix with a normal overlying endocervical epithelium. **B**, A mucicarmine stain shows these cells to contain intracytoplasmic mucin droplets. This neoplasm resembled the primary cancer in this patient's breast. The patient presented with simultaneous breast and cervical masses.

REFERENCES

1. Huffman JW: Mesonephric remnants in the cervix. *Am J Obstet Gynecol* 1948, 56:23–39.
2. Segal GH, Hart WR: Cystic endocervical tunnel clusters. *Am J Surg Pathol* 1990, 14:895–903.
3. Al-Nafussi A, Rahilly M: The prevalence of tubo-endometrial metaplasia and adenomatoid proliferation. *Histopathology* 1993, 22:177–179.
4. Greeley C, Schroeder S, Silverberg S: Microglandular hyperplasia of the cervix: a true "pill" lesion? *Int J Gynecol Pathol* 1995, 14:50–54.
5. Young RH, Scully RE: Atypical forms of microglandular hyperplasia of the cervix simulating carcinoma. *Am J Surg Pathol* 1989, 13:50–56.
6. Novak ER, Woodruff JD: In *Novak's Gynecologic and Obstetric Pathology*, edn 5. Philadelphia:WB Saunders Co; 1962.
7. Gloor E, Hurlimann J: Cervical intraepithelial glandular neoplasia (adenocarcinoma in situ and glandular dysplasia). *Cancer* 1986, 58:1272–1280.
8. Bertrand M, Lickrish G, Colgan TJ: The anatomic distribution of cervical adenocarcinoma in situ: implications for treatment. *Am J Obstet Gynecol* 1987, 157:21–25.
9. Benda JA, Lamoreaux J, Johnson SR: Artifact associated with use of strong iodine solutions (Lugol's) in cone biopsies. *Am J Surg Pathol* 1987, 11:367–374.
10. Davis JR, Steinbronn KK, Graham AR, Dawson BV: Effects of Monsel's solution in uterine cervix. *Am J Clin Pathol* 1984, 82:332–335.
11. Thomas PA, Zaleski S, Ohlhausen WW, *et al.*: Cytomorphologic characteristics of thermal injury related to endocervical brushing following loop electrosurgical excision procedure (LEEP). *Diagn Cytopathol* 1996, 14:212–215.
12. Staging announcement: FIGO Cancer Committee. Gynecol Oncol 1995, 58:157–158.
13. Benda JA, Platz CE, Buchsbaum H, Lifshitz S: Mucin production in defining mixed carcinoma of the uterine cervix: a clinicopathologic study. *Int J Gynecol Pathol* 1985, 4:314–327.
14. Platz CE, Benda JA. Female genital tract cancer. *Cancer* 1995, 75:270–294.

SELECTED BIBLIOGRAPHY

Benda JA: Histopathologic prognostic factors in early stage cervical carcinoma. National Institutes of Health Consensus Conference on Cervical Cancer. *J Nat Cancer Inst* 1996, 21:27–34.

Benda JA: Pathology of cervical carcinoma and its prognostic implications. In *Semin Onc* 1994, 21:3–11.

Kurman RJ, ed: *Blausteins's Pathology of the Female Genital Tract*, edn 4. New York: Springer-Verlag; 1994.

Kurman RJ, Norris HJ, Wilkinson E: *Atlas of Tumor Pathology: Tumors of the Cervix, Vagina, and Vulva*. Bethesda, MD: Armed Forces Institute of Pathology; 1992

CHAPTER 5

Endometrium

Richard J. Zaino

The endometrium represents a tissue of paradoxes to the gynecologist and pathologist. It is subject to the complex interplay of sex steroids and growth factors which dramatically modulate its growth and differentiation throughout life, yet manifestations of disease are generally restricted to one of the triad of abnormal bleeding, infertility, or occasionally, pain. The endometrium is one of the most widely sampled of tissues, with dilatation and curettage representing perhaps the most common operative procedure performed in the United States [1]. Nevertheless, at the microscopic level, it remains the source of incredible diagnostic challenges and frustration. Not only must one be familiar with the sequence of endogenous hormone actions on the endometrium resulting in daily cyclic changes, but the diagnostician must also recognize the morphologic alterations consequent to an astounding variety of agents used by millions of women each year for hormonal contraception, ovulation induction, or menopausal hormonal replacement. Consequently, it is no surprise that endometrial samples are not always greeted by diagnostic pathologists with enthusiasm. Only after the diagnostician has mastered this panoply of physiologic and iatrogenic histologic patterns, can he or she begin to comprehend the abnormal endometrium. For that reason, the histology of cycling and iatrogenically altered endometrium is presented in detail in this chapter before presentation of the pathologic processes.

Fortunately, there is a logical theme of an end-organ response to circulating sex hormones that is manifested morphologically in predictable fashion in most of these conditions. Even the majority of hyperplastic and malignant processes retain some degree of hormonal responsiveness. Thus, a rational scheme for the evaluation of the endometrium is possible, which can be used to guide one reliably to accurate diagnoses. This approach is based on a highly simplistic but reliable assertion that estrogenic compounds cause proliferation of the endometrial glands and stroma, while progestational agents induce their differentiation.

A method of data collection and analysis, briefly presented in the tables at the beginning of this chapter, is used throughout as a means to understand the diagnostic criteria.

It is helpful to maintain a methodical approach to consideration of the endometrial specimen, which includes the following steps: 1) assembly of a brief clinical history, 2) examination of the gross specimen, 3) collection of data at low and high magnification, 4) analysis of the data, and 5) synthesis of a diagnosis. The minimum history should include age, reproductive history, date of last menstrual period or menopause, and history of hormonal, cytotoxic, or radiation therapy. Since very few endometrial processes can be reliably recognized at the level of gross examination, and far more endometrial samples are obtained by biopsy or curettage than by hysterectomy, the emphasis is placed on microscopic features in this chapter.

COLLECTING THE DATA

VOLUME OF ENDOMETRIUM AS A DIAGNOSTIC AID

Scant	Intermediate	Great
Atrophy	Cycling	Disordered proliferative
Inactive	Endometritis	Hyperplasia
HRT		Carcinoma
Oral contraceptives		Polyp
		Gestation

FIGURE 5-1.
Volume of endometrium as a diagnostic aid. There is limited but important information available from gross inspection of the endometrium in curettage or hysterectomy specimens. During the normal menstrual cycle, the thickness of the endometrium varies from about 1 to 7 mm, and generally is soft and tan (*see* Figs. 5-5, 5-9, and 5-12). Only with marked proliferation, such as that associated with hyperplasia, carcinoma or other malignant neoplasms, is the endometrium characteristically more abundant, thicker, irregular in configuration, or necrotic (*see* Figs. 5-34 and 5-38). The one major exception is gestational endometrium, which usually does not represent a diagnostic challenge. HRT—hormone replacement therapy at menopause. (From Zaino, RJ. Interpretation of Endometrial Biopsies and Curettings. Lippincott-Raven, Philadelphia, PA, 1996.)

MICROSCOPIC COMPONENTS OF THE ENDOMETRIUM

- Glandular epithelium
- Surface epithelium
- Stromal cells and matrix
- Blood vessels (arterial and venous)
- Lymphocytes (stromal granulocytes)
- Other infiltrating cells (inflammatory or neoplastic)

FIGURE 5-2.
Microscopic components of the endometrium. Given the complexity of tissues and morphologic patterns, it is easy to be overwhelmed by the large quantity of data present in a histologic specimen. A systematic approach to the examination of the endometrium helps to ensure that all elements are explored and defined. In addition to the components listed, one must also determine whether the specimen is derived from the *functionalis* or *basalis*. The functionalis represents about the superficial two thirds of the endometrium, is responsive to sex hormones, and displays striking morphologic variation during the menstrual cycle. In contrast, the glands and stroma of the basalis are remarkably constant in their appearance. Similarly, the development of the lower uterine segment is relatively retarded chronologically and qualitatively compared with the fundus. (From Zaino, RJ. Interpretation of Endometrial Biopsies and Curettings. Lippincott-Raven, Philadelphia, PA, 1996.)

A. DEVELOPMENT OF THE ENDOMETRIUM

Uniform	Variable
Proliferative	Endometritis
Early or mid secretory	Late secretory
Oral contraceptive	Gestation
	Polyp
	Hyperplasia
	Carcinoma

B. GLAND:STROMA RATIO

<1:1	1:1	>1:1
Early proliferative	Mid proliferative	Mid secretory
Inactive	Late proliferative	Early secretory
Atrophy	Mid secretory	Hyperplasia
Progestin therapy	Disordered proliferation	Carcinoma
Secretory (after day 20)		Gestation
OCP		

FIGURE 5-3.
Microscopic features examined at low magnification. Although it is tempting to search for a highly characteristic feature at high magnification to make a diagnosis, discordant development of glands and stroma is common, and reliance on a single histologic feature is imprudent. Errors are best avoided by first concentrating efforts at low (4() magnification. This provides an overall perspective of each of the microscopic components and their relationships to one another. In particular, it is essential to assess the uniformity of development (**A**), gland:stroma ratio (**B**), glandular configuration (**C**), gland luminal diameter (**D**), variation in gland size or contour (**E**), and stromal character (**F**).

(*Continued on next page*)

C. GLAND CONFIGURATION

Straight	Coiled	Dilated	Serrated	Branching
Early proliferative	Late proliferative	Midsecretory	Gestation	Disordered proliferative
Mid proliferative	Early secretory	Polyp	Late secretory	Hyperplasia
OCP				Carcinoma
Progestin therapy				
Atrophy				

D. LUMEN DIAMETER

Narrow	Wide
Proliferative	Mid secretory
Early secretory	Late secretory
Disordered proliferation	Polyps (some)
Progestin therapy (late)	Progestin therapy (early)
Hyperplasia (some)	Hyperplasia (some)
Neoplasia (some)	Neoplasia (some)
OCP	
HRT	

E. VARIATION IN SIZE OR CONTOUR

Regular	Irregular
Cycling	Disordered proliferation
Endometritis	Hyperplasia
	Carcinoma
	Gestation

F. STROMAL CHARACTER

Spindle	Compact	Predecidua	Complete decidua
Menses (late)	Mid proliferative	Late secretory	Gestation
Early proliferative	Late proliferative	OCP	Progestin therapy
Endometritis (rare)	Early secretory	HRT	
	Mid secretory		
	Atrophy		

FIGURE 5-3. *(Continued)*
The principle which underlies this approach is that the proliferation of glands and stroma almost always reflects a response to estrogen exposure, whereas differentiation of glands and stroma occurs in estrogen-primed glands exposed to a progestin. Short, simple tubular glands grow in length and coil during the proliferative phase, and then dilate and fill with luminal product consequent to the secretion of apical cytoplasm. The stroma grows less rapidly than the glands during the proliferative phase (hence the coiling of glands), and then displays differentiation by the formation of edema and decidualization in the secretory phase. Similar but not identical responses also occur predictably when iatrogenic or pathologic alterations in the quantity or duration of steroid hormone exposure occurs. HRT—hormone replacement therapy; OCP—oral contraceptive pill. (From Zaino, RJ. Interpretation of Endometrial Biopsies and Curettings. Lippincott-Raven, Philadelphia, PA, 1996.)

MICROSCOPIC FEATURES EXAMINED AT HIGH MAGNIFICATION

- Epithelial cell stratification
- Epithelial cell cytoplasmic differentiation
- Nuclear morphology
- Mitotic activity
- Secretion (basal, apical, or luminal)
- Stromal infiltrates (inflammatory or neoplastic)
- Vascular development (arterial or venous)

FIGURE 5-4.

Microscopic features examined at high magnification. A careful examination at low magnification usually permits a tentative classification of the process involving the endometrium. Then it is appropriate to use the 20 or 40 objective lens to search for the corresponding features of proliferation or differentiation, which can be used to confirm the diagnosis. The proliferation induced by estrogen is expressed as nuclear stratification and enlargement in glands, and both glandular and stromal mitotic figures. In contrast, progestin causes the formation of a secretory product in the endoplasmic reticulum of the cytoplasm of glandular epithelium, which is initially basal, then apical, and ultimately discharged by apical secretion into the gland lumen. The development of spiral arterioles, stromal decidualization, and a marked increase in the density of stromal granulocytes are sequential hallmarks of stromal exposure to progestins.

THE CYCLING ENDOMETRIUM

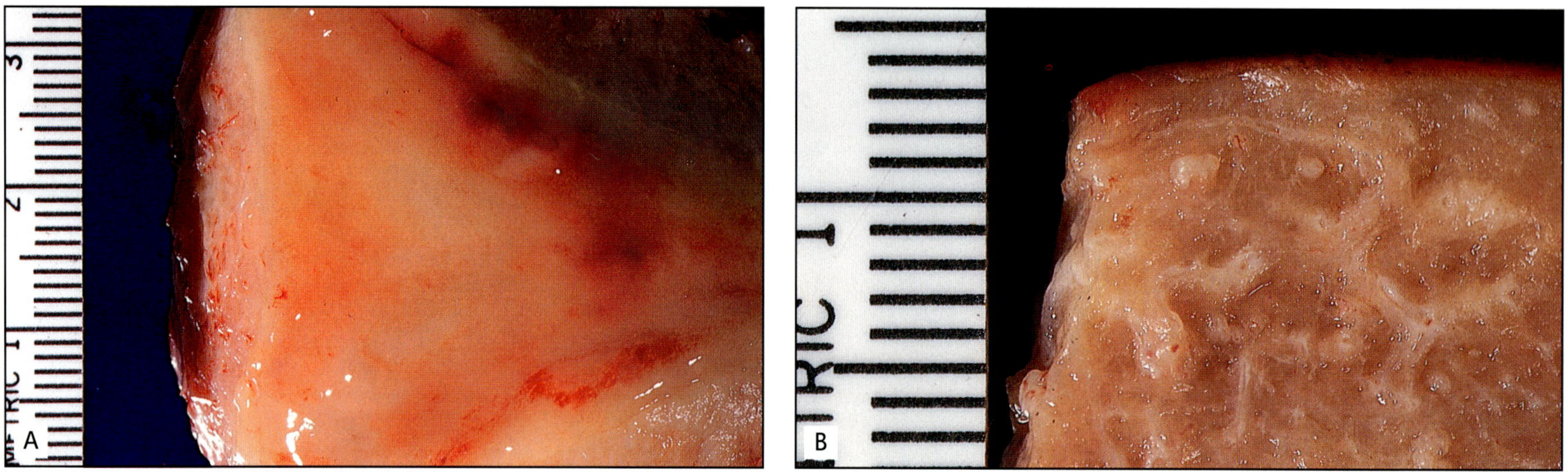

FIGURE 5-5.

The proliferative phase uterus. The hemisected uterus is lined by a triangularly shaped, smooth, tan, soft endometrium (**A**). This cross section of uterus removed during the proliferative phase demonstrates that the pink endometrial lining is surprisingly thin, only about 1 mm (**B**). The endometrial thickness typically varies from 1 mm in the early proliferative phase to about 4 mm in the late proliferative phase. The normal menstrual cycle has a modal length of 28 days. However, this represents only a statistical norm, and only about 15% of menstrual cycles are actually 28 days in length [2]. Although the proliferative phase of the typical menstrual cycle lasts about 14 days, it is generally possible to reliably distinguish only three broad categories of proliferative phase morphology, corresponding to the early, mid, or late proliferative phase.

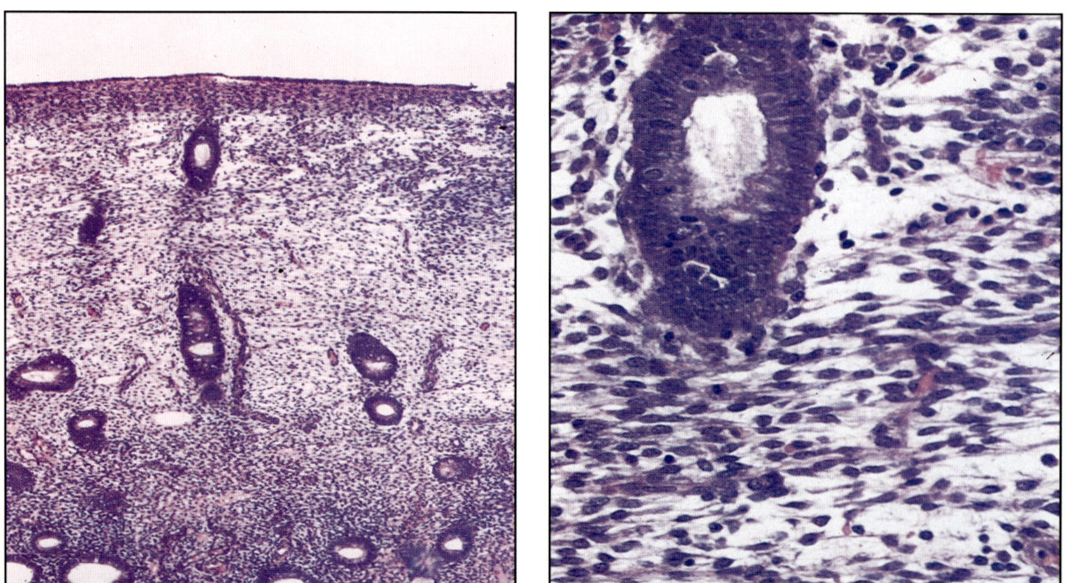

FIGURE 5-6.

Early proliferative phase endometrium. At low magnification, it is evident that the morphology is relatively uniform, the gland:stroma ratio is much less than 1:1, with glands that are straight, narrow tubules, surrounded by abundant stroma (**A**). The gland:stroma ratio is assessed most easily by estimating the proportion of the total area of endometrium in the section occupied by the silhouette of the glands. At high magnification, the lining epithelium is columnar, with mild stratification. The stroma, undergoing repair from the recent menses, resembles granulation tissue. Mitotic figures in the glands and stroma are caused by an estrogen-induced proliferation (**B**).

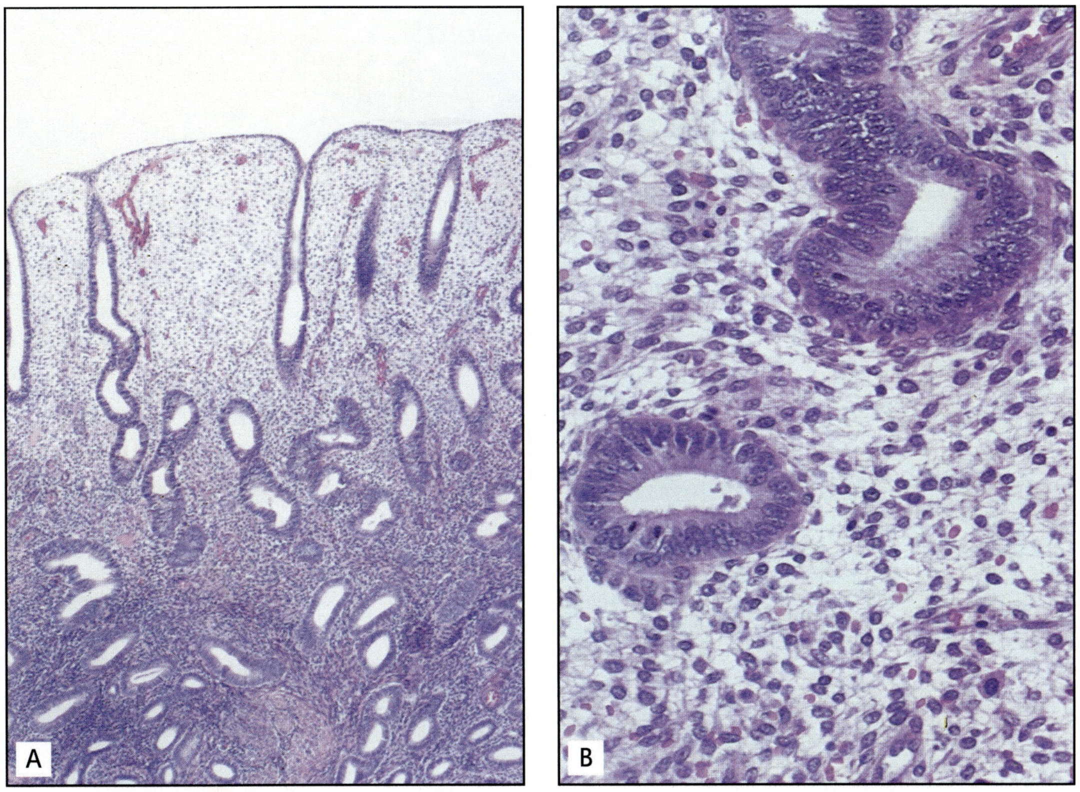

FIGURE 5-7.
Mid proliferative phase endometrium. At low magnification, the endometrium displays a uniform development, with a gland:stroma ratio of slightly less than 1:1, and glands that are straight and narrow, with a small lumen (**A**). At higher magnification, the estrogen-induced proliferation of glands and stroma is apparent, with stratification of nuclei in glands, and mitotic figures in both glands and stroma. The shared apical border of the glandular epithelium is characteristic of proliferative-type endometrium, and results in a sharply circumscribed or "punched out" lumen. The spindled cells of the regenerative stroma of the early proliferative phase have been replaced by compact polygonal stromal cells that possess scant cytoplasm (**B**).

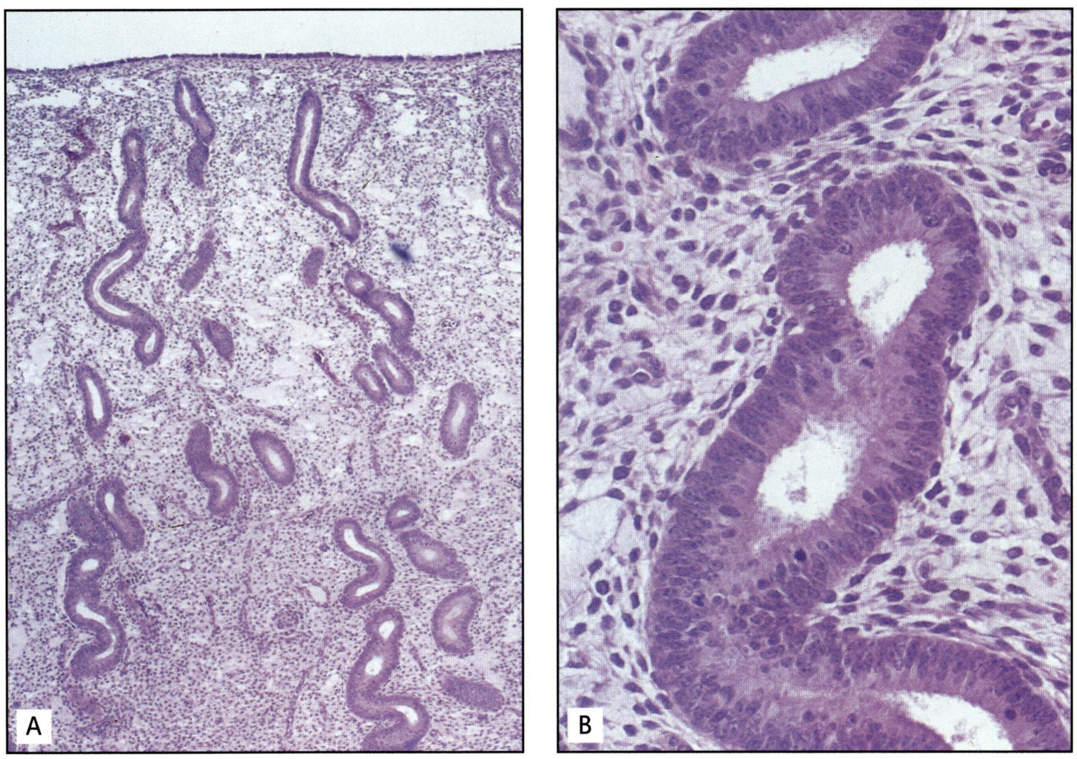

FIGURE 5-8.
Late proliferative phase endometrium. At low magnification, the volume can be noted to be greater than that of the early proliferative phase. The appearance is uniform, the gland:stroma ratio remains slightly less than 1:1, and the glands are narrow. However, in contrast to the early or mid proliferative phase endometrium, the gland configuration is coiled rather than straight. The coiling results in the repeated appearance and disappearance of the glands even in well-oriented sections (**A**). At high magnification, the proliferation caused by estrogen secreted by the developing ovarian follicle continues, with even greater stratification of nuclei and mitotic activity (**B**).

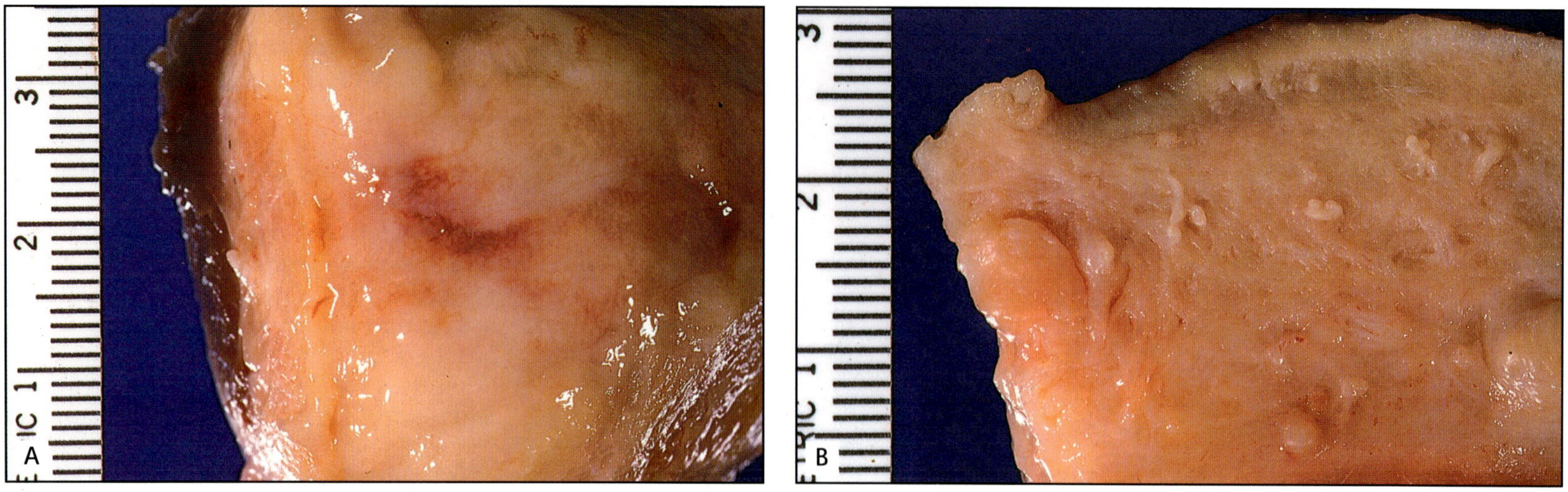

FIGURE 5-9.

The early secretory phase uterus. The hemisected uterus is lined by a soft, tan endometrium, which has a slightly variable thickness, resulting in a mildly ridged or undulating appearance (**A**). This cross section of an early secretory phase uterus displays a thickness of about 4 mm (**B**). The thickness of the endometrium typically varies from about 4 mm in the early secretory phase to a peak of about 7 mm on days 26 to 27. There is a slight reduction of thickness that occurs on the last day before the onset of menses. In contrast to proliferative phase endometrium, there is a sequence of distinctive histologic features in the glands or stroma that permit assignment of a specific date during the idealized 14-day secretory phase of the menstrual cycle. Examples of early, mid, and late secretory phase endometrium are depicted subsequently to illustrate intermediate steps in this continuum.

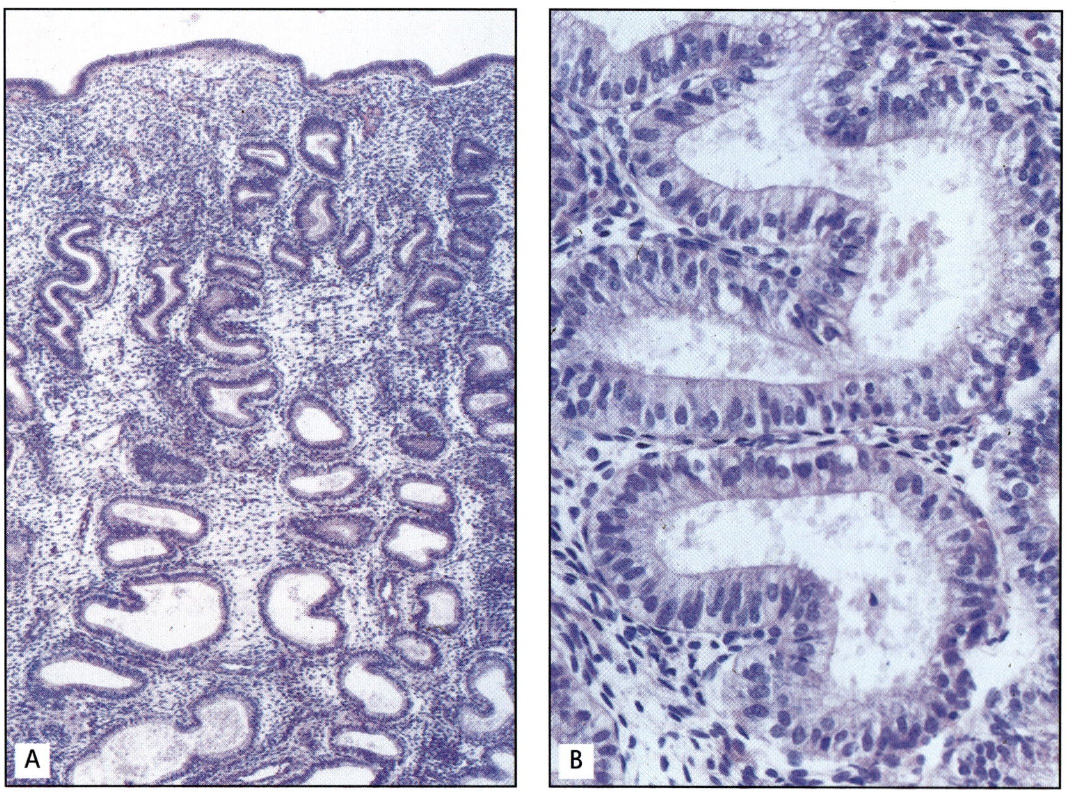

FIGURE 5-10.

Early secretory phase endometrium, about day 18 (postovulatory day 4). At low magnification, the endometrium is relatively uniform, with a gland:stroma ratio slightly greater than 1:1. The glands have a coiled tubular configuration, and vary from narrow (*upper portion*) to dilated (*lower portion*) (**A**). At higher magnification, it is evident that the glands are lined by a simple columnar epithelium, with a few persisting subnuclear vacuoles. However, most of the secretion has moved to the apical cytoplasm, which, in some areas, has resulted in the formation of apical blebs. Elsewhere, it has been shed as an apical secretion into the gland lumen (**B**). The process of glandular epithelial cell secretion is a manifestation of differentiation resulting from the action of a progestin on estrogen-primed cells.

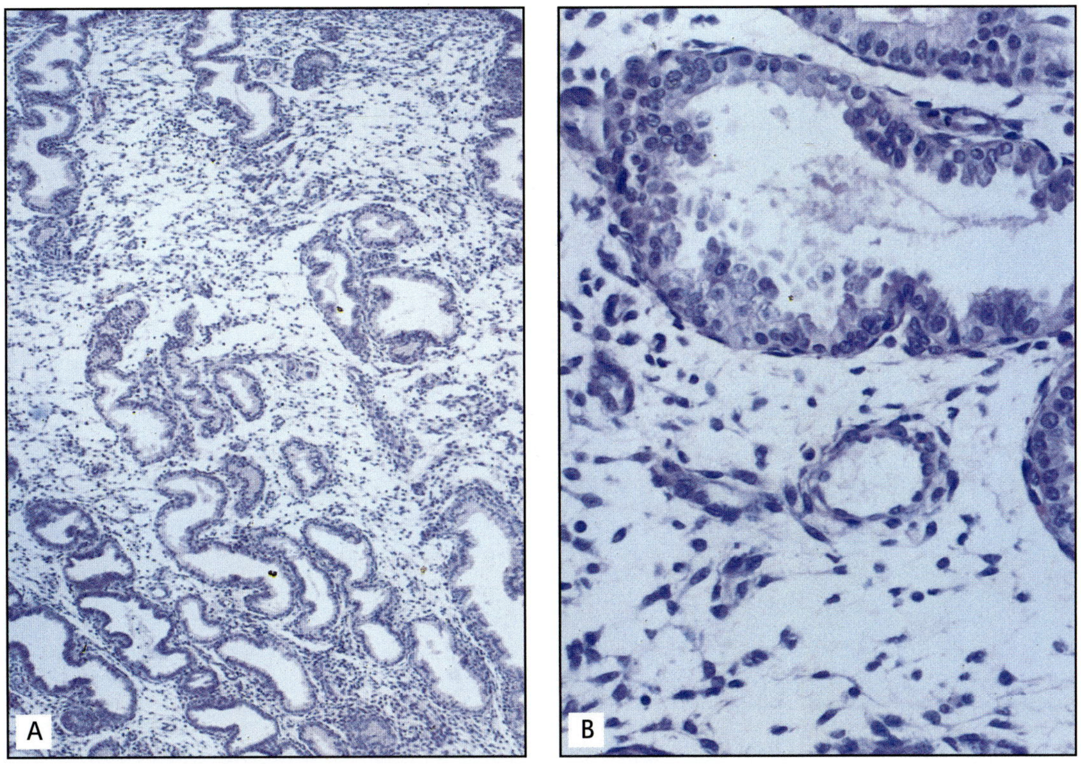

FIGURE 5-11.
Mid secretory phase endometrium, about day 21 (postovulatory day 7). At low magnification, the morphology is relatively uniform, with the gland:stroma ratio dropping to about 1:1, because of the increased stromal volume associated with the peak of stromal edema. The glands are dilated and coiled, with a wide luminal diameter (**A**). At high magnification, the irregular dilation of some gland lumens results in a complex architecture, with papillary infoldings of the epithelium. This may cause the epithelium to appear serrated, even though it is generally not stratified. As a consequence of secretion, the epithelial cells are of a short columnar configuration, with basal nuclei, apical cytoplasmic snouts, and variable vacuolation of cytoplasm. The gland lumens contain abundant, wispy secretion. Mitotic figures are absent. The stromal cells are small, with scant cytoplasm, and are separated from one another by optically clear matrix, representing the stromal edema (**B**).

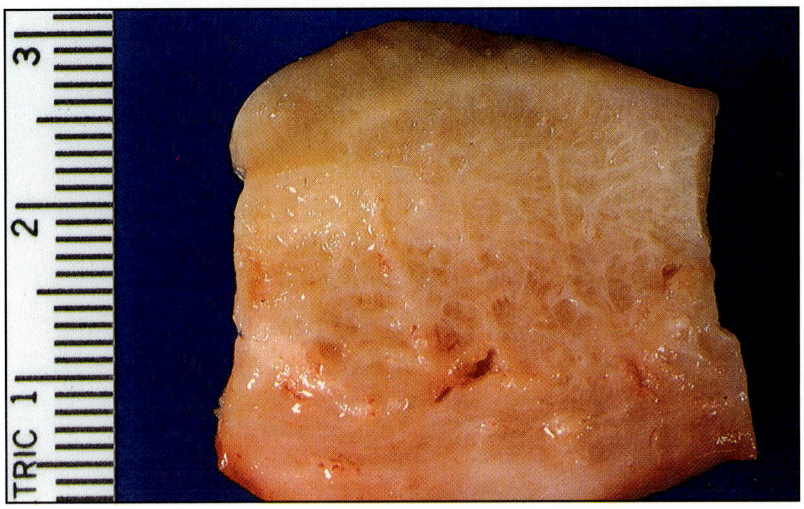

FIGURE 5-12.
The late secretory phase uterus. This cross section of uterus illustrates the relatively thick, soft, tan endometrium of the late secretory phase. The endometrium is about 5 mm in thickness, and is more easily distinguished from the firm, resilient myometrium by texture than by color.

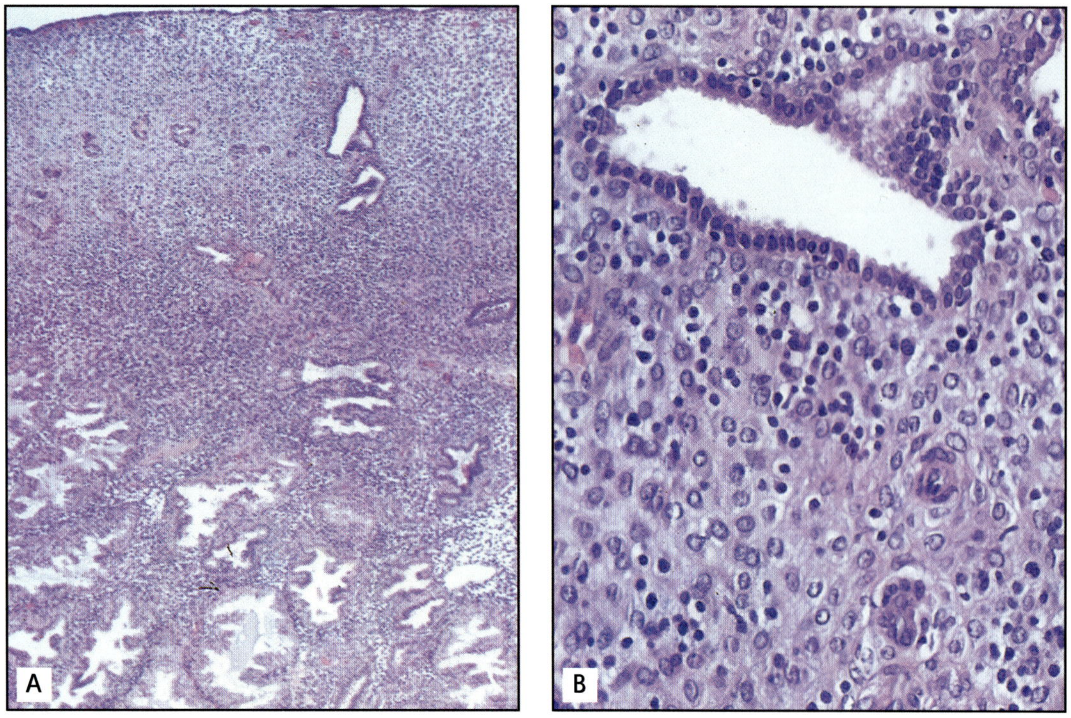

FIGURE 5-13.
Secretory phase endometrium, about day 26 (postovulatory day 12). There is variability in endometrial morphology, with a superficial zona compacta having a low gland:stroma ratio, and a deeper zona spongiosa, with a gland:stroma ratio that is greater than 1:1 (**A**). This variability reflects the confluent predecidualization that occurs in the superficial stroma accompanied by narrow exhausted glands, compared with the dilated secretion-filled deeper glands surrounded by a stroma with little decidual change. At higher magnification, the exhausted secretory glands of the zona compacta are noted to have a simple, low columnar epithelial lining, embedded in a stroma with spiral arterioles surrounded by partially decidualized cells (**B**). The decidual change of stromal cells is characterized by their acquisition of more abundant polygonal-shaped cytoplasm and distinct cell membranes. Stromal granulocytes, a unique population of large granular lymphocytes [3], increase in number throughout the secretory phase, and become a prominent component of the endometrium by days 25 to 26. The process of stromal decidualization results from progestin stimulation of estrogen primed stromal cells. The strength (quality and quantity) of the decidual change reflects both the amount and duration of the progestin exposure. The requirement for both estrogen and progestin to cause the complete sequence of proliferation and differentiation of the normal menstrual cycle is evident from the morphologic aberrations that are observed with endogenous and iatrogenic hormonal perturbations.

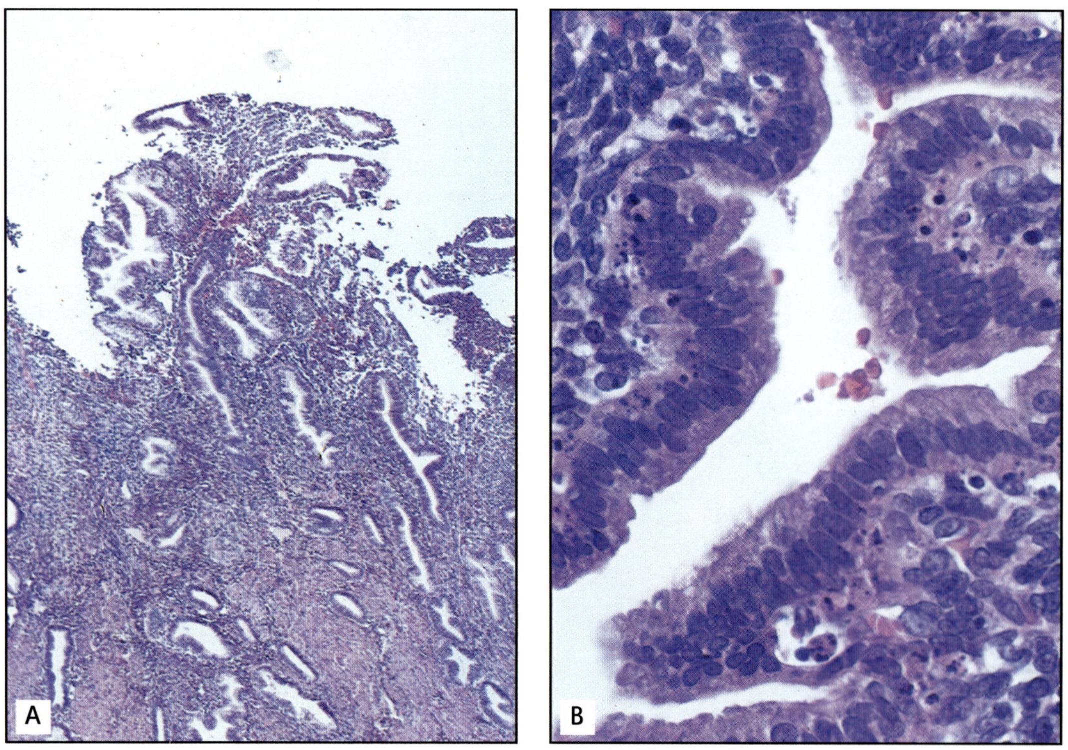

FIGURE 5-14.
Menstrual endometrium. The menstrual phase endometrium is characterized by variability, with a thickness of 1 to 4 mm, depending on the extent of shedding. The gross morphology is distinguished by a hemorrhagic lining to the uterus that is of irregular thickness and variable quantity. At low magnification, this variability persists, and regions devoid of stratum functionalis interdigitate with relatively intact areas (**A**). The gland:stroma ratio cannot be accurately assessed due to the loss of structural integrity. Fragments of glands at times seem to float within pools of blood, without obvious stromal attachment. At high magnification, there is a rapid loss of stromal decidual change, replaced by stromal condensation. The intact glands may appear either exhausted or have persistent vacuolization, the latter serving as a clue helpful in distinguishing menstrual from nonmenstrual shedding. Nuclear dust, representing fragments of disintegrating nuclei, may be found in the cytoplasm of intact epithelium with either menstrual or nonmenstrual shedding (**B**).

THE NORMAL, NONCYCLING ENDOMETRIUM

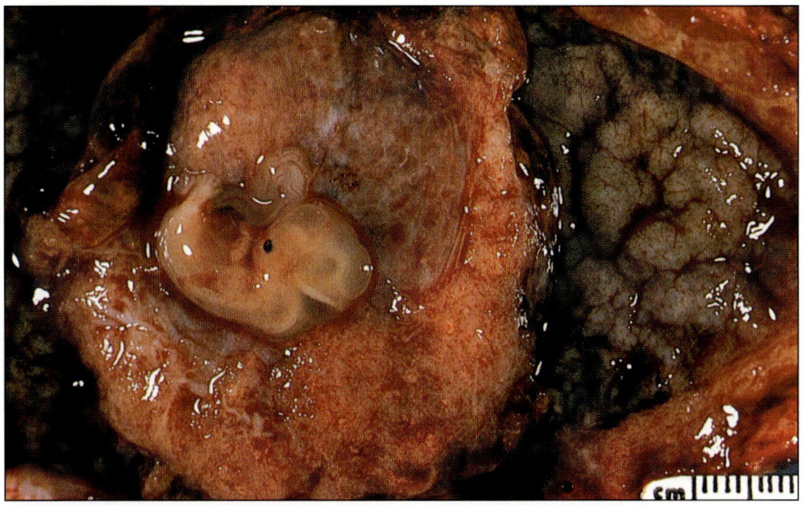

FIGURE 5-15.

The gravid uterus. This hemisected uterus contains a gestation of about 8 weeks. The amnionic sac has been opened to reveal a fetus with a crown-rump length of about 2 cm, and a distinct 5-cm-diameter placenta. The endometrium remote from the gestation has an irregular nodular-surface configuration.

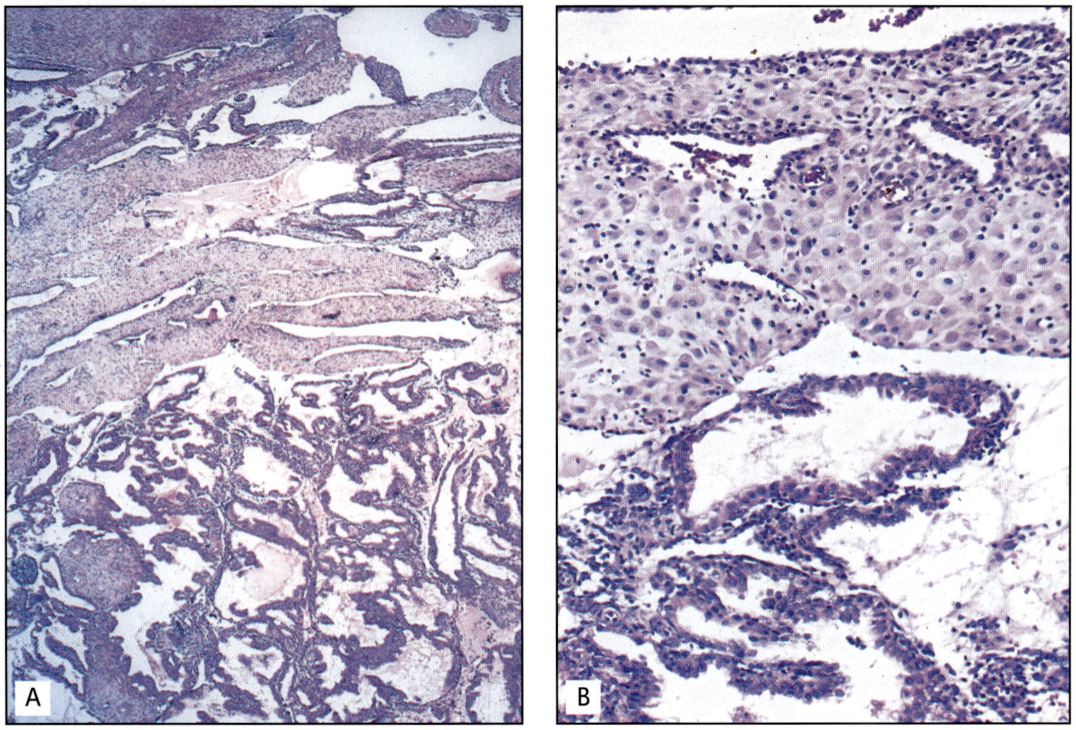

FIGURE 5-16.

Gestational endometrium. At low magnification, the variability of the endometrium is striking. This reflects the differences between the decidua basalis (the endometrium between the implanted chorionic vesicle and the myometrium), the decidua capsularis (the decidua overlying the implanted chorionic vesicle), and the decidua vera (endometrium distant from the site of implantation), and also the differences between the zona spongiosa and zona compacta. The random distribution of these tissues within curettage specimens results in a multitude of highly dissimilar fragments (**A**). At higher magnification, a fragment of zona compacta with fully decidualized stroma and exhausted glands is contrasted with zona spongiosa containing hypersecretory glands in a nondecidualized stroma (**B**).

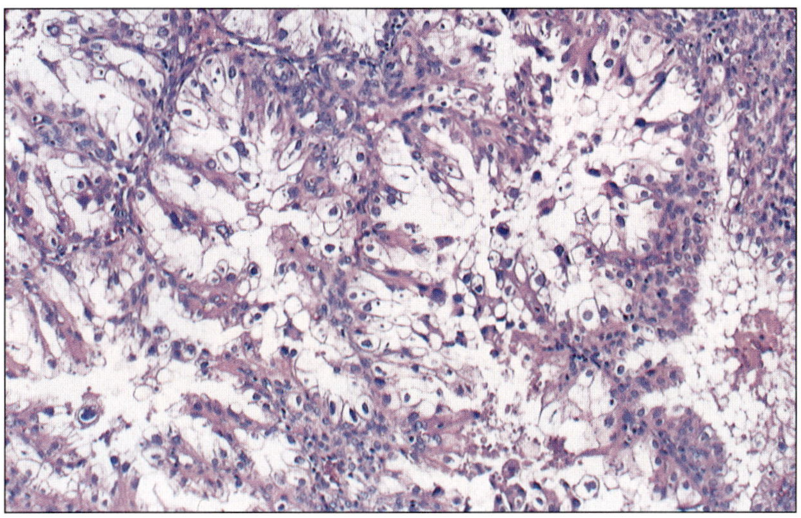

FIGURE 5-17.

Arias-Stella reaction in gestational endometrium. Nuclear enlargement of glandular epithelium coupled with some degree of either proliferative or more often secretory change constitutes the change described by Arias-Stella [4]. In its florid form, as depicted, there may be such pronounced nuclear pleomorphism and hyperchromasia accompanied by papillary tufting of an epithelium with cytoplasmic clearing that a diagnosis of clear cell carcinoma is entertained. Arrival at the correct diagnosis is facilitated by consideration of the clinical context, including a young age, and history of current gestation, as well as the presence of associated secretory or gestational changes in the endometrium. In contrast, clear cell carcinoma of the endometrium is typically found in menopausal women, with adjacent atrophic endometrium.

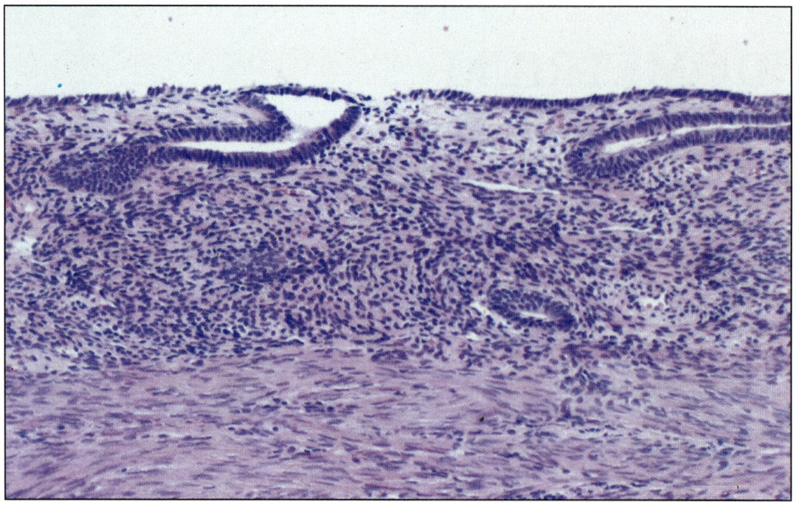

FIGURE 5-18.

Atrophy. Following menopause, the endometrium that is not exposed to estrogen progressively loses proliferative capacity and sequentially passes from patterns referred to as weakly proliferative to inactive to atrophic. There is a loss of glandular stratification and mitotic activity, and eventually the endometrium is reduced to a very thin lining of less than 1 mm, formed of sparse, short tubular glands, with a gland:stroma ratio of much less than 1:1. Atrophic endometrial gland epithelial nuclei are also typically smaller than those of cycling endometrium. The stroma frequently contains dilated, thin-walled veins that are fragile and may be the source of menopausal bleeding, in the absence of any other endometrial pathology.

ENDOMETRITIS

AN ABBREVIATED CLASSIFICATION OF ENDOMETRITIS

Neisserial
Chlamydial
Ureaplasmal
Cytomegalovirus
Herpes simplex virus
IUD associated
Postpartum
Postabortal
Granulomatous
Nonspecific, chronic

FIGURE 5-19.

A current, abbreviated classification of endometritis. Sexually transmitted diseases are epidemic in the United States, and pelvic inflammatory disease (PID) represents one of the more serious complications [5]. Endometrial biopsy is one of the most accurate methods by which to diagnose PID, with a sensitivity and specificity greater than 75%.

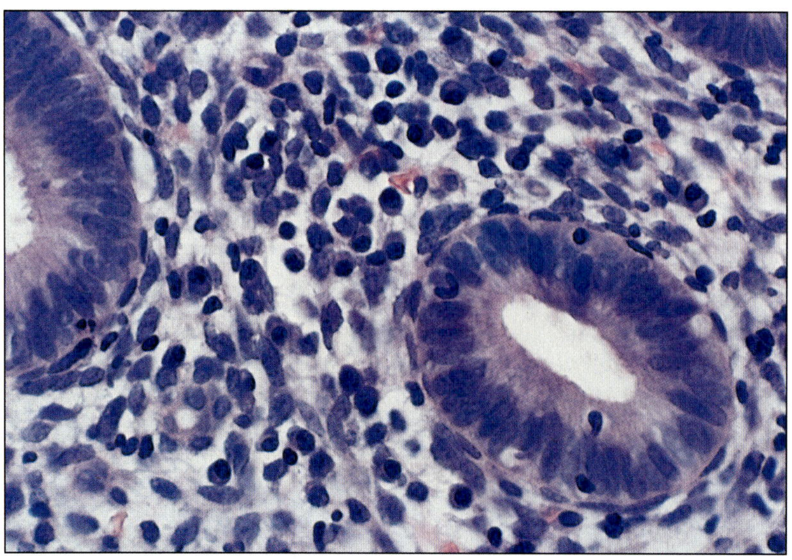

FIGURE 5-20.

Nonspecific, chronic endometritis. Because lymphocytes normally infiltrate the endometrium during the menstrual cycle, pathologists have sought the presence of other cells, such as the plasma cell, to establish the diagnosis of endometritis. Indeed, in some cases, such as the one illustrated, a multitude of plasma cells may provide evidence of a nonspecific, chronic endometritis. However, predecidualized stromal cells can resemble plasma cells, and clinically significant endometritis usually also contains other histologic manifestations of inflammation such as edema, vascular ectasia, neutrophils, dense collections of lymphocytes, hemorrhage, necrosis, and spindled stromal cells indicative of tissue repair. As a result of careful pathologic and microbiologic studies, it is now evident that other criteria (as depicted in Figs. 5-21 and 5-22) can provide clues to permit more specific diagnoses, with a suggested causative infectious agent.

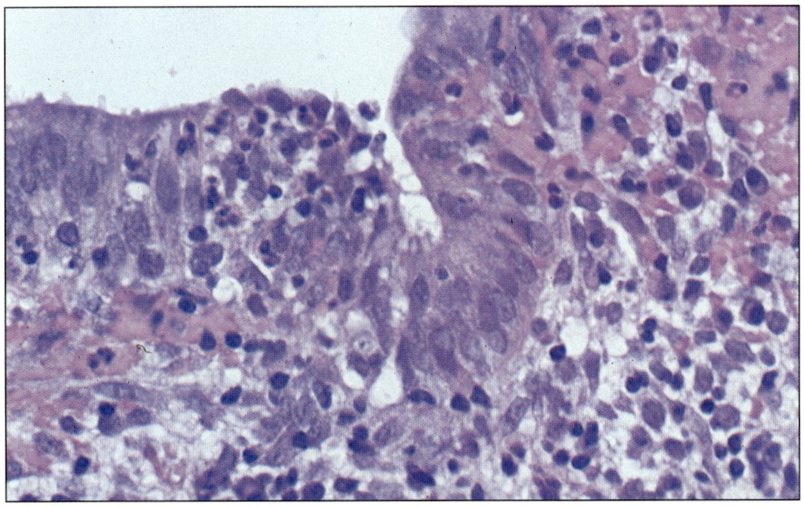

FIGURE 5-21.
Chlamydial or neisserial endometritis. In recent studies, the organisms most often associated with significant sexually transmitted infections of the upper genital tract have been *Chlamydia trachomatis* and *Neisseria gonorrhoeae* [6,7]. Histopathologic features strongly associated with the presence of these organisms include the following: the presence of one or more plasma cells per × 120 power field of endometrial tissue, and a concentration of five or more neutrophils per × 400 power field in the endometrial surface epithelium [6].

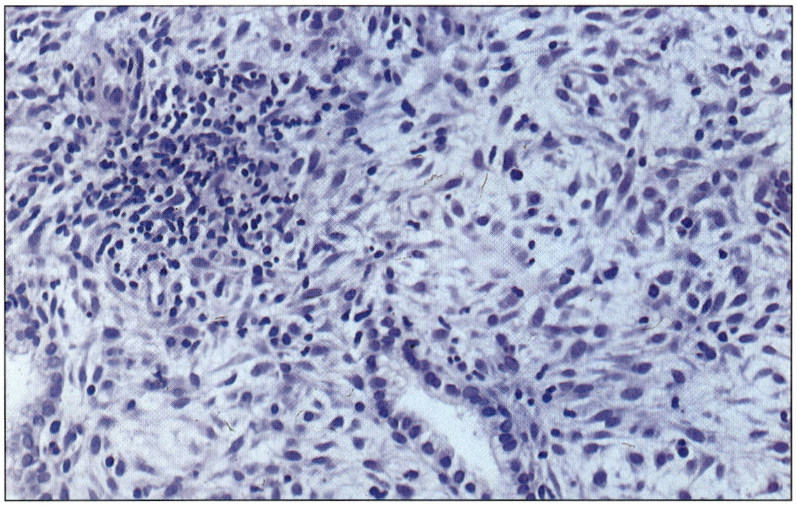

FIGURE 5-22.
Ureaplasmal endometritis. A chronic endometritis has been associated with infection by the T-mycoplasma, *Ureaplasma urealyticum*. The women have generally presented with infertility rather than symptoms of pelvic inflammatory disease. The histologic features include the following: 1) patchy, non-necrotizing inflammation; 2) small numbers of discrete, minute clusters of lymphocytes and histiocytes; and 3) a tendency for the inflammation to be concentrated immediately subjacent to the surface epithelium or near the stromal interface with glands [8]. There is often edema and spindling of the stroma, which suggests a reparative process. Plasma cells are generally not a conspicuous feature of ureaplasmal infection.

IATROGENIC CHANGES

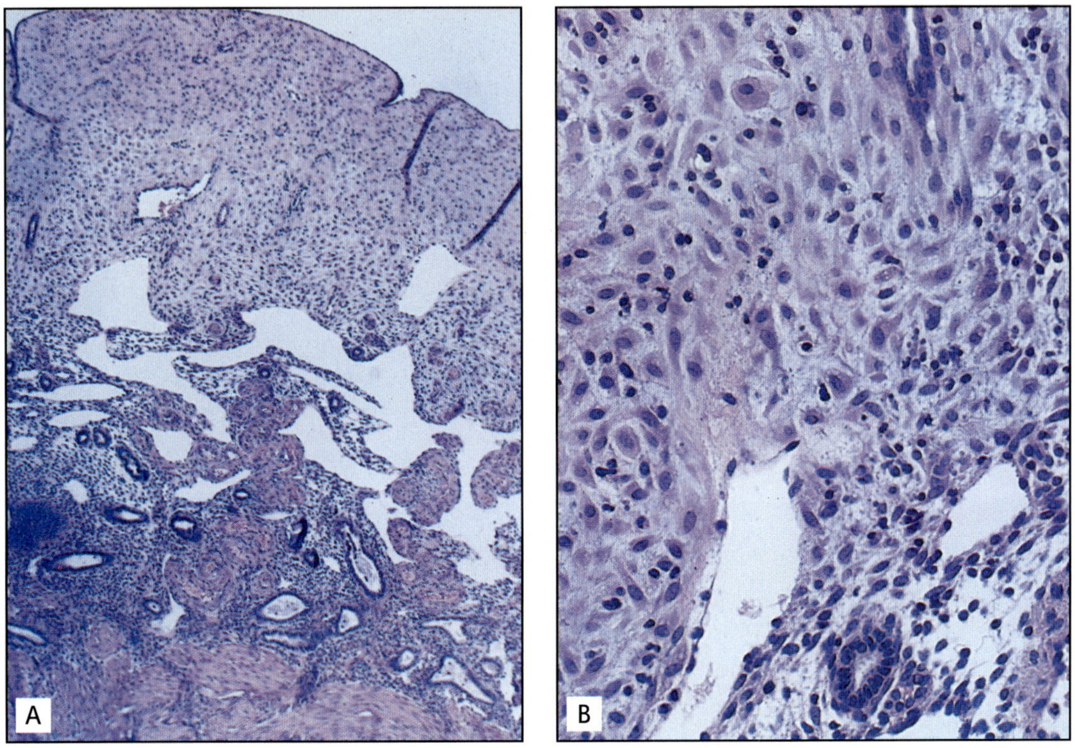

FIGURE 5-23.
Combined oral contraceptive effect. Oral contraceptives are among the most commonly prescribed medications in the United States, and have been in use for more than two decades. This patient had been treated with Enovid, (GD Searle & Co, Chicago IL.), which contains a relatively potent estrogen (mestranol) and progestin (norethynodrel). Consequently, there is a strong cumulative histologic effect, manifest at low magnification by extensive decidual change, and secretory exhaustion of glands. The gland:stroma ratio is consequently much less than 1:1, and the glands are simple tubes or narrow diameter, with no stratification or mitotic activity (**A**). In common with late secretory endometrium, there is extensive predecidualization of stromal cells, but in place of spiral arterioles there are numerous dilated veins (**B**).

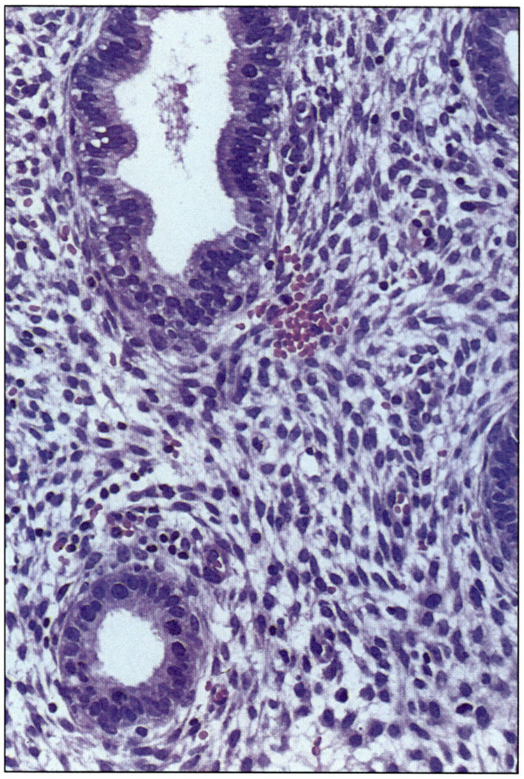

FIGURE 5-24.
Oral contraceptive effect. This patient had been treated with Desogen, (Organon Inc. West Orange, NJ), which contains only 30 μg of ethinyl estradiol per pill, thus providing very little proliferation or stimulation of progesterone receptor. Consequently, there is only weak proliferation and differentiation, which may be expressed simultaneously. The gland:stroma ratio is slightly less than 1:1, the glands have a tubular configuration, and they are lined by a weakly stratified epithelium, with scattered subnuclear vacuoles. The stroma has a very weak predecidual change, with acquisition of stellate shaped cytoplasm.

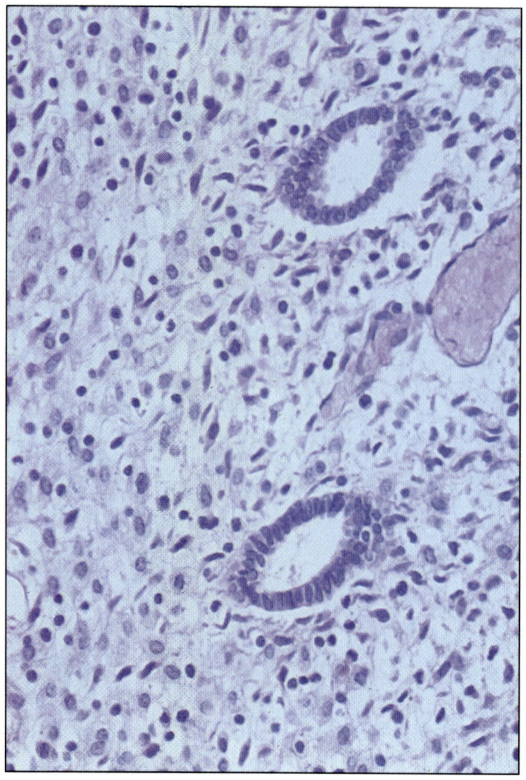

FIGURE 5-25.
Menopausal hormone replacement therapy. As with combined oral contraceptive therapy, the histologic effects of exogenous estrogen and progestin therapy on the endometrium vary according to the potency, duration, and quantity of hormone prescribed. With combined estrogen-progestin therapy, the endometrium usually is atrophic after a few months of therapy. With cyclic therapy, weak proliferation is followed about 3 days after the initiation of the progestational agent with weak secretion and then weak predecidual change. In this specimen, taken during the addition of the progestational agent, there is a very low gland:stroma ratio, no glandular secretory activity, and weak decidual change in the stroma.

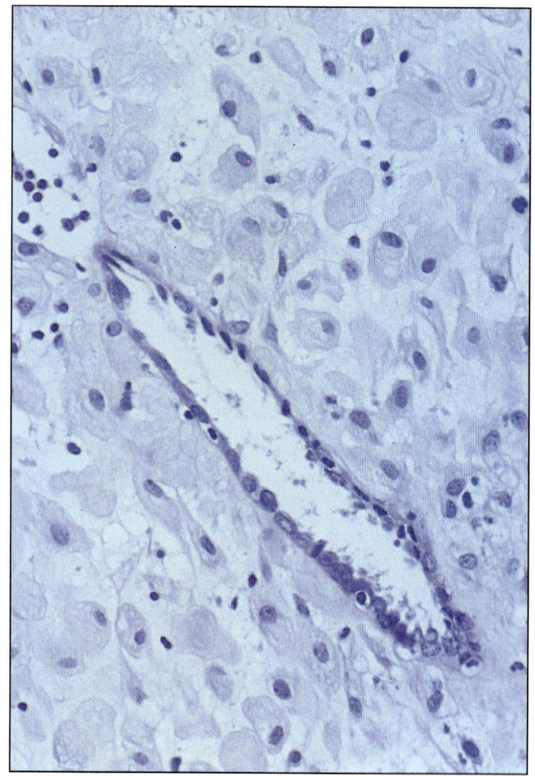

FIGURE 5-26.
Progestin therapy. Abnormal endometrial proliferations caused by unopposed estrogen stimulation may sometimes be hormonally reversed by high dose progestin therapy. In this case, a simple hyperplasia was successfully treated, with complete decidualization of the stroma and secretory exhaustion of glands, resulting in a morphology that resembles portions of the gravid endometrium (*see* Fig. 5-16).

POLYPS AND METAPLASIAS

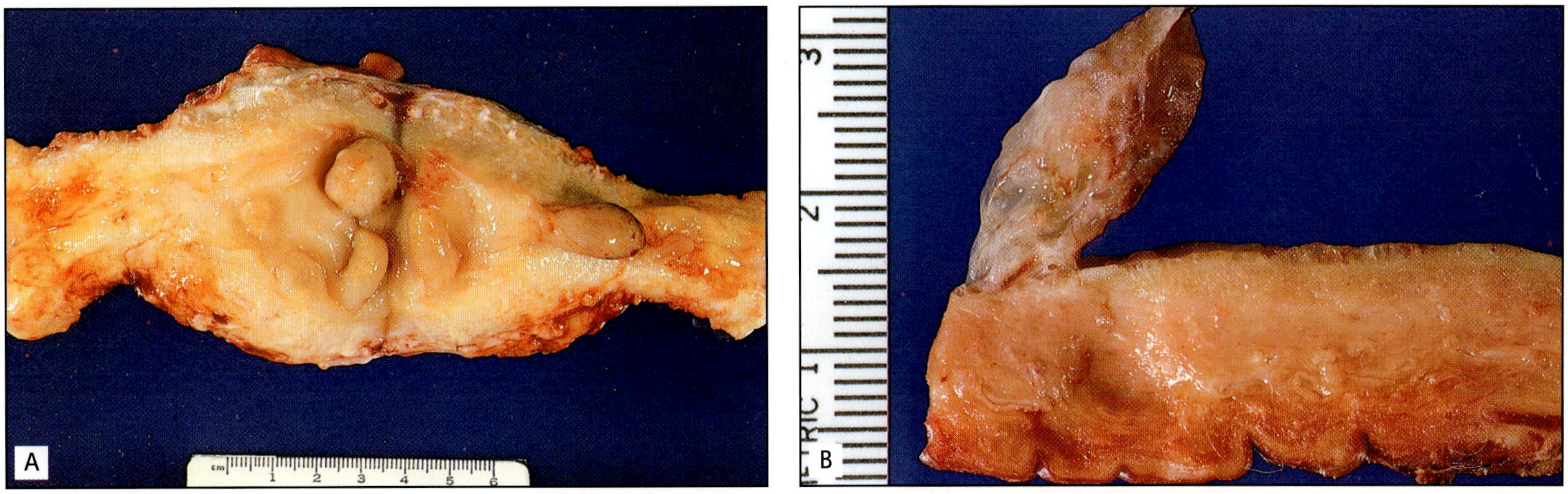

FIGURE 5-27.

Endometrial polyps. Endometrial polyps are relatively common, with a peak incidence in the fifth decade, and if symptomatic, usually cause abnormal uterine bleeding [9]. Their pathogenesis remains uncertain, and although it has been suggested that polyps arise from the basalis of the endometrium, there is no convincing evidence to support this assertion. It is even unclear whether they represent hamartomas, hormonally unresponsive endometrium, or neoplasms. They may be sessile or pedunculated, in the fundus or lower uterine segment, single or multiple, and vary from a few millimeters to several centimeters in diameter (**A**). On close inspection, areas of cyst formation can sometimes be seen, and the texture is often firm (**B**).

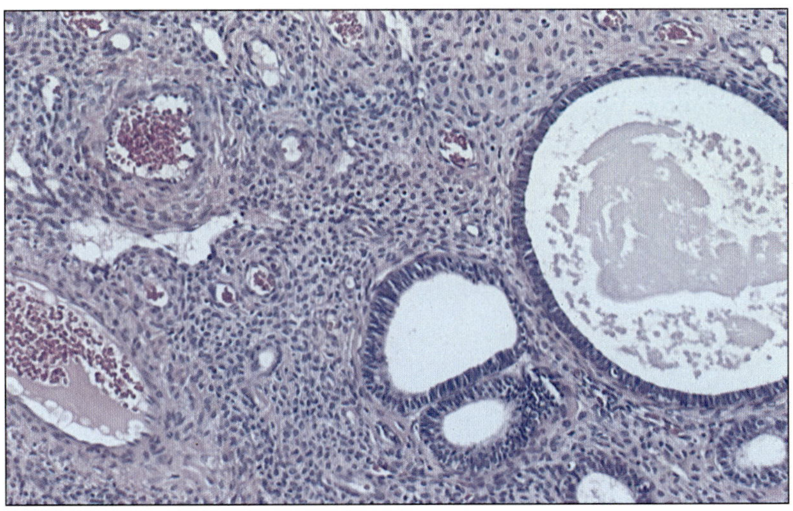

FIGURE 5-28.

Endometrial polyp. The endometrial polyp often contains the triad of a fibrous stroma, thick-walled or ectatic blood vessels, and an altered glandular pattern. In this example, two thick-walled blood vessels are present in a stroma that is more eosinophilic than cycling endometrium, indicative of the increased stromal collagen. The glands vary from small tubes to cystically dilated structures. However, variability is characteristic of endometrial polyps, and different portions of the same polyp may appear quite dissimilar. Hyperplasia may be present in a polyp, the biologic significance of which has often been considered minimal, but in truth remains unknown. Carcinoma may also be found confined to the tip of endometrial polyps.

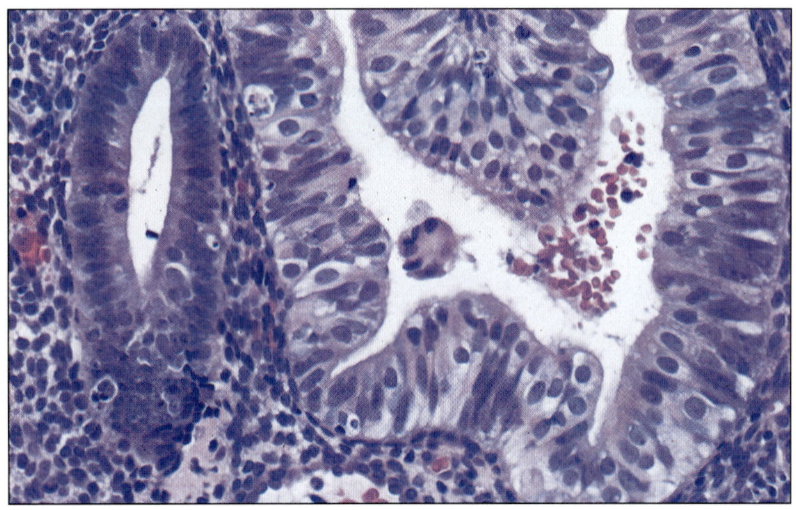

FIGURE 5-29.

Tubal metaplasia. Endometrial metaplasia is a relatively common finding, present in about 20% of specimens obtained from noncycling women, most frequently associated with uterine bleeding, endometrial carcinoma, or a history of recent estrogen therapy [10]. Seven forms of endometrial metaplasia have been well characterized histologically, as follows: ciliated (tubal), eosinophilic, squamous, papillary syncytial, mucinous, hobnail, and clear cell metaplasia. Ciliated or tubal metaplasia is the most common form of metaplasia, recognized by the presence of large cells, with pale or eosinophilic cytoplasm and apical cilia. In this case, only a few of the cells bear cilia. In their absence, this would be represent eosinophilic metaplasia, a closely related condition. An adjacent proliferative endometrial gland is included for comparison. Tubal metaplasia is essentially never found with secretory endometrium, but can be seen in about 20% of proliferative phase and the majority of hyperplastic endometria [11].

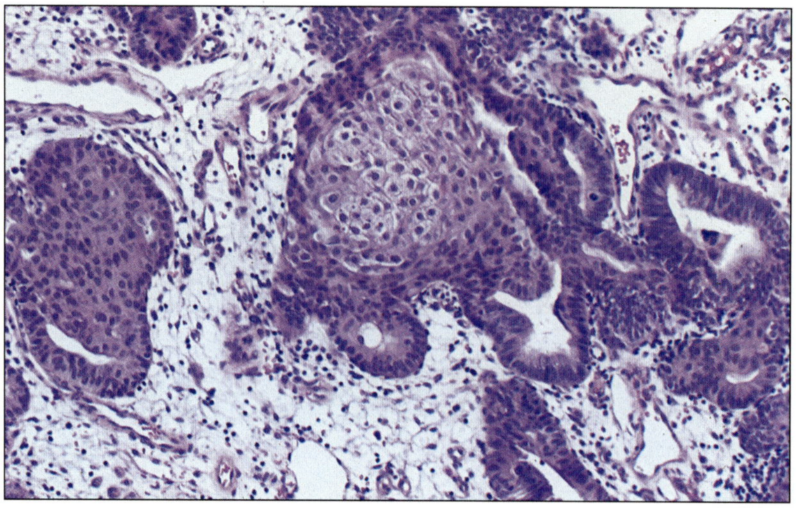

FIGURE 5-30.

Squamous metaplasia. A spectrum of morphologic changes extending from the intraglandular squamous morules of Dutra to large masses of keratinizing squamous cells with intercellular bridges and keratin debris comprise squamous metaplasia. It is a component of about one third of metaplastic endometrium, and it must be distinguished from the squamous differentiation that occurs within about 20% of adenocarcinomas of the endometrium. It often accompanies endometrial polyps or hyperplasia, and in this case partially fills the lumens of two hyperplastic glands.

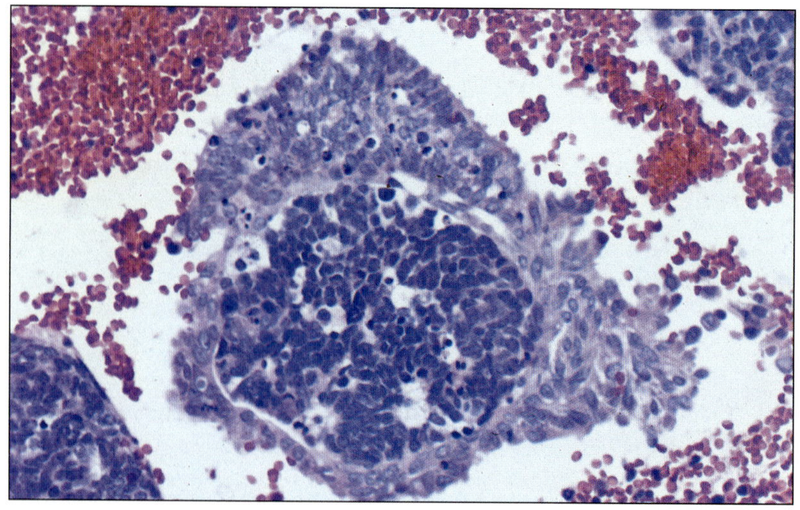

FIGURE 5-31.

Papillary syncytial metaplasia. Papillary syncytial change is almost always found in the context of endometrial shedding, whether menstrual or nonmenstrual. It is a component of about 10% of metaplasias, and can be found in the benign endometrium adjacent to carcinomas. It may represent either a retrogressive or reparative alteration of the surface epithelium [12]. True papillae with central fibrovascular cores are not a feature of this lesion. Instead, syncytial masses of epithelial cells with indistinct cytoplasmic membranes partially or totally cover aggregates of condensed stromal cells. The columnar shape of the glandular or surface epithelium is replaced by a stellate or polygonal configuration.

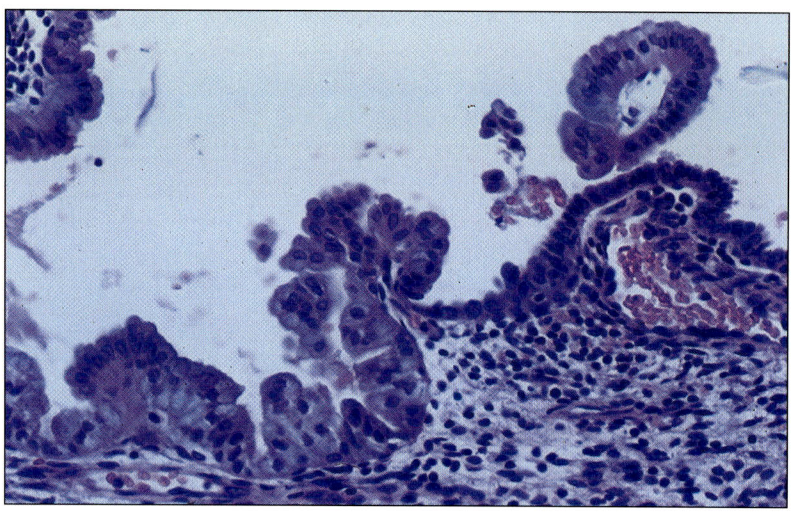

FIGURE 5-32.

Mucinous metaplasia. This is a relatively uncommon type of metaplasia, most commonly discovered in the postmenopausal endometrium or in association with polyps. It is easy to recognize, because the glands usually resemble those of the endocervix, with basal nuclei and relatively abundant, pale blue, vacuolated cytoplasm [13]. In the setting of hyperplasia, when the architecture is complex and papillary, with tufts of cells covering fibrovascular cores, it may be difficult to distinguish from mucinous adenocarcinoma.

DISORDERED PROLIFERATIVE AND HYPERPLASTIC ENDOMETRIUM

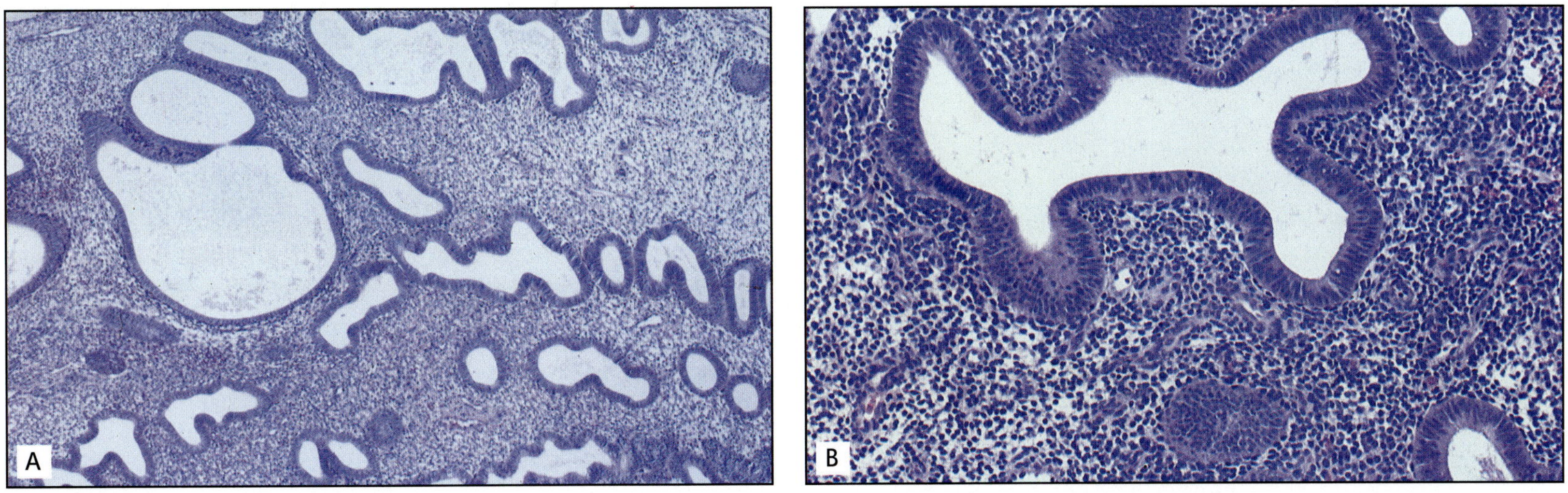

FIGURE 5-33.

Disordered proliferative endometrium. The disordered proliferative endometrium represents a caricature, an exaggeration of the normal proliferative phase, due to a physiologic response to unopposed estrogen-stimulated proliferation. It represents the extreme low end of the spectrum of hyperplasia, and is very commonly found in perimenopausal women with a history of abnormal uterine bleeding caused by anovulatory cycles. (Menarchal females also frequently have these changes, but fortunately are only rarely biopsied. The onset of ovulatory cycles then typically causes differentiation and shedding of the disordered proliferative endometrium.) In contrast to the proliferative endometrium, the appearance is variable, with normal glands interspersed among glands with architectural abnormalities. The gland:stroma ratio is about 1:1, but focally may deviate from this ratio. The glands may be straight or coiled, with budding and bifurcation. Some glands may be cystically dilated (**A**). Although the glandular epithelium is stratified, with interspersed mitoses, by definition there is no significant cytologic atypia (**B**). The stroma is usually compact, and foci of papillary syncytial metaplasia commonly occur in regions of nonmenstrual shedding.

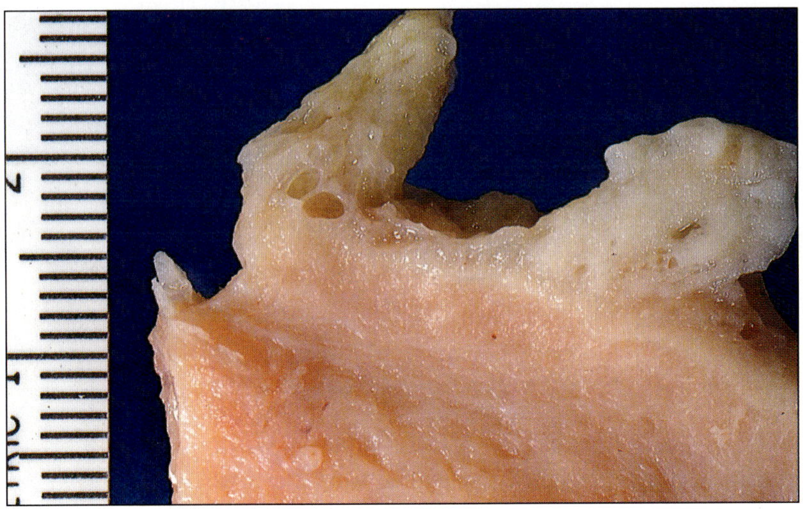

FIGURE 5-34.

Endometrial hyperplasia. A bewildering set of diagnostic terms has been suggested, abandoned, and reintroduced during the past 30 years, leaving both pathologists and gynecologists with a lexicon of remarkable length and obscurity. The International Society of Gynecological Pathologists has recently adopted the four designations of hyperplasia proposed by Kurman *et al.* [14], as follows: 1) simple hyperplasia (SH); 2) complex hyperplasia (CH); 3) atypical simple hyperplasia (ASH); and 4) atypical complex hyperplasia (ACH). The reproducibility and utility of this classification have not yet been justified in a prospective study. In most cases of hyperplasia, the volume of the endometrial tissue is increased, with either a diffuse or nodular thickening of the endometrium observed by ultrasound examination or gross inspection. Obviously, there is no extension of the process to the underlying myometrium, but one would be unable to distinguish grossly whether this hysterectomy specimen contained hyperplasia or an adenocarcinoma confined to the endometrium.

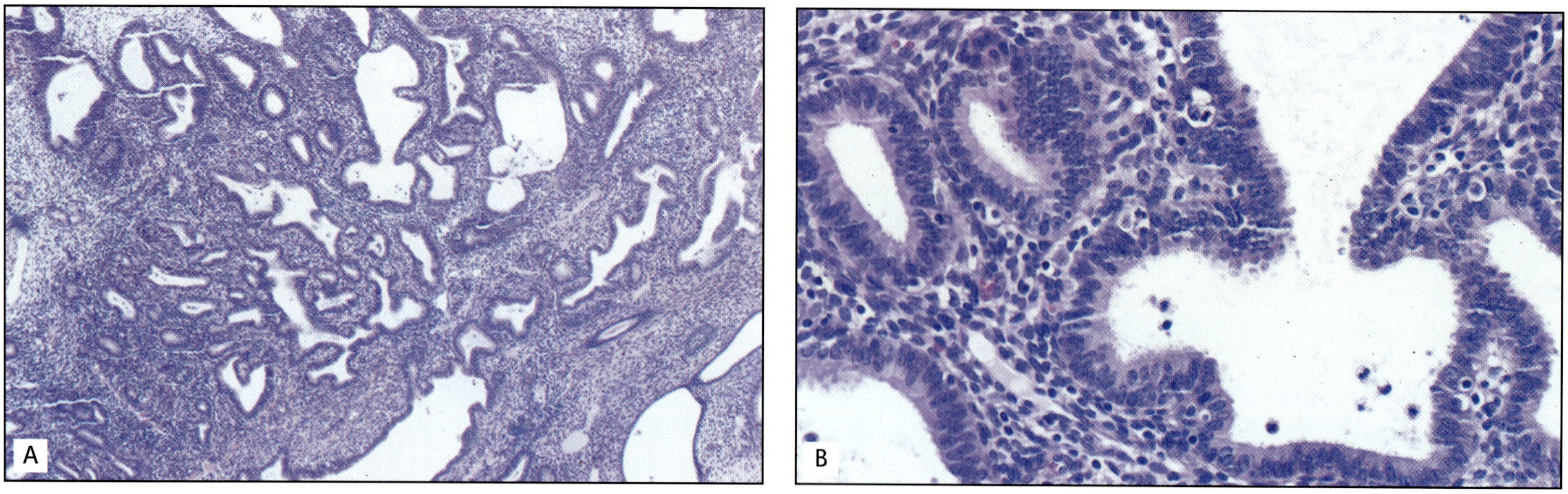

FIGURE 5-35.

Simple hyperplasia. Simple hyperplasia is defined as an increase in the number of endometrial glands, which may be dilated with little crowding, or have an irregular outline and exhibit some crowding. In this example, the volume is increased, and there is variability from one area to another. The gland:stroma ratio is greater than 1:1, and the glands have irregular configurations that can be described using simple geometric terms. Extensive branching and budding is characteristic (**A**). The surrounding stroma is compact, unless there are foci of nonmenstrual shedding where condensation of stroma and syncytial metaplasia are found. At higher magnification, excessive proliferation is manifest by stratification and mitotic figures in glands. There is no significant cytologic atypia such as nuclear enlargement, pleomorphism, or the presence of macronucleoli (**B**). Contrast the cytologic features with those present in Figure 5-36B.

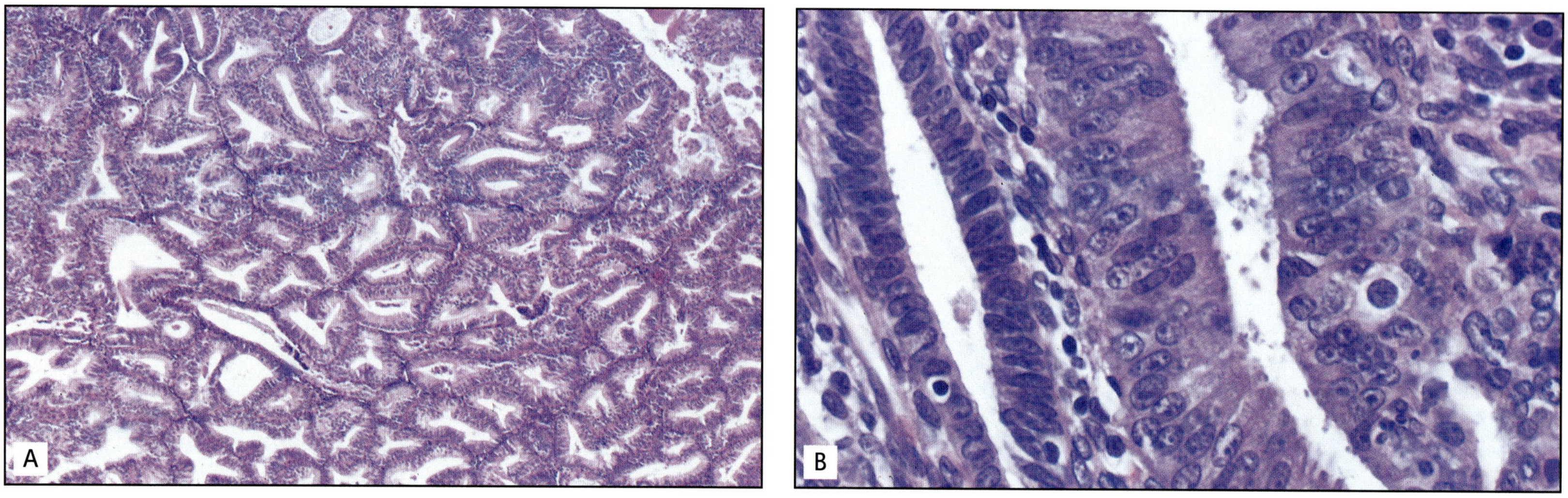

FIGURE 5-36.

Complex atypical hyperplasia. Complex hyperplasia is characterized by glands with irregular outlines, marked structural complexity, and back-to-back crowding. In this example, the gland:stroma ratio is greater than 10:1, and only small foci of stroma can be identified among the densely packed, architecturally complex glands (**A**). Atypical hyperplasia is used to designate a proliferation of glands exhibiting cytologic atypia. The cytologic atypia is recognized as nuclear enlargement and replacement of the typically highly elliptical gland nuclei by those that approximate a round configuration. The chromatin may be evenly or irregularly dispersed. Nucleoli may be either inconspicuous or prominent. In this example, the degree of cytologic atypia approaches that seen in well-differentiated adenocarcinoma, with vesicular chromatin and prominent nucleoli. The atypic nuclei can be contrasted with those lining an adjacent gland not involved by the process (**B**).

MALIGNANT ENDOMETRIAL NEOPLASMS

CORPUS CANCER STAGING—FIGO, 1988 REVISION

Stages

IA G123	Tumor limited to endometium
IB G123	Invasion to <1/2 myometrium
IC G123	Invasion to >1/2 myometrium
IIA G123	Endocervical glandular involvement only
IIB G123	Cervical stromal invasion
IIIA G123	Tumor invades serosa and/or positive peritoneal cytology
IIIB G123	Vaginal metastases
IIIC G123	Metastases to pelvic and/or para-aortic lymph nodes
IVA G123	Tumor invasion of bladder and/or bowel mucosa
IVB G123	Distant metastases including intra-abdominal and/or inguinal lymph node

Histopathology—Degree of Differentiation

Cases of carcinoma of the corpus should be grouped with regard to the degree of differentiation of the adenocarcinoma as follows:

G1 = 5% or less of a nonsquamous or nonmorular solid growth pattern

G2 = 5–50% of a nonsquamous or nonmorular solid growth pattern

G3 = more than 50% of a nonsquamous or nonmorular solid growth pattern

Notes on Pathological Grading

1. Notable nuclear atypia, inappropriate for the architectural grade, raises a grade 1 or grade 2 tumor by one grade
2. In serous adenocarcinomas, clear cell adenocarcinomas, and squamous cell carcinomas, nuclear grading takes precedence
3. Adenocarcinomas with squamous differentiation are graded according to the nuclear grade of the glandular component

FIGURE 5-37.

The 1998 International Federation of Gynecology and Obstetrics (FIGO) staging of malignant neoplasms of the uterus [15]. Adenocarcinoma is the most common malignant neoplasm of the uterus, and currently is the most common invasive malignant neoplasm of the entire female genital tract, with about 31,000 cases diagnosed each year in the United States [16]. The overall 5-year survival rate is about 75%. The current FIGO scheme for staging is based on the pathologic findings at surgery, and is much more accurate than the previously used clinical staging method. A series of studies has validated the significance of the staging criteria, including spread, depth of myometrial invasion, architectural and nuclear grade, and cell type as independent prognostic indicators [17–23]. (*Data from* Mikuta [16].)

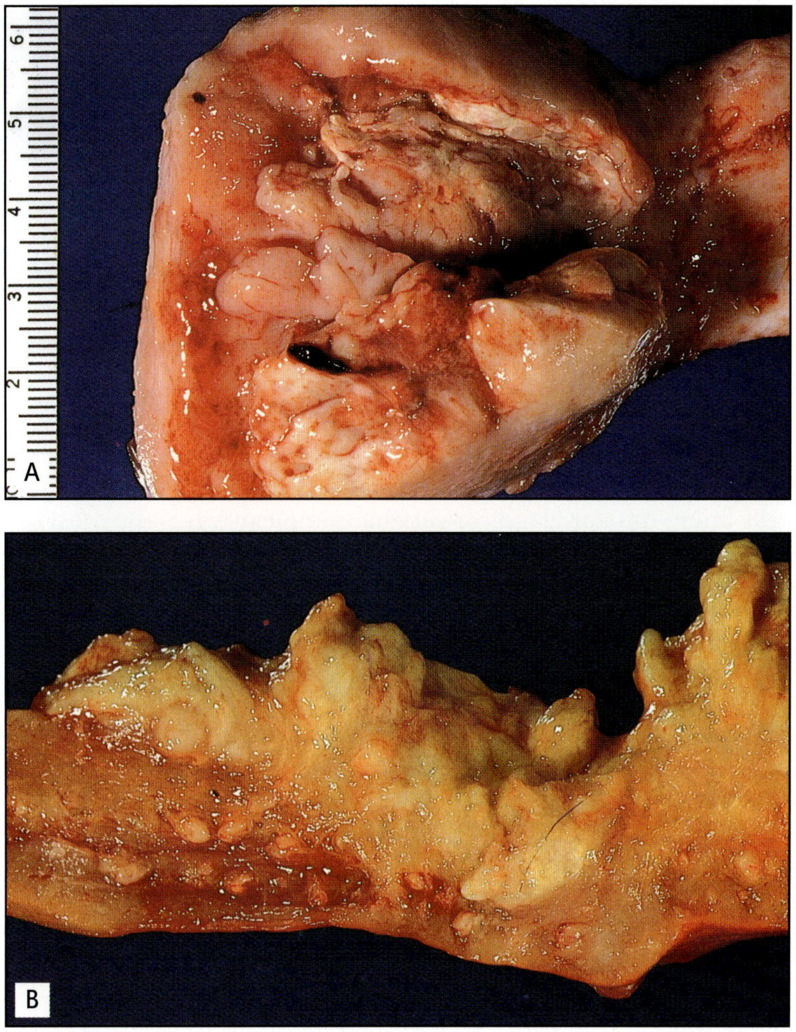

FIGURE 5-38.

Endometrial adenocarcinoma. This hemisected uterus contains a large, polypoid, soft, tan neoplasm that almost completely fills the endometrial cavity (**A**). However, the gross morphology of endometrial adenocarcinomas are quite variable, and the tumors may be focal, multifocal, or diffuse, ulcerated, flat, nodular, or papillary, solid, necrotic or hemorrhagic, and may be located in either the fundus or lower uterine segment. Assessment of the depth of invasion is critical in helping to establish the prognosis, because it is one of the most important predictors of outcome for tumors confined to the uterus. Numerous, parallel sections should be made in the uterus to identify the region of greatest tumor penetration. In this case, there is a relatively small region of invasion into the outer third of the myometrium, identifiable in the center of the field (**B**).

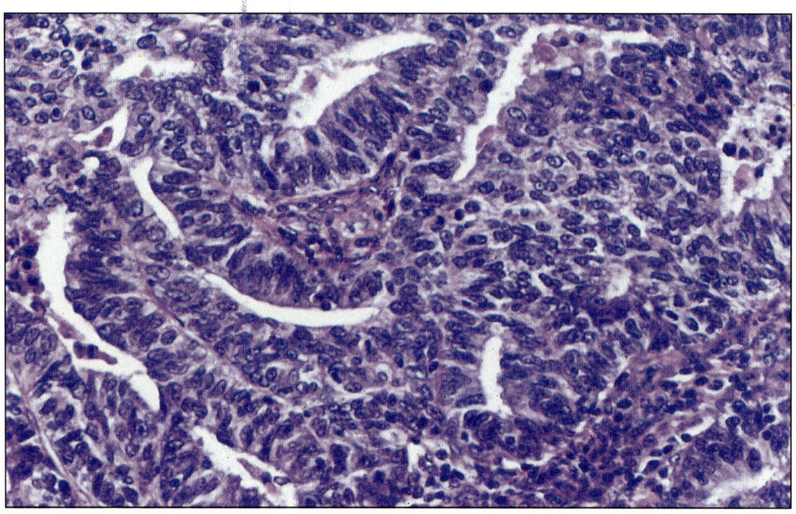

FIGURE 5-39.
Endometrioid adenocarcinoma. The prototypical histologic type of endometrial adenocarcinoma is referred to as endometrioid, reflecting its retention of the basic architectural arrangement of epithelial cells lining tubular glands of variable complexity. It is the most common cell type, representing about 75% of endometrial adenocarcinomas, and is frequently found in the setting of endometrial hyperplasia and unopposed estrogen stimulation. The glands are usually small and relatively uniform, but they may be branching or undulating in configuration. Decreasing differentiation is characterized by diminishing lumen formation, with replacement by solid masses of neoplastic cells. The cells lining the glands are characteristically cuboidal to columnar and share a common apical border that results in a smooth oval luminal contour.

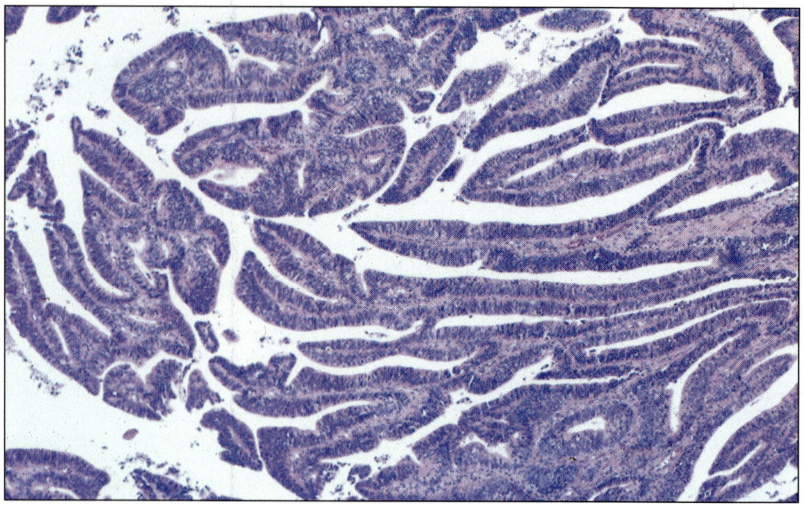

FIGURE 5-40.
Villoglandular carcinoma. This common variant of endometrioid adenocarcinoma often represents the superficial portion of otherwise typical endometrioid adenocarcinomas. It is characterized histologically by tall thin papillae, with a central fibrovascular core covered by columnar cells sharing a smooth apical border. The age at diagnosis, stage, depth of invasion, and clinical outcome for this tumor appears to resemble that of endometrioid adenocarcinoma [24–26]. The importance of recognition of this cell type is in its potential confusion with papillary serous carcinoma, a much more highly virulent tumor.

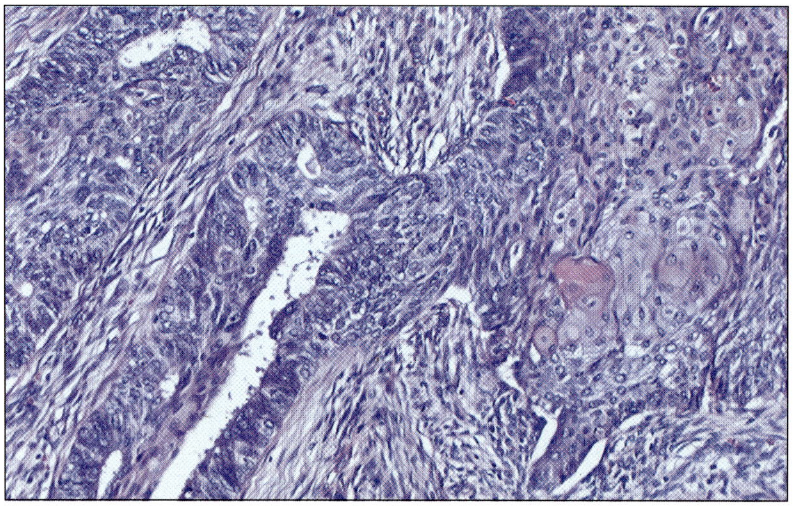

FIGURE 5-41.
Endometrioid adenocarcinoma with squamous differentiation. About 20% of endometrial adenocarcinomas contain regions of squamous differentiation. Recent studies have demonstrated that their behavior is similar to that of endometrioid adenocarcinomas lacking squamous differentiation, and that the grade of the glandular component is a better indicator of prognosis than the grade of the squamous portion [27]. Usually, the squamous differentiation is easy to recognize, with sheets of keratin, isolated cell keratinization, or obvious intercellular bridges connecting neoplastic cells. Occasionally, the identifiable features are limited to sheets of cells with abundant, eosinophilic, polygonal cytoplasm, and distinct cell membranes. In this case, the latter features are predominant, but note the presence of a small cluster of squamous cell with intensely eosinophilic cytoplasm in the center left of the field.

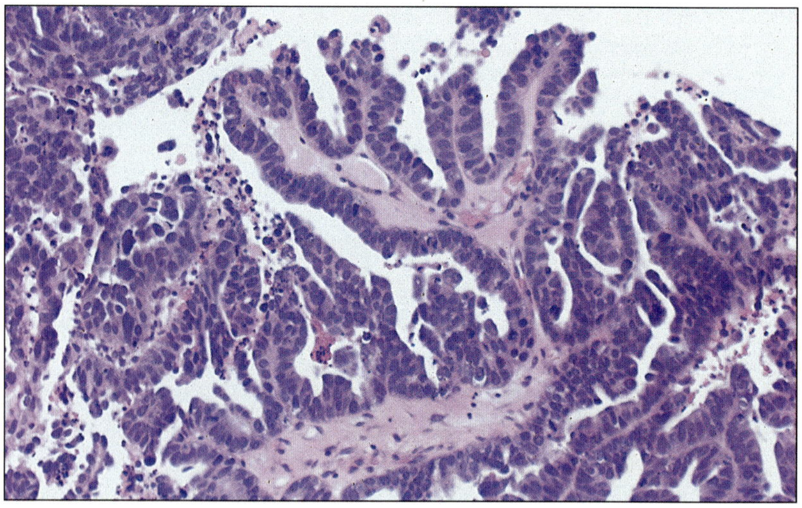

FIGURE 5-42.
Papillary serous carcinoma. This highly aggressive form of endometrial carcinoma is most often found in women of advanced age, not associated with hyperplasia or hyperestrinism [28,29]. Although the tumors are often of advanced stage at the time of diagnosis, even tumors confined to the endometrium may prove lethal. Serous carcinoma is recognized by branching, complex papillae formed of fibrovascular cores that may be thick and hyalinized, covered by eosinophilic, cuboidal cells, which often have a scalloped apical border and very pleomorphic nuclei. Detached tufts of epithelial cells and psammoma bodies are commonly present.

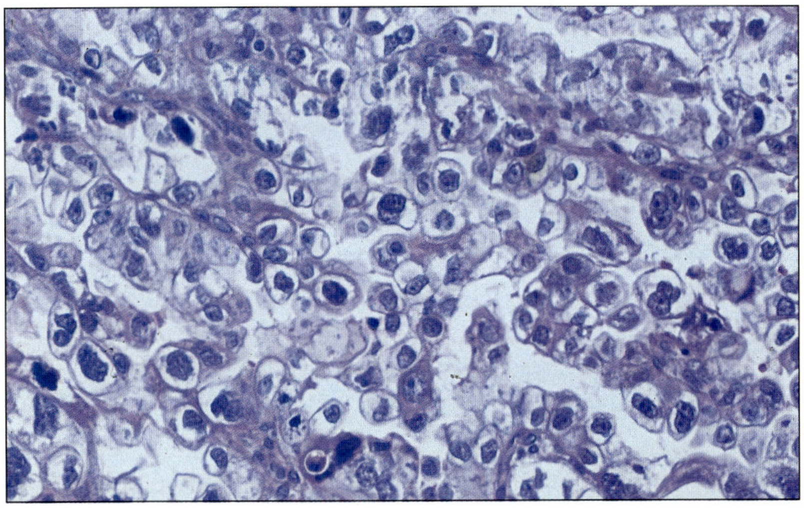

FIGURE 5-43.

Clear cell adenocarcinoma. This relatively rare type of tumor is recognized by the presence of optically clear cytoplasm in neoplastic cells growing in a solid, cystic, tubulocystic, or papillary architectural configuration. Its distinction from serous carcinoma may be difficult, and the two cell types also share the features of relatively advanced stage at diagnosis and biologic aggressiveness [30,31]. The neoplastic cells usually have large, pleomorphic nuclei, distinct cytoplasmic membranes, and a scalloped apical border. In some cases the nucleus protrudes into the luminal aspect of the cell and consequently bears a resemblance to the cobbler's hobnail.

REFERENCES

1. Division of Health Care Statistics: *Data from the 1985 National Hospital Discharge Summary*. Hyattsville, MD: National Center for Health Statistics; 1988.
2. Vollman R: The menstrual cycle. In *Major Problems in Obstetrics and Gynecology*. Edited by Friedman E. Philadelphia: WB Saunders, 1977:78–98.
3. Bulmer JN, Hollings D, Ritson A: Immunocytochemical evidence that endometrial stromal granulocytes are granulated lymphocytes. *J Pathol* 1987, 153:281–288.
4. Arias-Stella J. Normal and abnormal mitoses in the atypical endometrial change associated with chorionic tissue effect. *Am J Surg Pathol* 1994, 18:694–701.
5. Washington A, Arno P, Brooks M: The economic cost of pelvic inflammatory disease. *JAMA* 1986, 255:1735–1738.
6. Kiviat N, Wolner-Hanssen P, Eschenbach D, *et al.*: Endometrial histopathology in patients with culture-proved upper genital tract infection and laparoscopically diagnosed acute salpingitis. *Am J Surg Pathol* 1990, 14:167–175.
7. Paavonen J, Teisala K, Heinonen PK, *et al.*: Microbiological and histopathological findings in acute pelvic inflammatory disease. *Br J Obstet Gynaecol* 1987, 94:454–460.
8. Horn H, Hertig A, Kundsin R, *et al.*: Subclinical endometrial inflammation and T-mycoplasma: a possible cause of reproductive failure. *Int J Fertil* 1973, 18:265–270.
9. Van Bogaert LJ: Clinicopathologic findings in endometrial polyps. *Obstet Gynecol* 1988, 71:771–773.
10. Hendrickson M, Kempson R: Endometrial epithelial metaplasias: proliferations frequently misdiagnosed as adenocarcinoma. *Am J Surg Pathol* 1980, 4:525–542.
11. Fruin A, Tighe J: Tubal metaplasia of the endometrium. *J Obstet Gynaecol Br Commonw* 1967, 74:93–97.
12. Zaman SS, Mazur MT: Endometrial papillary syncytial change: a nonspecific alteration associated with active breakdown [see comments]. *Am J Clin Pathol* 1993, 99:741–745.
13. Demopoulos R, Greco M: Mucinous metaplasia of the endometium: ultrastructural and histochemical characteristics. *Int J Gynecol Pathol* 1983, 1:383–390.
14. Kurman R, Kaminski P, Norris H: The behavior of endometrial hyperplasia: a long-term study of "untreated" hyperplasia in 170 patients. *Cancer* 1985, 56:403–411.
15. Creasman W: Announcement. FIGO stages–1988 revision. *Gynecol Oncol* 1989, 35:125–127.
16. Mikuta JJ: International Federation of Gynecology and Obstetrics staging of endometrial cancer, 1988. *Cancer* 1993, 71(suppl 4):1460–1463.
17. Abeler V, Kjørdstad K, Berle E: Carcinoma of the endometrium in Norway: a histopathological and prognostic survey of a total population. *Int J Gynecol Cancer* 1992, 2:9–22.
18. Zaino R, Silverberg S, Norris H, *et al.*: The prognostic value of nuclear versus architectural grading in endometrial adenocarcinoma: a GOG study. *Int J Gynecol Path* 1994; 13:29–36.
19. Zaino R, Kurman R, Diana K, Morrow C: The utility of the revised International Federation of Gynecology and Obstetrics histologic grading of endometrial adenocarcinoma using a defined nuclear grading system. *Cancer* 1995, 75:81–86.
20. Zaino R: Pathologic indicators of prognosis in endometrial adenocarcinoma. *Pathol Annu* 1995, 30(part 1):1–28.
21. Zaino R, Kurman R, Diana K, Morrow C: Pathologic model to predict outcome for women with endometrial adenocarcinoma. *Cancer*, 1996; 77:1115–1121.
22. Mittal KR, Schwartz PE, Barwick KW. Architectural (FIGO) grading, nuclear grading, and other prognostic indicators in stage I endometrial adenocarcinoma with identification of high-risk and low-risk groups. *Cancer* 1988, 61:538–545.
23. Kadar N, Malfetano J, Homesly H. Determinants of survival of surgically staged patients with endometrial carcinoma histologically confined to the uterus: implications for therapy. *Obstet Gynecol* 1992, 80:655–659.
24. Ambros R, Ballouk F, Malfetano J, Ross J: Significance of papillary (villoglandular) differentiation in endometrioid carcinoma of the uterus. *Am J Surg Pathol* 1994, 18:569–575.
25. Chen J, Trost D, Wilkinson E: Endometrial papillary adenocarcinomas: two clinicopathologic types. *Int J Gynecol Pathol* 1985, 4:279–288.
26. Ward BG, Wright RG, Free K: Papillary carcinomas of the endometrium. *Gynecol Oncol* 1990, 39:347–351.
27. Zaino RJ, Kurman R, Herbold D, *et al.*: The significance of squamous differentiation in endometrial carcinoma: data from a Gynecologic Oncology Group study. *Cancer* 1991, 68:2293–2302.
28. Lee KR, Belinson JL: Papillary serous adenocarcinoma of the endometrium: a clinicopathologic study of 19 cases. *Gynecol Oncol* 1992, 46:51–54.
29. Abeler VM, Kjørdstad KE: Serous papillary carcinoma of the endometrium: a histopathological study of 22 cases. *Gynecol Oncol* 1990, 39:265–271.
30. Abeler VM, Kjørdstad KE: Clear cell carcinoma of the endometrium: a histopathological and clinical study of 97 cases. *Gynecol Oncol* 1991, 40:207–217.
31. Carcangiu M, Chambers J: Early pathologic stage clear cell carcinoma and uterine papillary serous carcinoma of the endometrium. *Int J Gynecol Pathol* 1995, 14:30–38.

CHAPTER 6

Mesenchymal Tumors

Teri A. Longacre and Michael R. Hendrickson

The topic of this chapter is the varied group of pure mesenchymal and mixed mesenchymal-epithelial proliferations that occur in the uterus. Some members of this group are among the most common of gynecologic problems (leiomyomas and adenomyosis), whereas others are extremely rare.

The malignant members of this group are generically referred to as uterine sarcomas and their rarity and the refractoriness of the more common varieties to current therapy make these difficult diagnostic and therapeutic challenges [1,2].

This chapter touches on some of the difficulties facing pathologists in diagnosing proliferations in this group. Predicting clinical behavior for many of these neoplasms is often difficult and involves the careful evaluation of several histopathologic features [3,4].

CLASSIFICATION AND STAGING

CLASSIFICATION OF MESENCHYMAL AND MIXED EPITHELIAL-MESENCHYMAL PROLIFERATIONS IN TERMS OF DIFFERENTIATED FEATURES

Pure mesenchymal proliferations
- Endometrial stromal differentiation without sex cord elements, with sex cord-like elements
- Smooth muscle differentiation
- Heterologous differentiation (bone, cartilage, skeletal muscle, fat)
- Undifferentiated sarcoma

Mixed müllerian neoplasms

FIGURE 6-1.
Classification of mesenchymal and mixed epithelial-mesenchymal proliferations of the uterus.

CONVENTIONAL STAGING OF UTERINE SARCOMA

Stage	Characteristic
I	Sarcoma confined to the uterine corpus
II	Sarcoma confined to uterine corpus and cervix
III	Sarcoma confined to the pelvis
IV	Extrapelvic sarcoma

FIGURE 6-2.
The staging of uterine sarcomas. There is no special staging system for uterine sarcomas. It is conventional to employ the former clinical staging system for endometrial carcinoma to stage uterine sarcomas.

ENDOMETRIAL STROMAL NEOPLASMS

A. CLASSIFICATION OF ENDOMETRIAL STROMAL NEOPLASMS

I. Endometrial stromal nodule
II. Endometrial stromal sarcoma (a low-grade malignancy)
III. Undifferentiated uterine sarcoma (a high-grade malignancy)
IV. Uterine tumours resembling ovarian sex cord tumours

FIGURE 6-3.
A, The classification of endometrial stromal neoplasms. Endometrial stromal neoplasms exhibit differentiation that strongly resembles the stroma of normal proliferative endometrium. Specifically, these tumors are composed of a monomorphous population of blunt, spindled to oblong cells with scanty cytoplasm and relatively small uniform nuclei. A highly characteristic feature of endometrial stromal neoplasms is the delicate arborizing vasculature. In the author's view, neoplasms that depart from this pattern in terms of marked cytologic atypia and an absence of the characteristic arborizing vasculature should be separately classified as "undifferentiated stromal sarcomas"; these are clinically high-grade malignancies.

(*Continued on next page*)

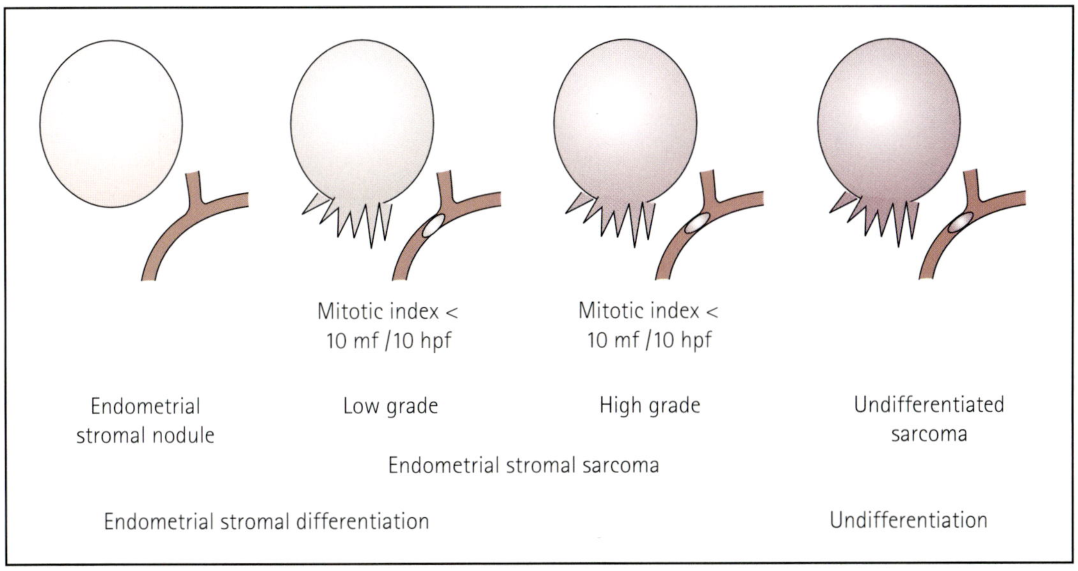

FIGURE 6-3. *(Continued)*
B, The distinction between benign and malignant lesions exhibiting endometrial stromal differentiation is based on the relationship of the proliferation to surrounding normal structures. A stromal nodule features at most minimal interdigitation with surrounding normal myometrium and an absence of vascular involvement. Stromal sarcoma is distinguished from a stromal nodule by virtue of the presence of myometrial invasion and/or vascular invasion in the former. It has been conventional since the initial studies of stromal sarcoma to distinguish between high-grade and low-grade lesions based on an evaluation of the mitotic index. A mitotic index of greater than or equal to 10 mitotic figures per 10 high-power fields in this scheme is diagnostic of high-grade stromal sarcoma, whereas the lower mitotic indices are diagnostic of low-grade stromal sarcoma. In the author's experience, while it is true that high-grade stromal sarcoma (defined on the basis of mitotic index and excluding undifferentiated sarcoma) tends to present at higher stage than low-grade stromal sarcoma, no prognostic insight is provided in low-stage cases by the mitotic index. Undifferentiated sarcoma is represented at the extreme right. The malignant neoplasm lacks the characteristic plexiform vasculature of endometrial stromal sarcoma and is composed of highly atypical and pleomorphic cells. Myoinvasion is typically present and frequently there is vascular invasion [5].

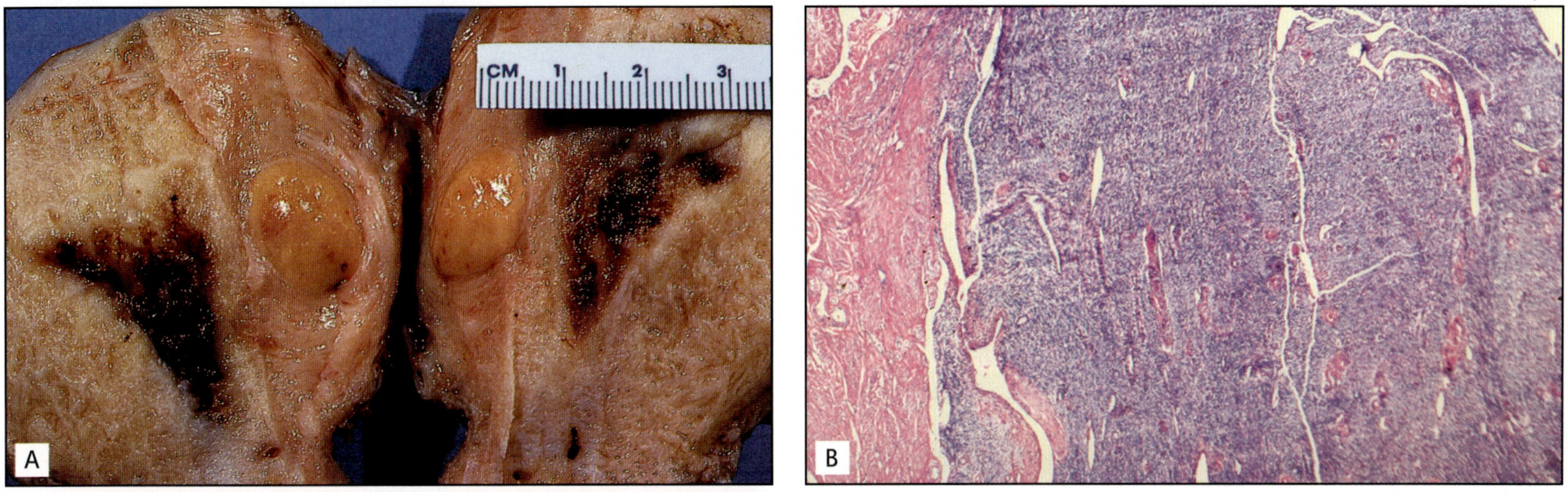

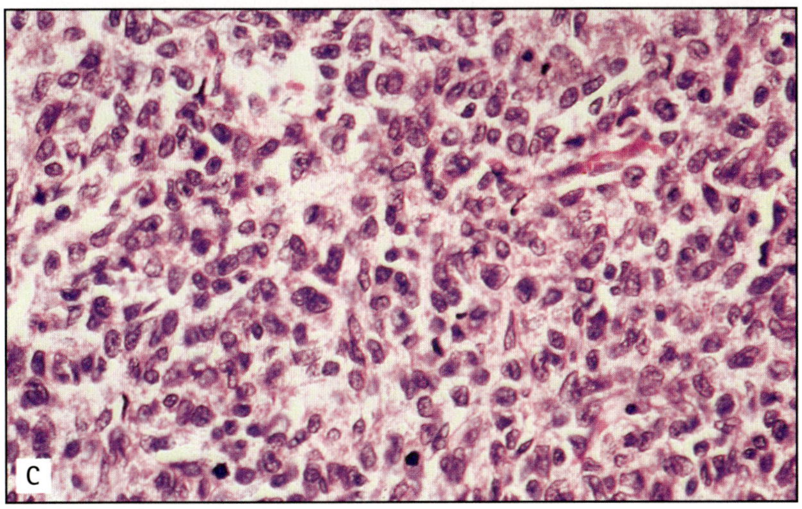

FIGURE 6-4.
Endometrial stromal nodule. **A**, Grossly, a well-circumscribed, yellow, soft intramural nodule is present. **B**, The scanning power view shows the nodule to be hypercellular and to have a circumscribed compressive interface with the surrounding myometrium. **C**, The characteristic microscopic features of endometrial stromal differentiation are seen: uniform, blunt, spindled cells with indistinct cytoplasm and an arborizing vaculature.

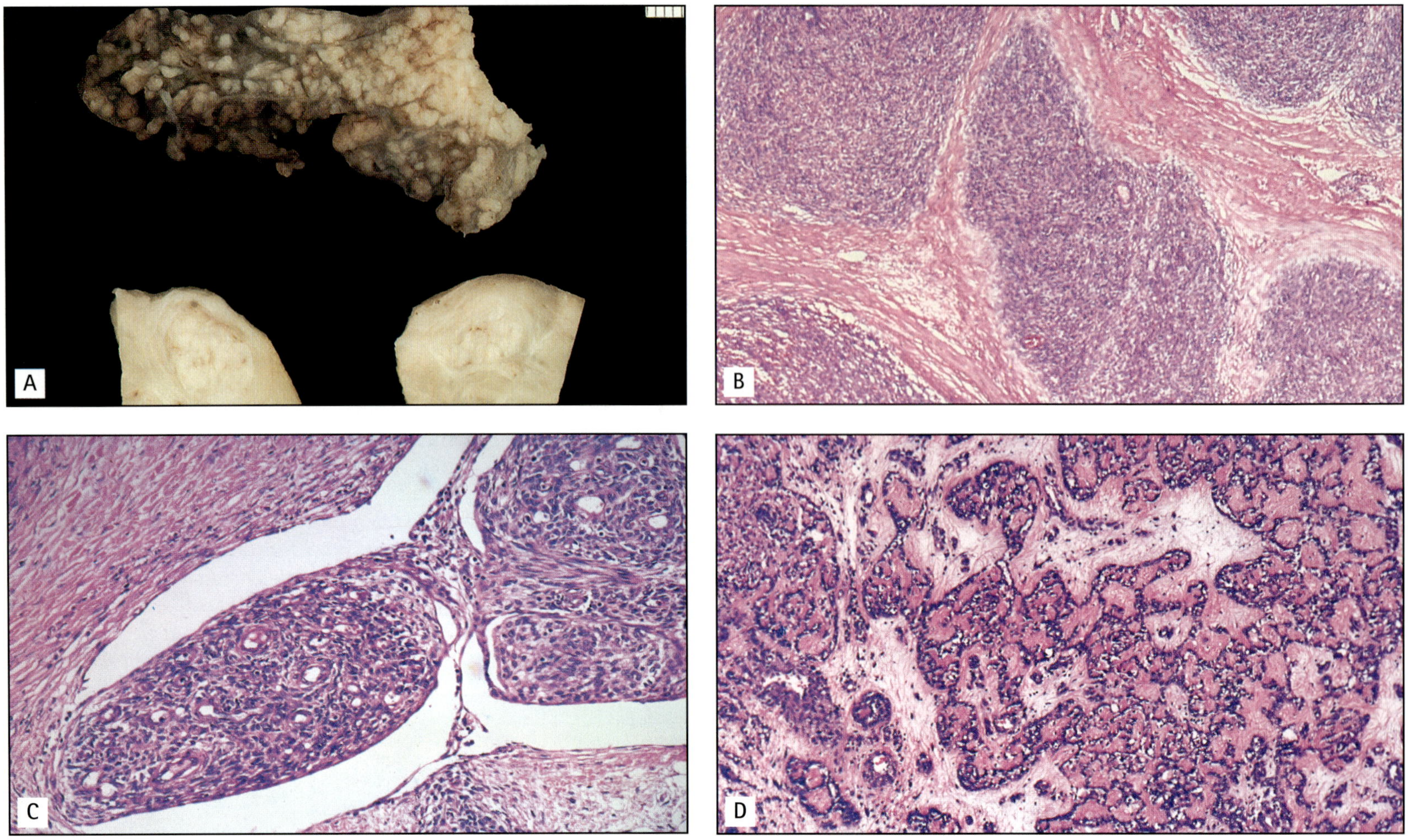

FIGURE 6–5.

Endometrial stromal sarcoma. **A**, Two gross sections of myometrium (*bottom*) and a portion of the broad ligament (*top*) are seen. The myometrial sections feature a vague nodularity with an extension of yellowish wormlike masses into the normal myometrium (*bottom portion of the myometrial sections*). **B**, This low-power photomicrograph shows islands of hypercellular tumor infiltrating the myometrium. Some islands are associated with a lighter-appearing fibroblastic host response to the invasive sarcoma. **C**, A vascular channel contains a wormlike extension of sarcoma. **D**, Sex cord–like elements in endometrial stromal sarcoma. Some endometrial stromal sarcomas and endometrial stromal nodules exhibit formations resembling the sex cord elements encountered in the specialized gonadal stromal tumors of the ovary. Stromal sarcomas may also contain well-formed glands producing a pattern that resembles endometriosis focally.

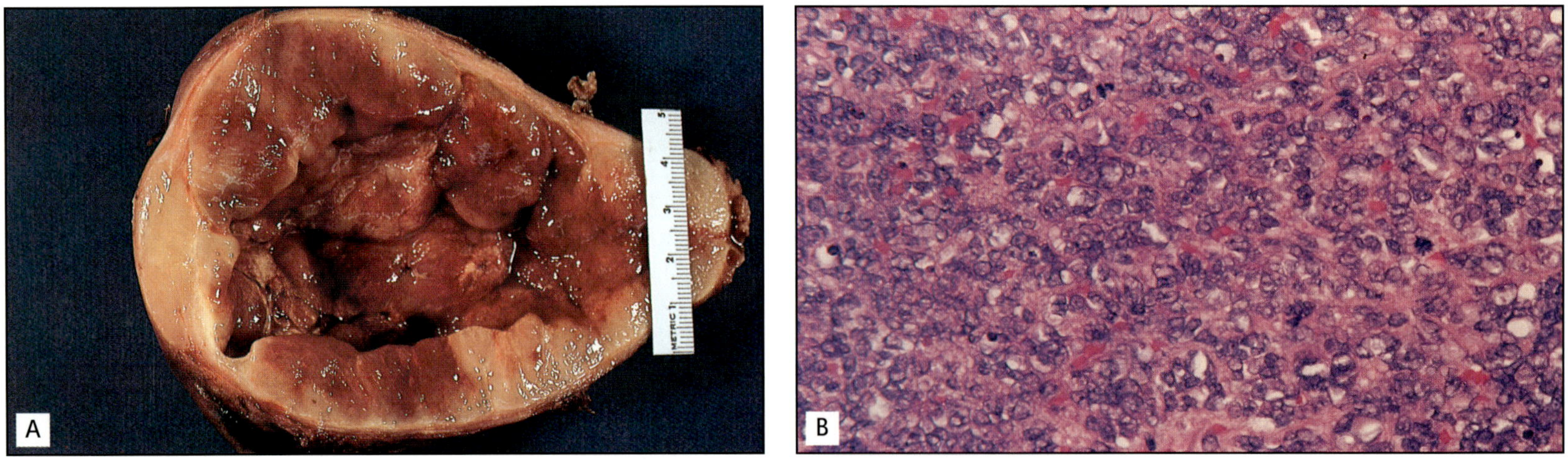

FIGURE 6–6.

Undifferentiated sarcoma. **A**, In contrast to endometrial stromal sarcoma, undifferentiated uterine sarcomas present as extensive hemorrhagic and necrotic neoplasms that largely replace the uterus. In this gross photograph, the ruler lies over the cervix, and the entire uterine corpus is infiltrated by necrotic neoplasm. The natural history of undifferentiated sarcoma is strikingly different from the clinically indolent endometrial stromal sarcoma and more closely resembles that of the high-grade malignancies, carcinosarcoma and leiomyosarcoma. **B**, This neoplasm is composed of anaplastic cells that have a high mitotic index and frequently encountered abnormal mitotic figures. The overall appearance is that of the undifferentiated sarcomatous component of some malignant mixed müllerian tumors.

MIXED MÜLLERIAN NEOPLASMS

CLASSIFICATION OF MIXED MÜLLERIAN NEOPLASMS

Normal Proliferations

The normal endometrium (glands + stroma)

Hyperplastic Proliferations

Endometrial hyperplasia, endometrial polyps

Adenomyoma, typical and atypical

Neoplastic Proliferations

Stroma	Epithelium: Benign	Epithelium: Malignant
Benign	Adenofibroma	Carcinofibroma
Malignant	Adenosarcoma	Carcinosarcoma

FIGURE 6–7.

The classification of mixed müllerian neoplasms. The highly varied group of tumors subsumed under the heading of mixed müllerian neoplasms is currently classified in accordance with the histologic appearance of the glandular elements on the one hand, and the mesenchymal elements on the other. This classification is conveniently depicted in a 2 x 2 table. Proliferations featuring benign stromal components admixed with benign glandular components include adenofibroma and adenomyosis in its various forms. Of particular note is atypical polypoid adenomyoma, which is sometimes confused histologically with endometrial carcinoma. Neoplasms featuring malignant stroma and benign glands are termed adenosarcoma. Among other things, the mitotic index of the stromal components serves to distinguish adenosarcoma from adenofibroma (*see* Fig. 6-8). Neoplasms featuring malignant stroma and malignant epithelium (sarcoma plus carcinoma) are variously designated as carcinosarcomas or malignant mixed müllerian tumors. Neoplasms featuring carcinoma and a prominent benign stromal component have been termed carcinofibromas by some, although it must be emphasized that many müllerian neoplasms, particularly in the ovary, are conventionally considered epithelial neoplasms but in reality feature a prominent benign stromal component. Such neoplasms occasionally occur in the endometrium.

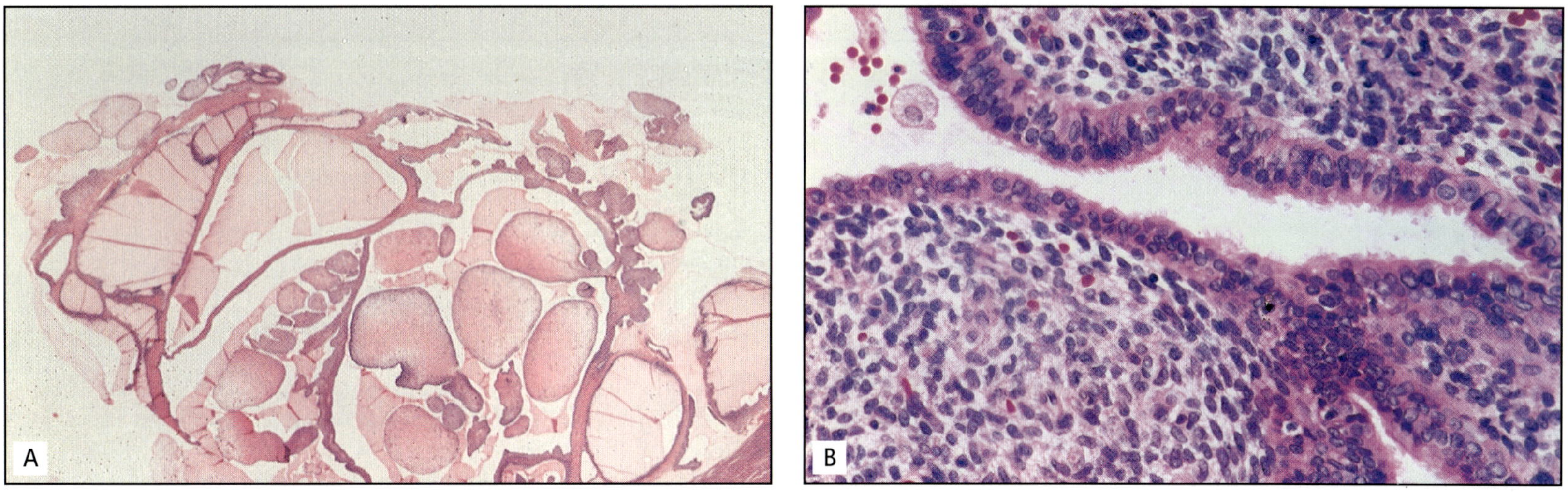

FIGURE 6–8.

Adenofibroma. **A**, Adenofibromas of the endometrium are extremely uncommon. They are approximately one tenth as common as the relatively rare adenosarcoma [6]. They have a low-power appearance very reminiscent of the very common adenofibroma of the ovary with papillary structures inserted into cystic spaces. The underlying myometrium is normal. **B**, The epithelium of adenofibromas is benign, and although the underlying stroma may be cellular, the mitotic index is low. Some authors have used a mitotic index of 4 mitotic figures per 10 high-power fields for separating adenofibroma and adenosarcoma, while others have employed a threshold of 2 per 10 high-power fields [6,7].

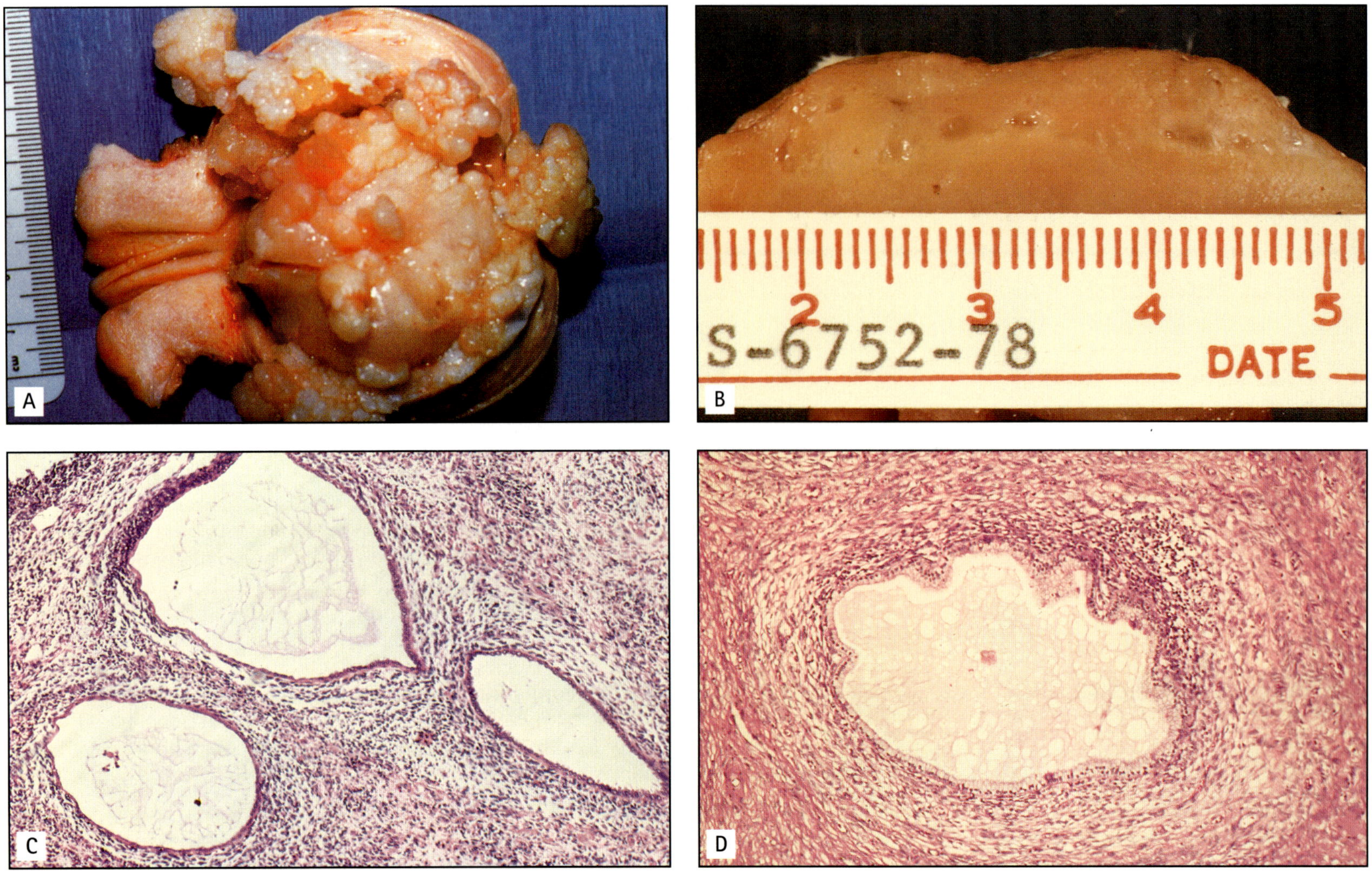

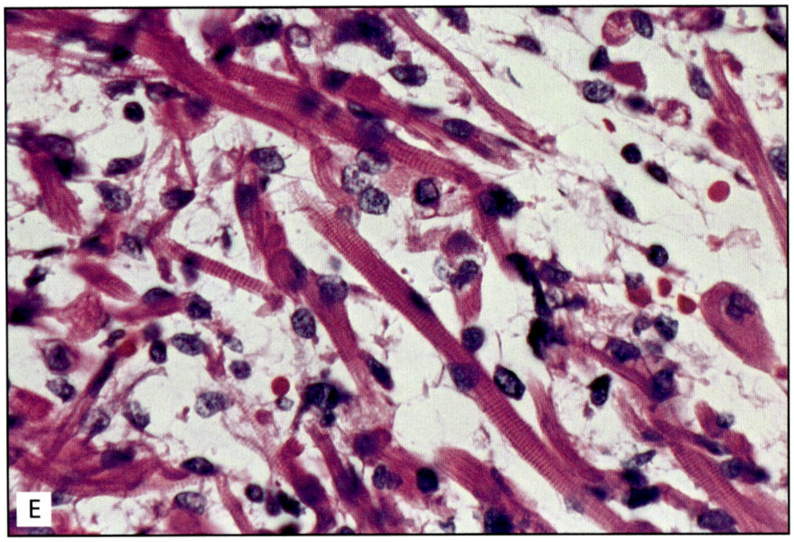

FIGURE 6-9.

Adenosarcoma. **A**, A large polypoid mass fills and distends the uterine cavity; its papillary architecture is evident. **B**, A cross section of another example of adenosarcoma shows the characteristic cystic glands with a circumferential accentuation of stroma. **C**, The histologic hallmark of this neoplasm is the cystically dilated gland with a circumferential cuff of cellular stroma. **D**, A higher-power view of a gland with its characteristic cuffing of stroma. The epithelial lining of the gland is mucinous; it is characteristic of adenosarcomas that they exhibit a range of müllerian epithelial types. **E**, Adenosarcoma with stromal overgrowth. One of the poor prognostic features of adenosarcoma is the presence of stromal overgrowth. On occasion, this stroma exhibits heterologous differentiation (*ie*, differentiation not native to the uterus, such as bone, cartilage, or skeletal muscle). In this example, a field of rhabdomyosarcoma is present. The bright pink cytoplasm of many cells features cross-striations.

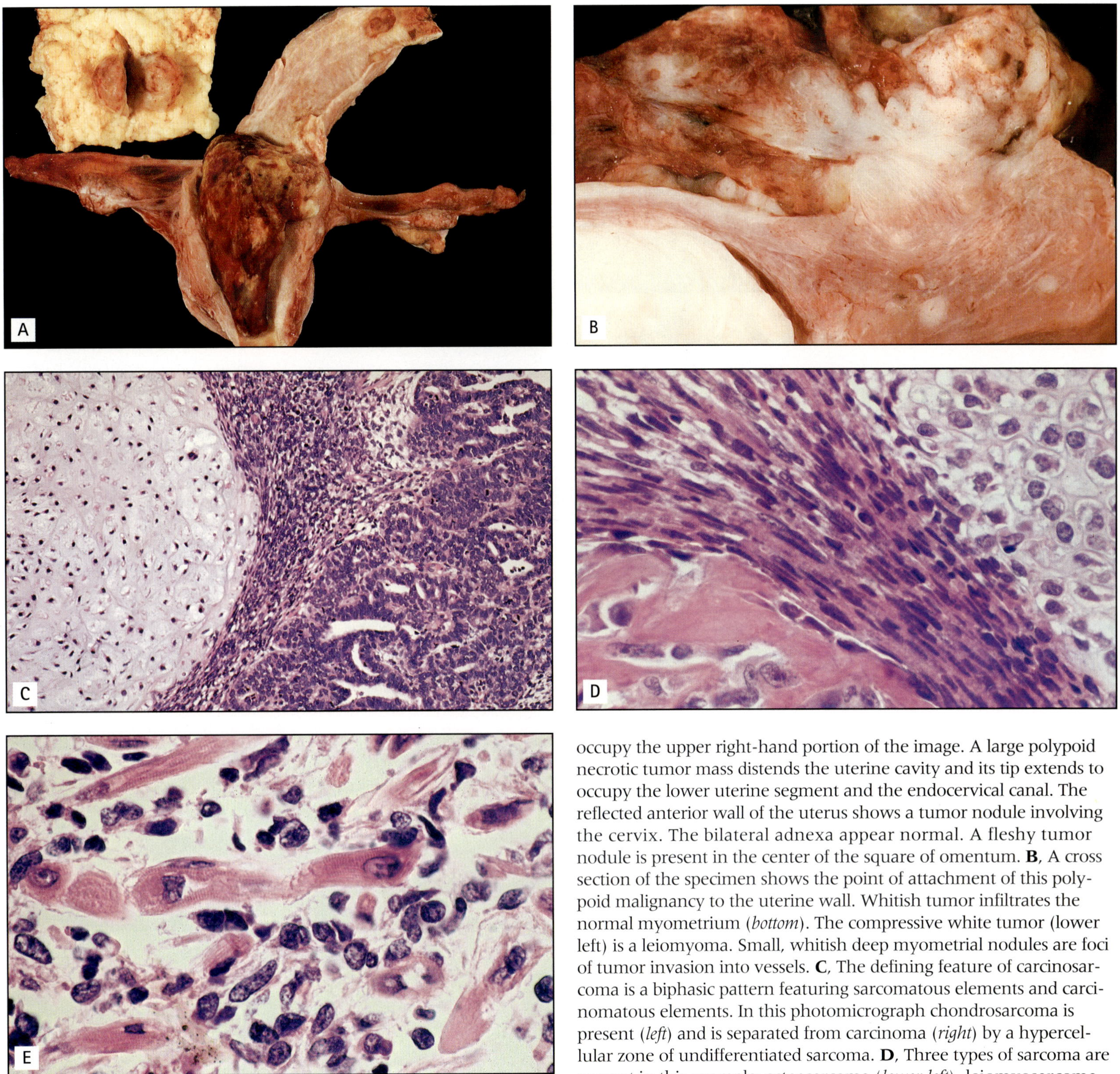

FIGURE 6-10.

Carcinosarcoma. **A**, This composite gross picture shows the uterus and bilateral adnexa and a square of omentum containing a tumor nodule (*upper left*). The anterior wall of the uterus is reflected to occupy the upper right-hand portion of the image. A large polypoid necrotic tumor mass distends the uterine cavity and its tip extends to occupy the lower uterine segment and the endocervical canal. The reflected anterior wall of the uterus shows a tumor nodule involving the cervix. The bilateral adnexa appear normal. A fleshy tumor nodule is present in the center of the square of omentum. **B**, A cross section of the specimen shows the point of attachment of this polypoid malignancy to the uterine wall. Whitish tumor infiltrates the normal myometrium (*bottom*). The compressive white tumor (lower left) is a leiomyoma. Small, whitish deep myometrial nodules are foci of tumor invasion into vessels. **C**, The defining feature of carcinosarcoma is a biphasic pattern featuring sarcomatous elements and carcinomatous elements. In this photomicrograph chondrosarcoma is present (*left*) and is separated from carcinoma (*right*) by a hypercellular zone of undifferentiated sarcoma. **D**, Three types of sarcoma are present in this example: osteosarcoma (*lower left*), leiomyosarcoma (*diagonal zone*), and chrondrosarcoma (*upper right*). **E**, This example shows extensive pleomorphic rhabdomyosarcoma elements. Large multinucleated cells with bandlike eosinophilic cytoplasm containing cross-striations are evident.

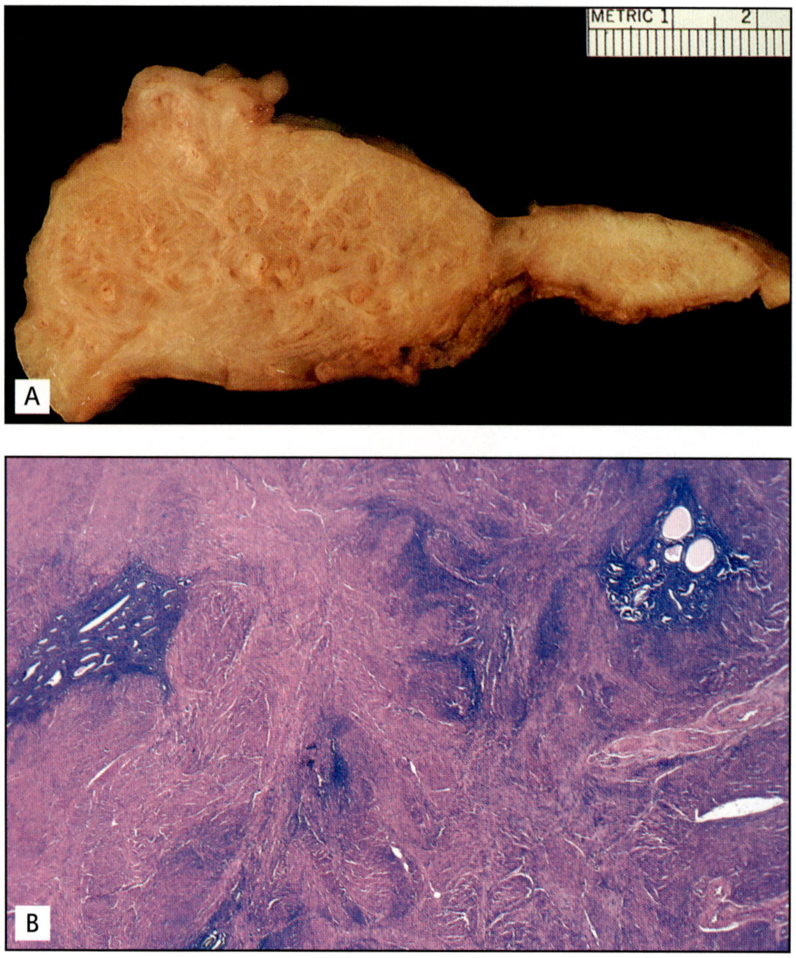

FIGURE 6-11.

Adenomyosis. **A**, Adenomyosis may focally involve the uterine corpus (adenomyoma) or may diffusely involve the entire uterus. In the latter circumstance, a characteristic globoid configuration of the uterus is produced; this is a gross cross section of such a case. The cervix is on the *right*, the thickened uterine corpus is present on the *left*, and the endometrium is at the *top*. A characteristic feature of adenomyosis is the coarse trabeculation of the myometrium; it is the myometrial hypertrophy that is largely responsible for the gross appearance of adenomyosis. **B**, The diagnostic features of adenomyosis include the presence of endometrial glands and stroma deep within the myometrium delivered by struts of hypertrophied smooth muscle [8].

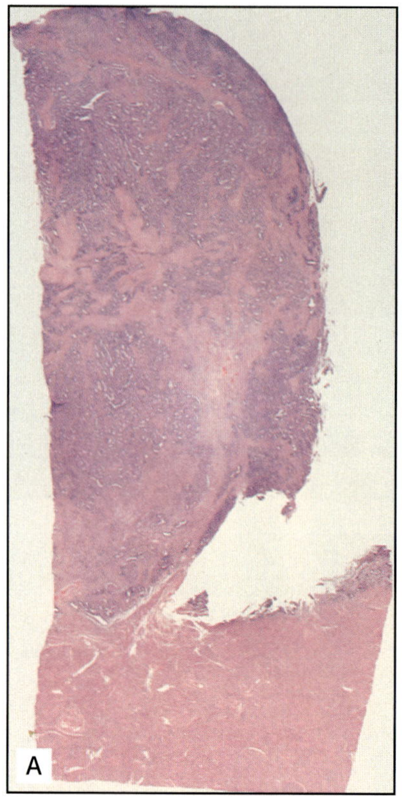

FIGURE 6-12.

Atypical polypoid adenomyoma. **A**, This low-power photomicrograph shows the characteristic polypoid appearance of this lesion, which is commonly mistaken for adenocarcinoma. Typical polypoid adenomyomas occur in women of reproductive years and feature nodules of architecturally complex glands separated by struts of smooth muscle. The interface with the underlying myometrium is typically compressive. The lesion characteristically arises in the lower uterine segment. **B**, Architecturally complex glands lined by cytologically mildly atypical epithelium. An almost invariable feature of this proliferation is the presence of morular or squamous differentiation [9].

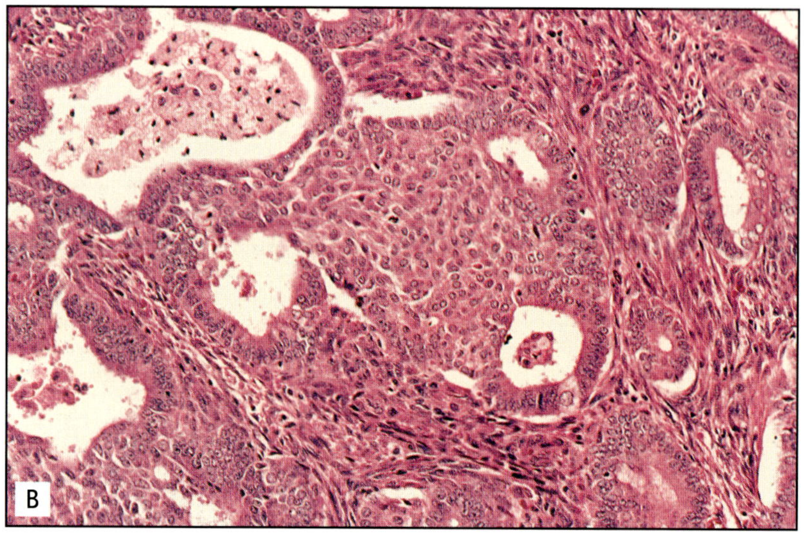

UTERINE SMOOTH MUSCLE NEOPLASMS

CLASSIFICATION OF UTERINE SMOOTH MUSCLE PROLIFERATIONS

I. Smooth muscle tumors with usual differentiation
   - A. Usual leiomyoma and leiomyoma with increased mitotic figures
   - B. Leiomyosarcoma

II. Smooth muscle tumors with unusual histologic patterns
   - A. Atypical leiomyoma (symplastic leiomyoma)
   - B. Epithelioid smooth muscle tumors
   - C. Myxoid stroma
   - D. Lipoleiomyoma
   - E. Neurilemmoma-like leiomyoma
   - F. Leiomyoma with tubules or glands
   - G. Leiomyoma with benign heterologous elements

III. Unusual growth patterns
   - A. Infiltrating leiomyoma including leiomyomatosis
   - B. Disseminated peritoneal leiomyomatosis
   - C. Benign metastasizing leiomyoma
   - D. Parasitic leiomyoma
   - E. Leiomyoma with vascular intrusion
   - F. Intravascular leiomyomatosis

FIGURE 6-13.

Classification of uterine smooth muscle proliferations. Smooth muscle proliferations of the uterus are extraordinarily common. Indeed, the ordinary leiomyoma is the most common neoplasm in women. The vast majority of these neoplasms are easily recognized surgically and microscopically and occasion no diagnostic difficulties for the pathologist. The malignant counterpart of the leiomyoma, leiomyosarcoma, is rare but comprises between a third and a half of uterine sarcomas. Again, the usual case of leiomyosarcoma is easily recognized surgically and microscopically. Diagnostic problems arise because intrauterine masses may exhibit gross features that suggest malignancy (necrosis, hemorrhage, and so on) and/or microscopic appearances that suggest malignancy (cytologically atypical cells, a high mitotic index, high cellularity, nonstandard differentiation) [3,10]. In addition, smooth muscle proliferations of the uterus may be associated with extrauterine smooth muscle deposits that raise the possibility of malignancy. However, on rare occasions, clinically benign smooth muscle neoplasms of the uterus may have an intravascular component, either confined to the uterus or present in extrauterine sites (intravenous leiomyomatosis) or may diffusely involve the uterus (leiomyomatosis) or may be associated with bland smooth muscle nodules in the lung (benign metastasizing leiomyoma). These processes are either clinically benign or clinically low grade and are important to recognize and distinguish from the fully malignant and clinically aggressive leiomyosarcoma.

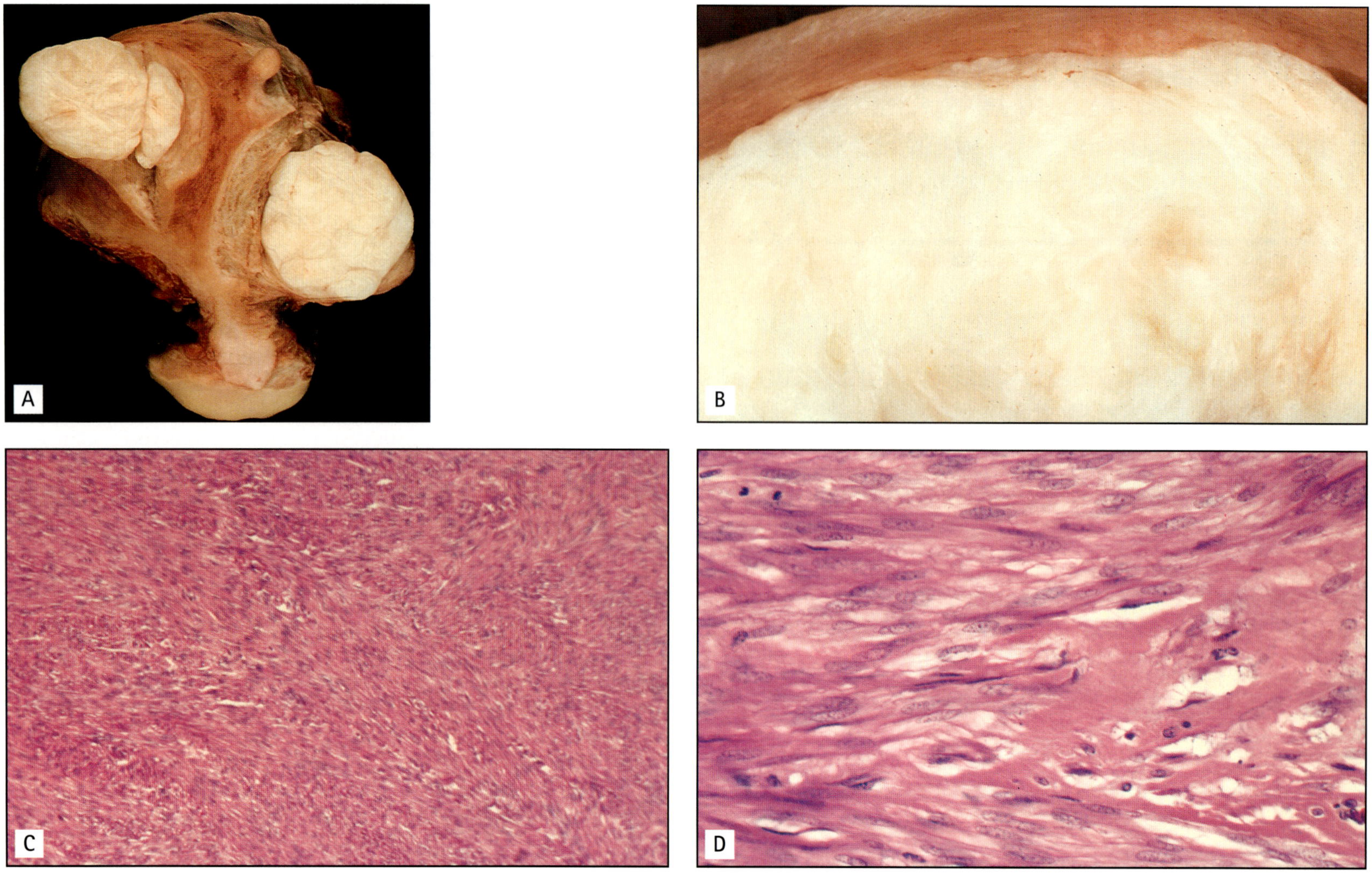

FIGURE 6-14.

Leiomyomas. **A**, This is a fairly typical appearance of a uterus harboring multiple leiomyomas. These benign smooth muscle tumors are easily shelled out from the surrounding compressed normal myometrium. They may occur in a subserosal or intramural location. Submucous leiomyomas are common and present as polypoid masses in the uterine cavity and may on occasion infarct, and patients present clinically with acute pain and hemorrhage. **B**, The sharply defined compressive interface of a leiomyoma with the normal myometrium is seen. In addition, the characteristic whorled, fibrous white appearance of the typical leiomyoma is depicted. **C**, The usual leiomyoma is composed of bundles of smooth muscle cells interdigitating in a gently curving fashion. **D**, The constituent cells closely resemble those of the normal myometrium. They possess fusiform nuclei surrounded by abundant eosinophilic cytoplasm with ill-defined cytoplasmic margins. A mitotic figure is present in the *upper left-hand corner* of the image.

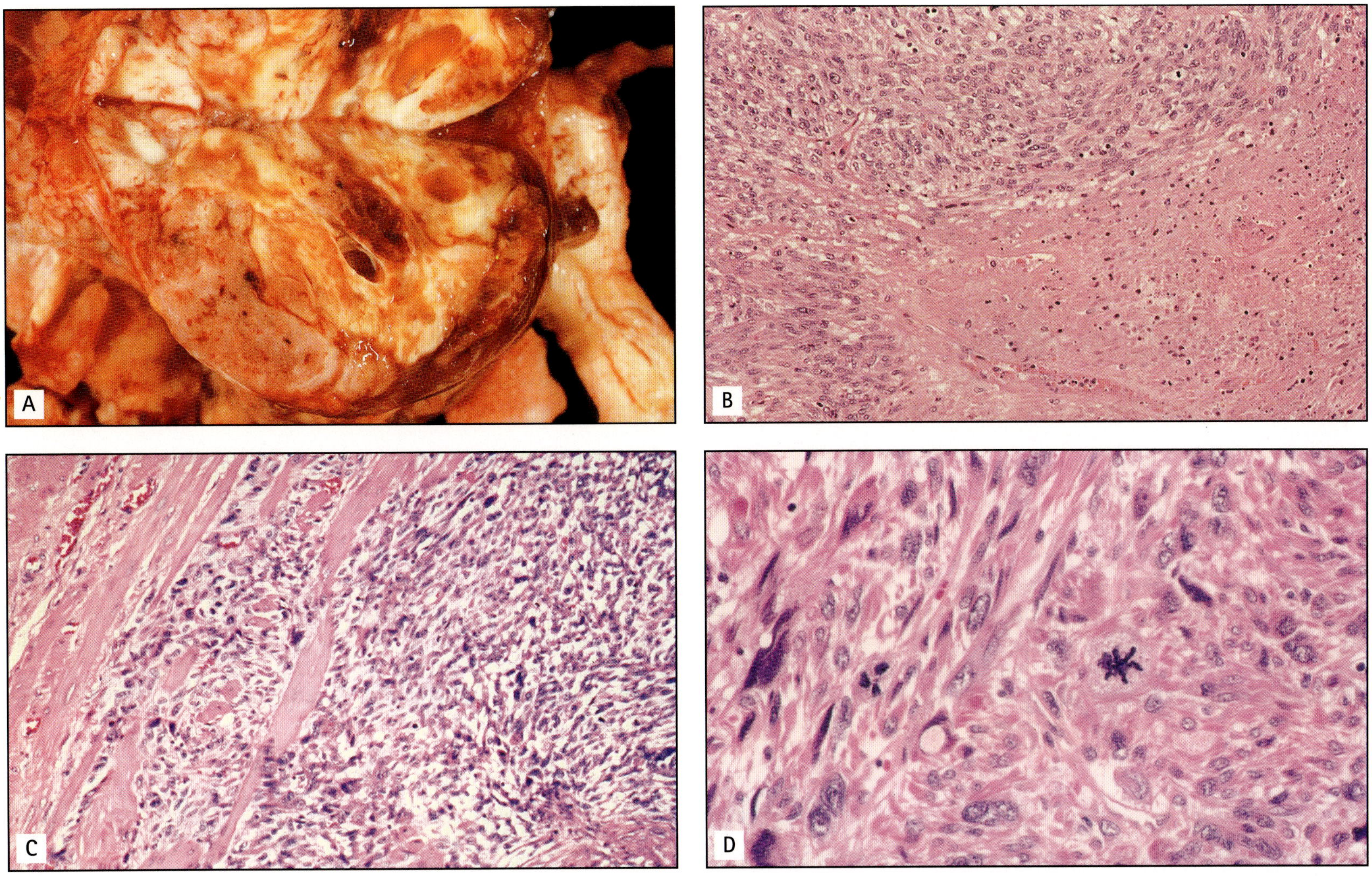

FIGURE 6–15.

The usual leiomyosarcoma. **A**, Leiomyosarcoma as defined using current morphologic definitions is a highly malignant neoplasm. The gross appearance is that of a typical high-grade sarcoma and features fleshy masses of tumor infiltrating the surrounding myometrium. Geographic zones of hemorrhage and necrosis are common. In this example the uterus (*extreme right*) is overshadowed by a large necrotic neoplasm. The uterine cervix is present in the *lower right-hand corner* of the image. **B**, This low-power photomicrograph shows a hypercellular spindle-cell neoplasm (*upper left*) immediately adjacent to a zone of coagulative tumor cell necrosis. **C**, Neoplastic cells (*right*) infiltrate the surrounding myometrium (*upper left*). **D**, The cells exhibit the usual features of malignancy: nuclear pleomorphism, nuclear hyperchromasia, individual cell necrosis, and abnormal mitotic figures (spiderlike object, *center*).

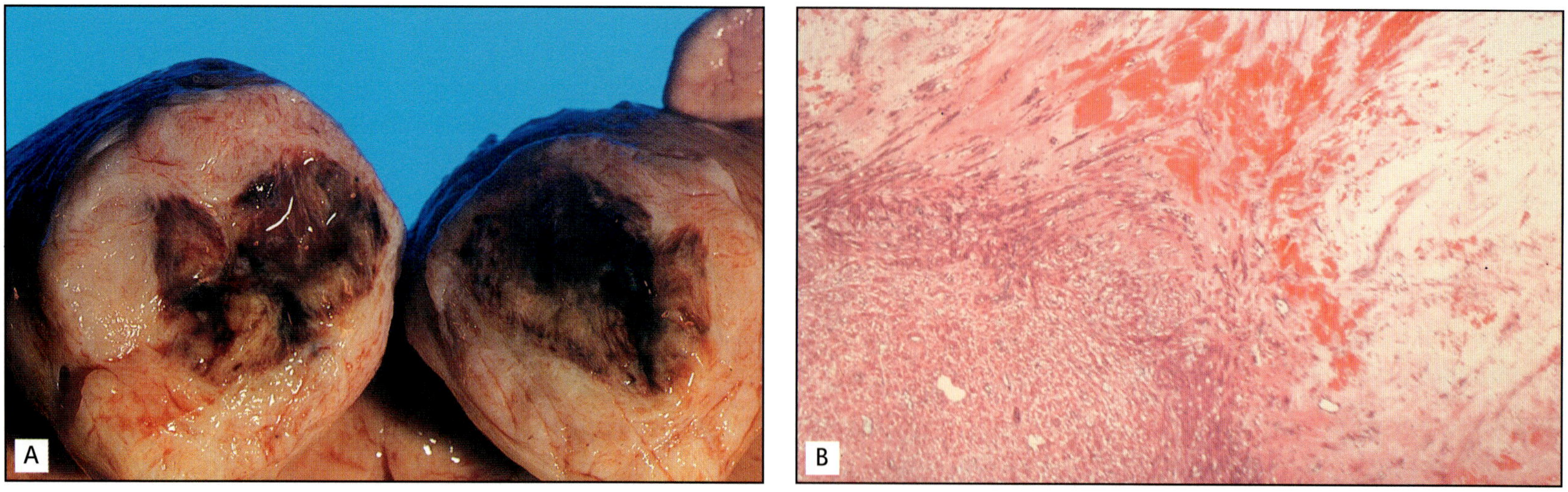

FIGURE 6-16.

Hemorrhagic infarction in a leiomyoma. **A**, The gross appearance of clinically benign smooth muscle tumors may mimic malignancy in a variety of ways. These collectively have been termed "degenerations." This example exhibits central hemorrhagic infarction of an otherwise typical leiomyoma. This change may occur during pregnancy or after the administration of progestational agents. A normal ovary is present at *upper right*. **B**, Leiomyoma with organizing hemorrhagic infarction. Leiomyomas may exhibit the full range of reparative processes seen in infarctions elsewhere in the body. In this example, the zone of hemorrhagic granulation tissue is forming at the interface of the necrotic portion of the leiomyoma and the viable remaining leiomyoma (*lower left*). The gross appearance of this process may suggest malignancy, and this impression may be reinforced by the frequent finding of mitotic figures in this actively proliferating granulation tissue. Recognition of this phenomenon is usually sufficient to avoid misdiagnosing this process as leiomyosarcoma.

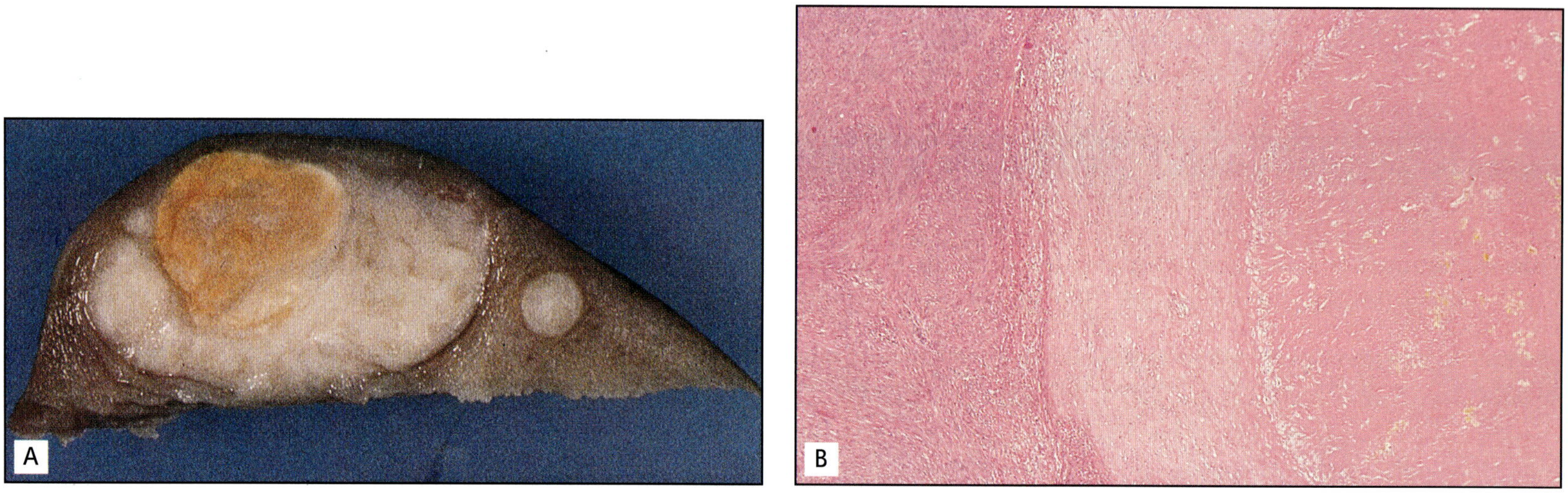

FIGURE 6-17.

Hyaline necrosis in a leiomyoma. **A**, The complete resolution of an acute ischemic episode may result in a leiomyoma with yellow central necrosis. In this example, the center of this subserosal leiomyoma is occupied by a yellowish, sharply marginated zone. The smaller myoma is present to the *right* of the specimen. **B**, In this example, viable leiomyoma is present (*left*) and is separated by a collagenized zone (*center*) from mummified necrotic remnants of the infarcted leiomyoma (*right*). This pattern of necrosis is important to distinguish from coagulative tumor cell necrosis characteristic of leiomyosarcoma.

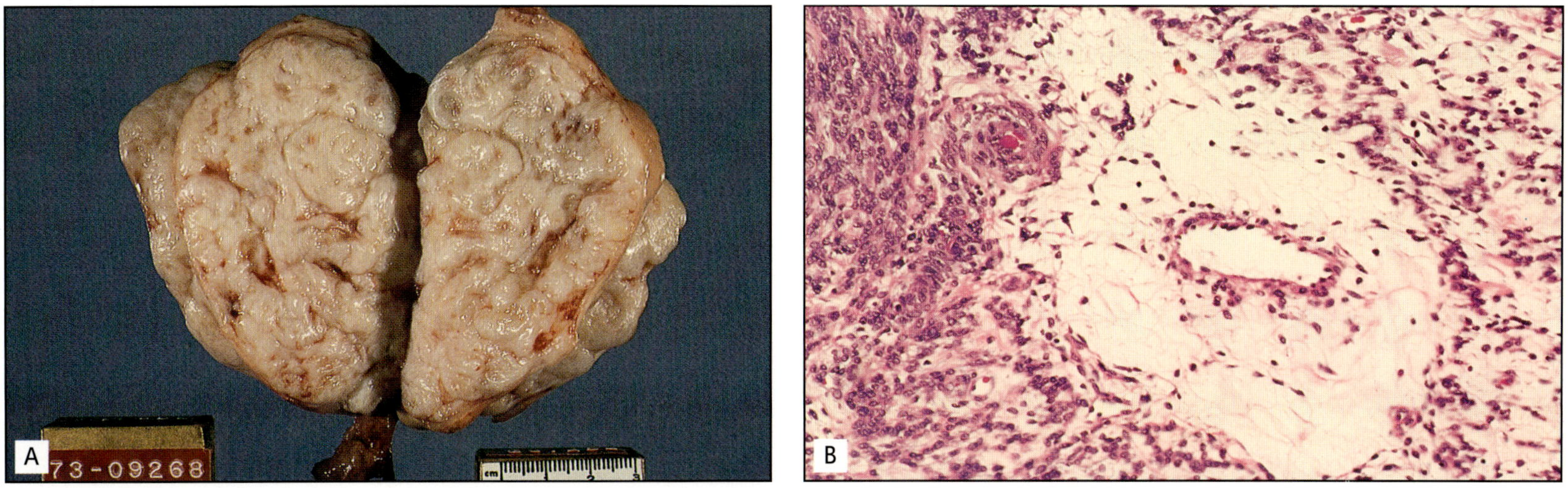

FIGURE 6-18.

Perihydropic nodular change in leiomyoma. **A**, This gross specimen illustrates another characteristic change that leiomyomas may undergo. Nodules of fibromuscular tissue are delimited by depressed zones of myxoid connective tissue. **B**, Leiomyoma with perinodular hydropic change. The distinguishing feature of the myxoid areas in this process is the large-calibered muscular vessels suspended in the myxoid tissue. Both the gross and microscopic appearances are quite distinct from myxoid leiomyosarcoma (*see* Fig. 6-21).

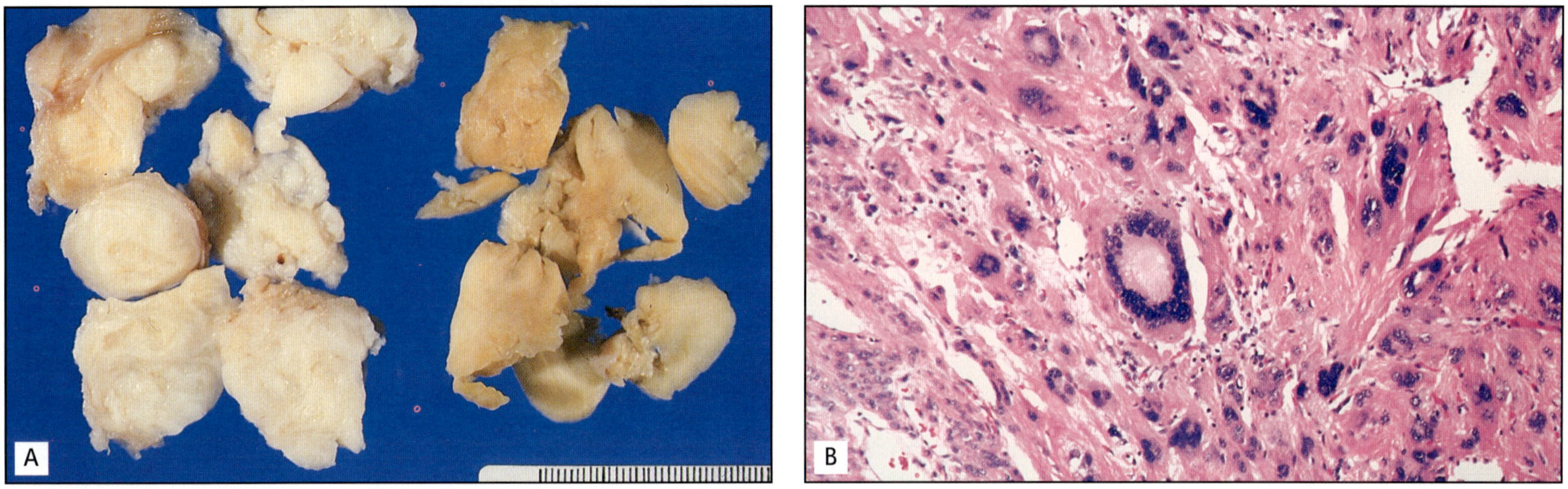

FIGURE 6-19.

Leiomyoma with atypical cytology. **A**, Multiple fragments of uterine smooth muscle tumors have been removed laparoscopically. Those on the *left* have the firm white, whorled fibrous appearance of typical leiomyomas. Those on the *right* have a slightly yellowish cast. **B**, The yellowish leiomyomas are composed largely of atypical cells, seen in this high-power photomicrograph. No necrosis and no mitotic figures are identified. These neoplasms have been variously designated in the literature as symplastic leiomyomas or atypical leiomyomas with low potential for recurrence. Thorough sampling and compulsive attention to the presence of tumor cell necrosis and/or mitotic figures is imperative before making this diagnosis. Unlike this case, most examples of the leiomyomas of this type are grossly unremarkable.

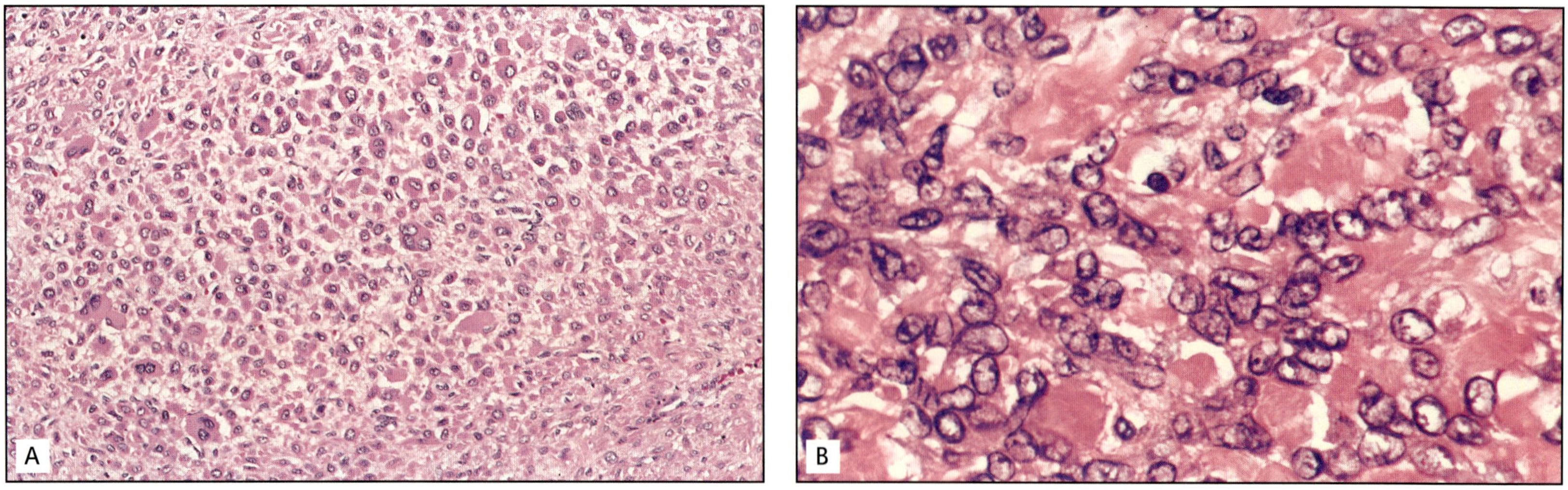

FIGURE 6-20.

Epithelioid leiomyosarcoma. **A**, Some smooth muscle proliferations may deviate from the usual appearance of smooth muscle neoplasms in that the cells become rounded and acquire an appearance reminiscent of epithelium. Smooth muscle neoplasms exhibiting epithelioid differentiation are unusual, and the rules for dividing them into benign, low-grade, and malignant differ from those used for neoplasms with standard smooth muscle differentiation. **B**, Another pattern of epithelioid smooth muscle differentiation is depicted in this high-power photomicrograph. The cords and trabeculae of rounded cells have eosinophilic cytoplasm and are embedded in collagen. No tumor cell necrosis is present, and no significant cytologic atypia is evident. Mitotic figures are absent. These neoplasms behave in a clinically benign fashion.

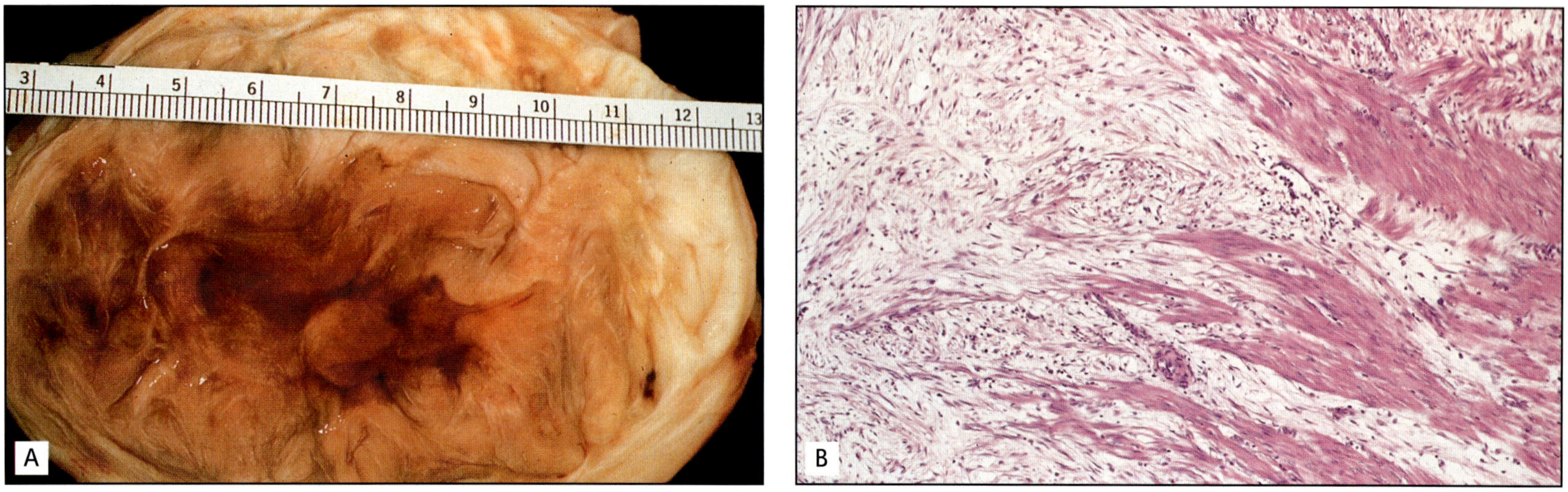

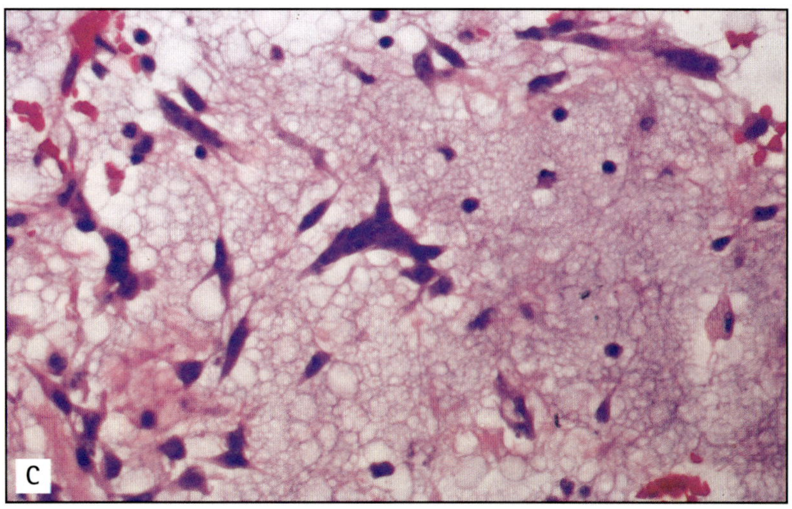

FIGURE 6-21.

Myxoid leiomyosarcoma. **A**, This large necrotic myxoid lesion has extensively distended and replaced the uterine corpus. Myxoid leiomyosarcomas are rare but occur at all ages. **B**, The hallmark of myxoid leiomyosarcoma is its infiltrative interface with the normal myometrium. This is in contrast to perihydropic nodular change (*see* Fig. 6-18), which occurs in leiomyomas having a compressive interface with the surrounding myometrium. **C**, The constituent cells of this malignancy are relatively bland but occasional cells show malignant features (*center of field*). Mitotic figures may be very difficult to find in clinically malignant lesions. This is in contrast to the usual leiomyosarcoma which characteristically has a high mitotic index.

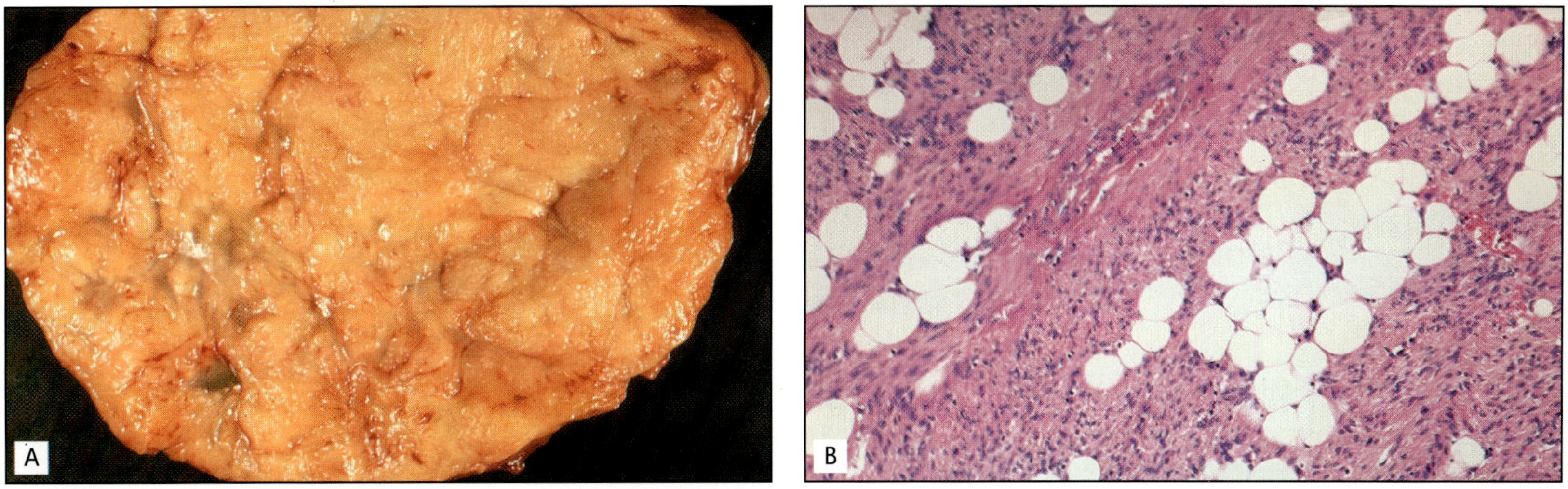

FIGURE 6-22.

Lipoleiomyoma. **A**, Another unusual leiomyoma variant is depicted here. On rare occasions, extensive mature fat may be present within an otherwise typical leiomyoma. Most smooth muscle tumors with this pattern of differentiation are benign, but rarely liposarcomas may be encountered. **B**, Microscopically, the distinctive admixture of typical smooth muscle cells with large mature adipocytes is characteristic of this benign neoplasm.

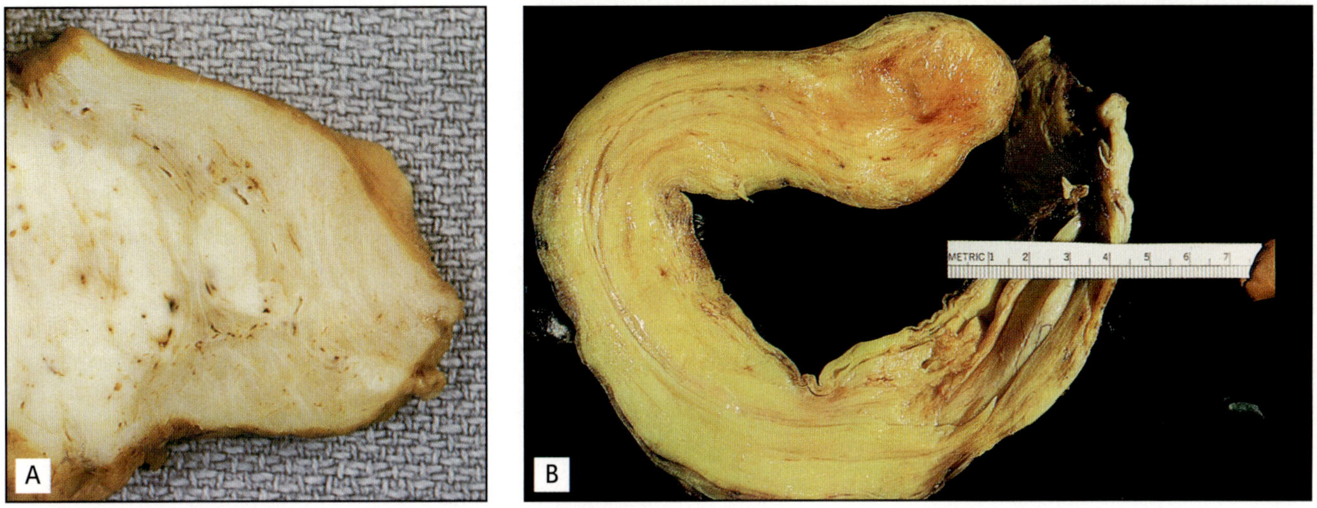

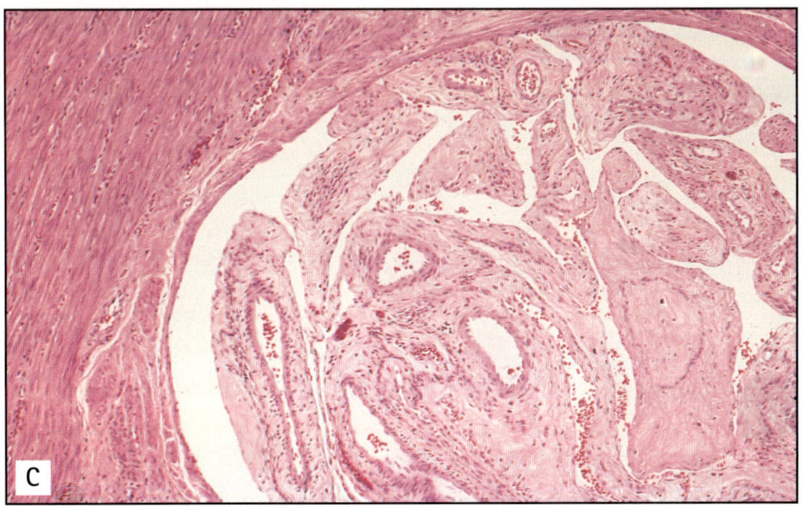

FIGURE 6-23.

Intravenous leiomyomatosis. **A**, A poorly defined nodule of neoplastic smooth muscle is present on the *left* and a plug of similar tissue extrudes toward the *right*. Most instances of intravenous leiomyomatosis are confined to the uterus, but on occasion, these plugs of tumor may extend into the broad ligament and beyond. **B**, A large tubular mass of smooth muscle distended the vena cava in this case. The patient presented with congestive heart failure and was found to have extensive involvement of the right heart and vena cava by intravenous leiomyomatosis. Intravenous leiomyomatosis is a clinically benign proliferation that causes hemodynamic difficulties when the right heart is involved by the process. **C**, Microscopically, large plug of vascularized smooth muscle distends an intramyometrial venous channel (*lower right*).

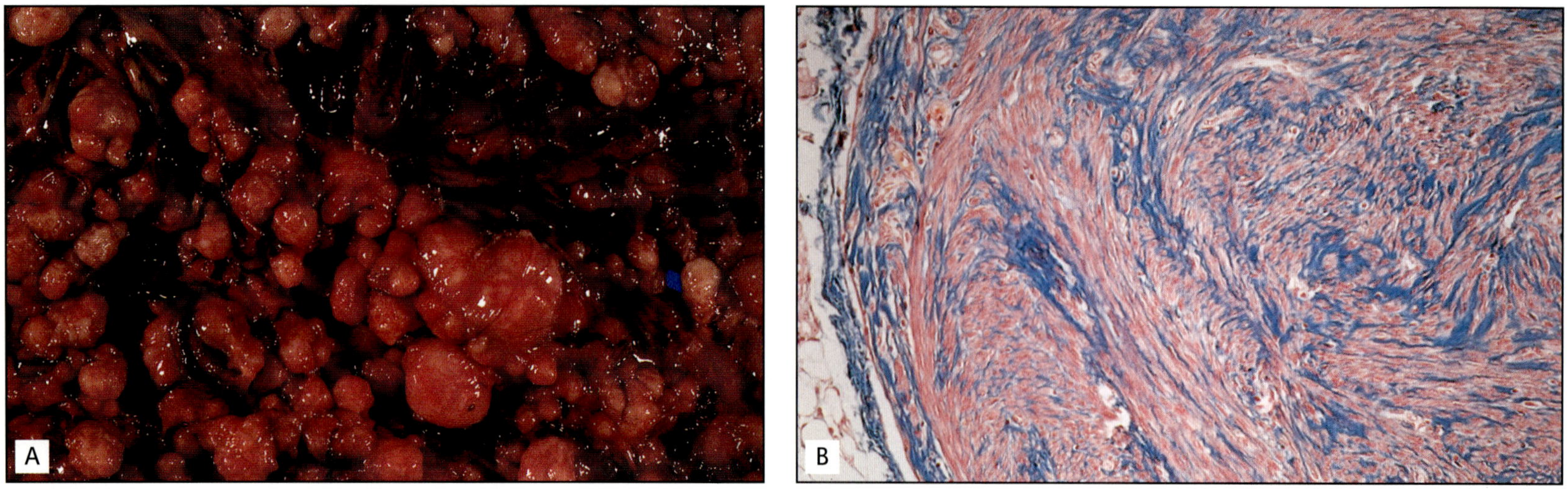

FIGURE 6-24.

Disseminated peritoneal leiomyomatosis. **A**, This rare and peculiar smooth muscle proliferation extensively involves the omentum. Nodules ranging from 0.2 to 1.5 cm extensively involve the omentum. Most patients with this condition have either been pregnant or have been receiving hormonal medication of some sort. Whether this is neoplastic or hyerplastic is unclear. Unless there is extensive involvement of the peritoneal surfaces, this lesion is clinically benign and often regresses after withdrawal of the associated hormonal stimulus. **B**, This trichrome stain shows the focal collagenization (*blue*) of this smooth muscle proliferation. In some instances, smooth muscle merges with what appears to be decidual reaction.

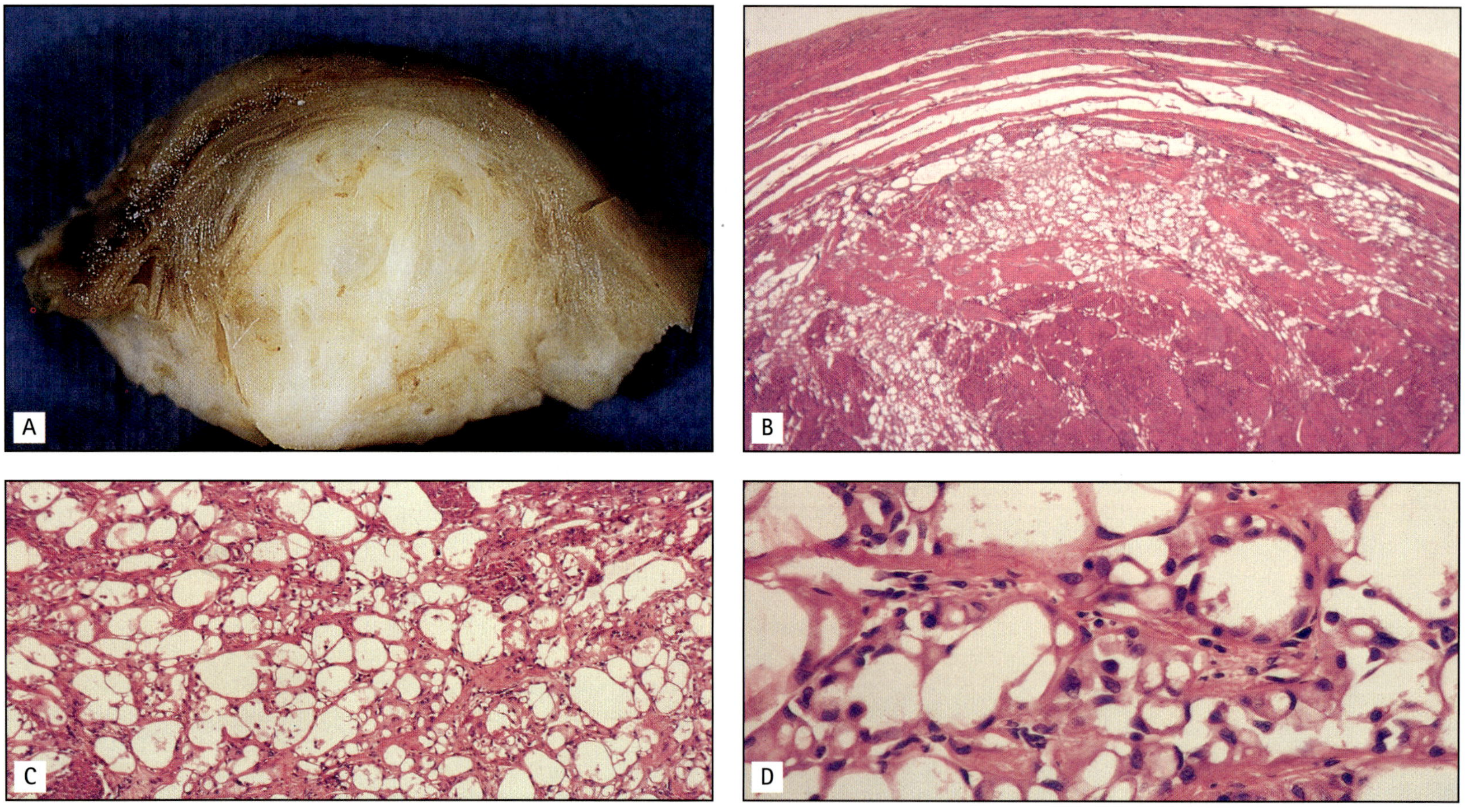

FIGURE 6-25.

Adenomatoid mesothelioma. **A**, This benign neoplasm most commonly occurs in the fallopian tube but less frequently may arise in the cornua of the uterus. The gross appearance is essentially that of a leiomyoma. Some neoplasms have a yellowish cast, reflecting the elastic tissue they often contain. **B**, A scanning power view shows expanded normal myometrium (*top*) and a nodular proliferation punctuated by innumerable cleared spaces. **C** and **D**, A honeycomb pattern of empty spaces lined by flattened cells resembling mesothelium is evident. When the spaces become very distended (*C*), they may resemble lymphangioma. When the lining cells become plump and have an epithelioid appearance (*D*), the possibility of invasive carcinoma is raised.

REFERENCES

1. Hannigan E, Curtin J, Silverberg S, et al.: Corpus: mesenchymal tumors. In *Principles and Practice of Gynecologic Oncology*. Edited by Hoskins WJ, Perez CA, Young RC. Philadelphia: JB Lippincott; 1992:695–714.
2. Morrow C, Curtin J, Townsend D: *Synopsis of Gynecologic Oncology*, edn 4. New York: Churchill Livingstone; 1993.
3. Hendrickson M, Kempson R: Pure mesenchymal neoplasms of the uterine corpus. In *Obstetrical and Gynaecological Pathology*. Edited by Fox H. New York: Churchill Livingstone; 1995:519–586.
4. Hendrickson M, Kempson R: The uterine corpus. In *Diagnostic Surgical Pathology*, edn 2. New York: Raven Press; 1994:2091–2193.
5. Chang K, Crabtree G, Lim-Tan S, *et al.*: Primary uterine endometrial stromal neoplasms: a clinicopathologic study of 117 cases. *Am J Surg Pathol* 1990, 14:415–438.
6. Clement P, Scully R: Mullerian adenosarcoma of the uterus: a clinicopathologic analysis of 100 cases with a review of the literature. *Hum Pathol* 1990, 21:363–381.
7. Zaloudek C, Norris H: Adenofibroma and adenosarcoma of the uterus: a clinicopathologic study of 35 cases. *Cancer* 1981, 48:354–366.
8. Hendrickson M, Kempson R, Longacre T: Endometriosis and adenomyosis. In *Haines and Taylor's Obstetrical and Gynecological Pathology*, edn 2. Edited by Fox H. London: Churchill Livingstone; 1995.
9. Longacre TA, Chung MH, Rouse RV, Hendrickson MR. Atypical polypoid adenomyofibromas (atypical polypoid adenomyomas) of the uterus: a clinicopathologic study of 55 cases. *Am J Surg Pathol* 1996, 20:1–20.
10. Bell SW, Kempson RL, Hendrickson MR: Problematic uterine smooth muscle neoplasms. a clinicopathologic study of 213 cases. *Am J Surg Pathol* 1994, 18:535–558.

CHAPTER 7

Fallopian Tube

Howard G. Muntz

The two fallopian tubes lie on each side of the uterus, and measure about 10 cm in length. Though relatively small, they play a central role in normal human reproduction, being responsible for the transport of ova and spermatozoa. Fertilization occurs within the ampullary portion of the fallopian tube, after which the preimplantation conceptus must be transported by the fallopian tube into the endometrial cavity. From a reproductive biology perspective, any condition that disrupts this process of fertilization and transportation is pathologic. Examples include severe endometriosis, tubal infection, and the sequelae of these processes, including hydrosalpinx and ectopic pregnancies. These conditions are covered extensively in this chapter.

In addition, the practicing gynecologist will encounter a number of structural anomalies and both benign and malignant tumors of the fallopian tube. Representative examples are included in the chapter.

NORMAL FALLOPIAN TUBE

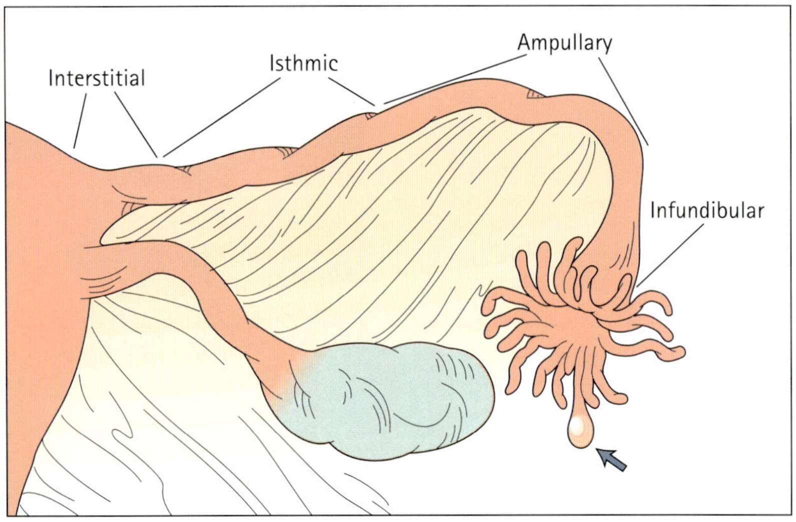

FIGURE 7-1.
Anatomic divisions of the normal fallopian tube. The interstitial portion lies within the uterine wall. It has a relatively simple lumen, surrounded by smooth muscle (*see also* Fig. 7-2). The isthmic portion of the tube begins immediately external to the uterine cornua, and forms approximately the medial third of the fallopian tube. It is rounded, muscular, and firm, and has a narrow lumen with only a few longitudinal mucosal folds supported by prominent surrounding muscularis (*see* Fig. 7-3). The luminal architecture becomes much more complex moving from the isthmic portion of the tube into the ampullary region, which comprises approximately the lateral one half of the tube. The ampulla has a larger overall diameter, with a thinner external wall, and a complex inner lumen filled with multiple papillary fronds (*see* Fig. 7-4). The infundibular portion is the fimbriated end of the fallopian tube. This part of the tube is shaped like a funnel, and is lined by multiple fimbriae, each of which is covered by ciliated epithelium (*see* Fig. 7-5). The cilia beat toward the ampulla, which facilitates capture of the unfertilized ovum from the ovary, and its transportation through the lumen of the fallopian tube. Hydatid cysts of Morgagni (*arrow*) commonly occur on the fimbria or arise from the adjacent broad ligament. These small, pedunculated cysts are a normal variant of tubal anatomy.

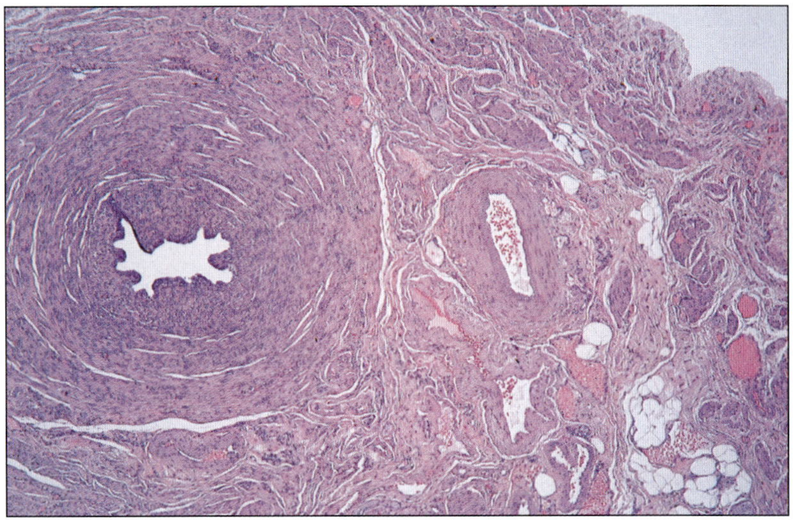

FIGURE 7-2.
Interstitial portion of the fallopian tube. The tubal cross section is to the left, with smooth muscle of the uterine cornu also visible in this photomicrograph. (*Courtesy of* John Bolen, MD.)

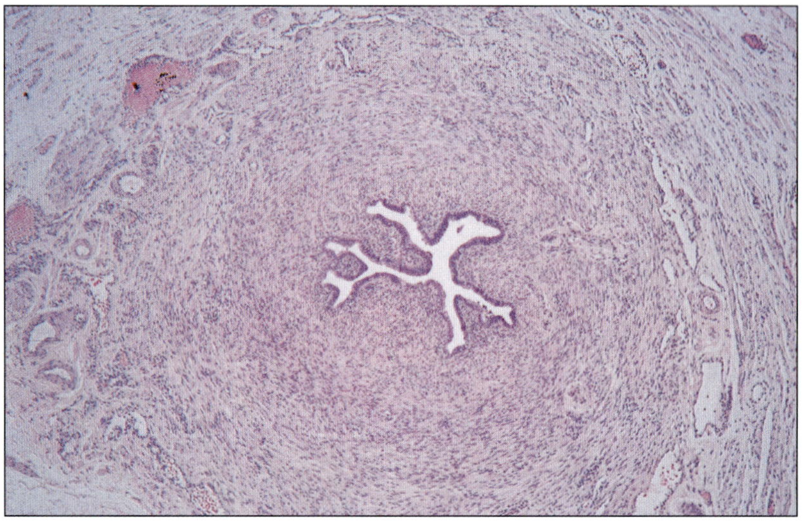

FIGURE 7-3.
Isthmic portion of fallopian tube (cross section). (*Courtesy of* John Bolen, MD.)

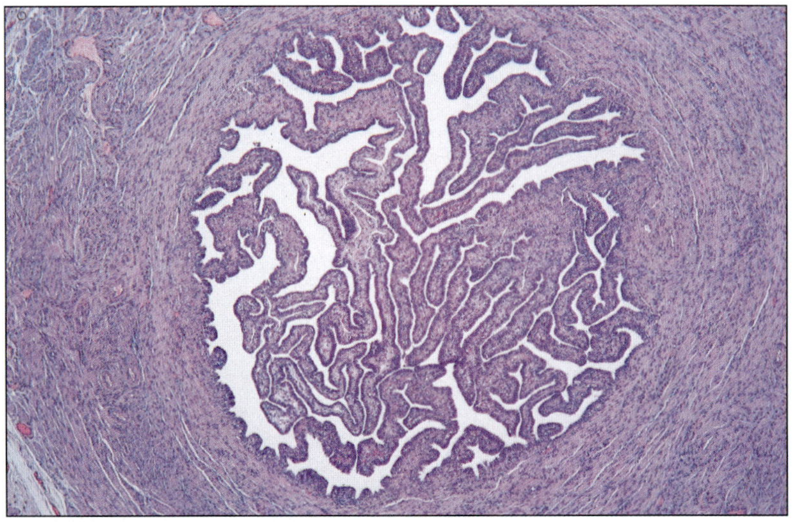

FIGURE 7-4.
Ampullary portion of fallopian tube (cross section). (*Courtesy of* John Bolen, MD.)

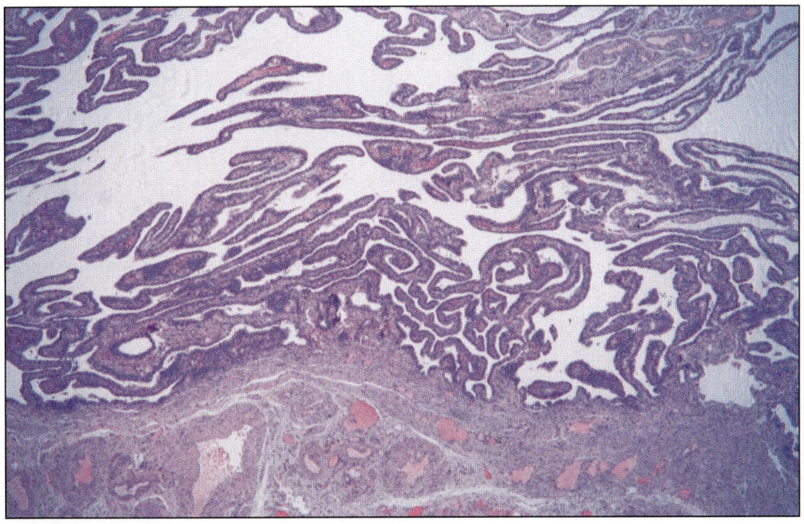

FIGURE 7-5.
Fimbriated end, or infundibular portion, of the fallopian tube. This longitudinal section illustrates the complex, predominantly linear arrangement of the fimbriae. The tubal wall is at the bottom of the frame. (*Courtesy of* John Bolen, MD.)

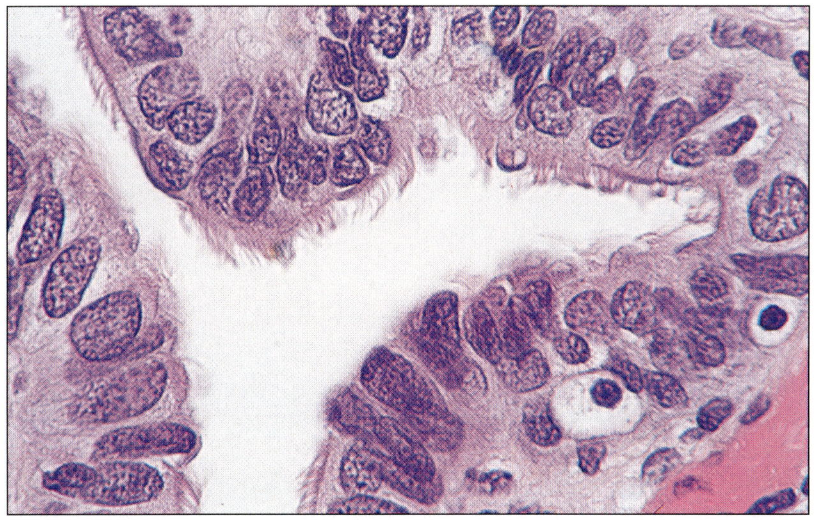

FIGURE 7-6.
Ciliated cells of tubal epithelium. This high-power photomicrograph demonstrates the numerous cilia present within the ampullary portion of the tube. Interestingly, women with the rare immotile cilia syndrome are able to conceive, suggesting that muscular movements of the tube are chiefly responsible for ova and spermatozoa transport. Patches of ciliated cells are separated in areas by protruding secretory cells. These secretory cells are also important for normal reproductive function because the zygotes and products of conception must be maintained in an appropriate fluid environment for survival. (*Courtesy of* David Dail, MD.)

PARATUBAL CYSTS AND BENIGN TUMORS OF THE FALLOPIAN TUBE

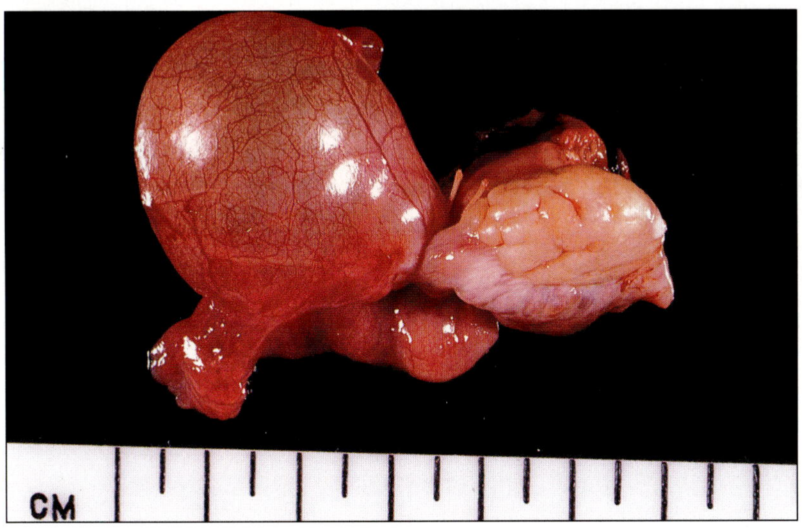

FIGURE 7-7.
Typical paratubal cyst. Paratubal (or para-ovarian) cysts commonly occur in the broad ligament between the fallopian tube and ovary. These arise from embryonic remnants of müllerian duct (paramesonephric) or wolffian duct (mesonephric) structures, or develop from peritoneal (mesothelial) inclusions.

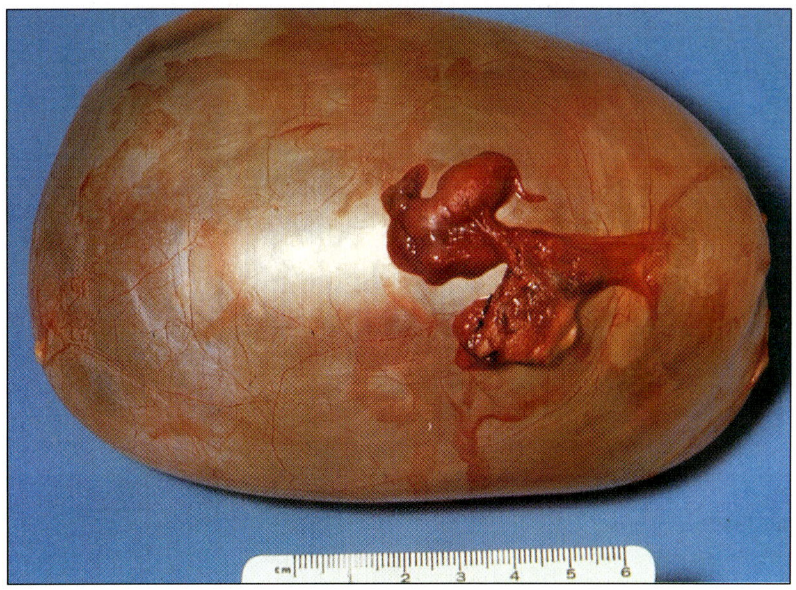

FIGURE 7-8.
Large paratubal cyst. This large paratubal cyst was excised from a 28-year-old woman who presented with complaints of pelvic pressure and frequent urination.

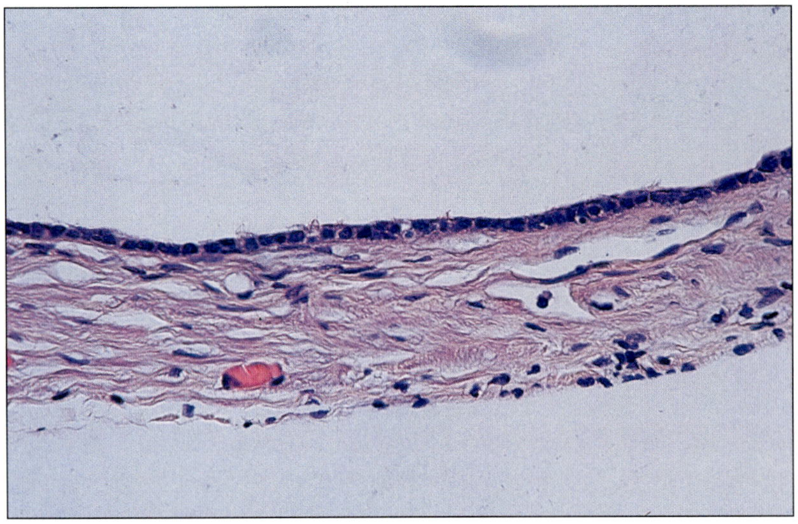

FIGURE 7-9.
Histology of typical paratubal cyst. Most paratubal cysts are lined by a single layer of benign epithelium, irrespective of the embryonic tissue of origin.

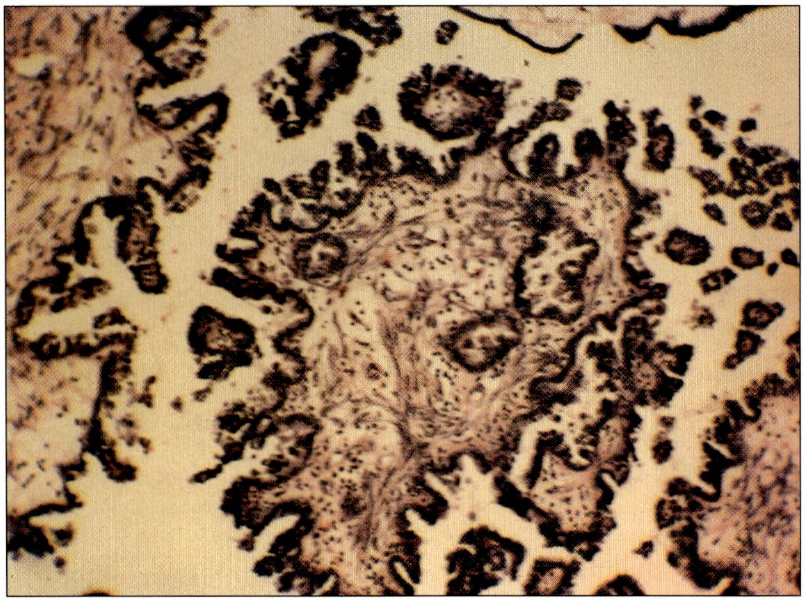

FIGURE 7-10.
Paratubal cyst of low malignant potential. Approximately 2% to 3% of paratubal cysts will be malignant. Typically, malignant cysts are large with diameters exceeding 5 cm. Any paratubal cyst with sonographic evidence of internal papillations should be considered a neoplasm, requiring intact removal similar to an ovarian neoplasm. The majority of cases involve tumors of low malignant potential, or "borderline" histology as demonstrated by this example, although frankly invasive malignancies have been reported. (*Courtesy of* Donald Bauermeister, MD.)

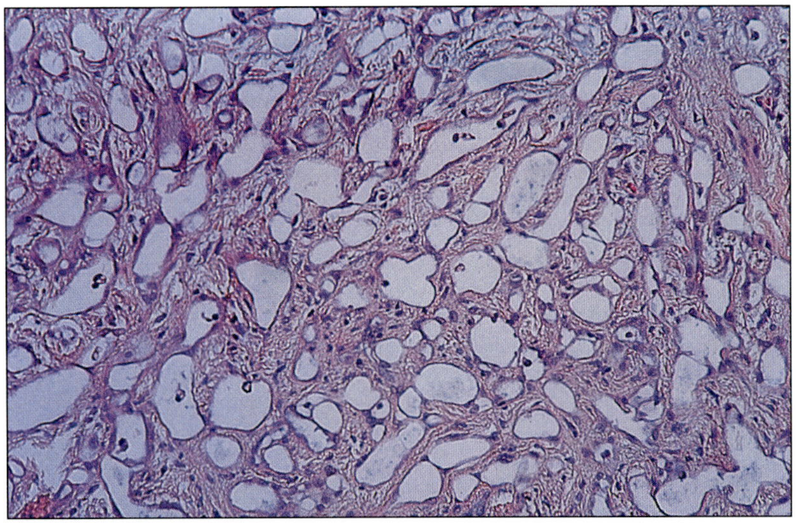

FIGURE 7-11.
Adenomatoid tumor. The most common tubal tumor is the benign adenomatoid tumor. Grossly, it appears as a firm, white or yellowish nodule, is usually relatively small, and detected incidentally at surgery. Microscopically (as shown), it consists of cleftlike spaces lined by mesothelial epithelium, embedded in a loose stroma.

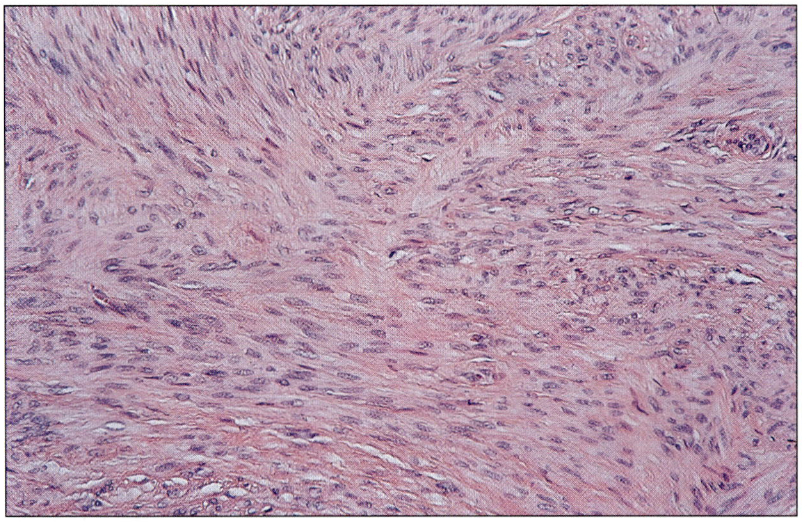

FIGURE 7-12.
Leiomyoma. This benign smooth muscle tumor can occur anywhere in the female genital tract. This tissue section from a small tubal myomyoma was an incidental finding in a woman undergoing a hysterectomy for multiple large uterine leiomyomas.

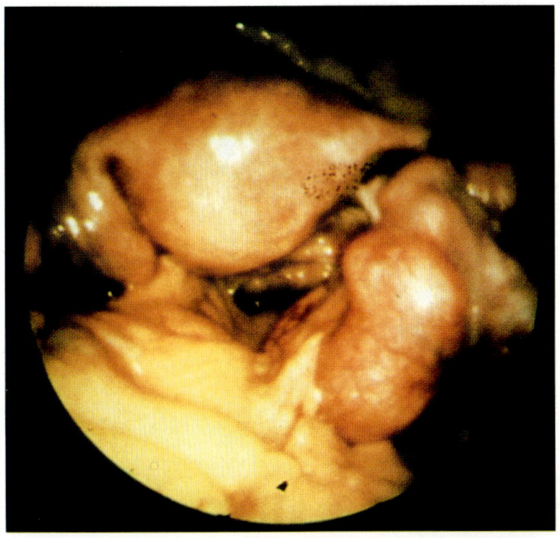

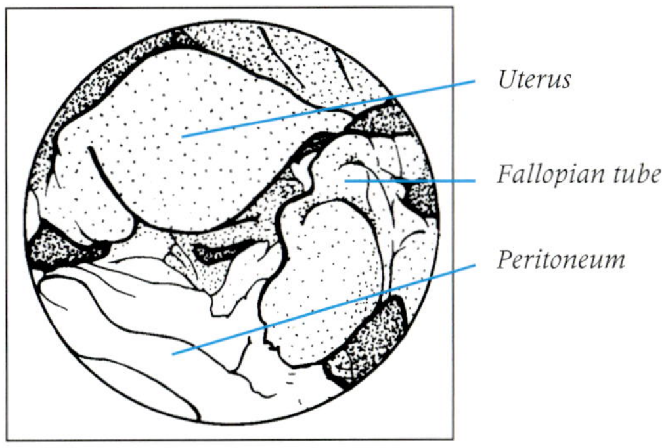

FIGURE 7-19.
Laparoscopic view of acute salpingitis. An erythematous and swollen right fallopian tube was visualized during laparoscopy performed in the evaluation of a young woman with signs and symptoms of pelvic inflammatory disease. (*From* Mardh PA, Moller B, Paavonen J, *et al.*: Pelvic inflammatory disease. Edited by Mandell G. Philadelphia: Current Medicine; 1996.)

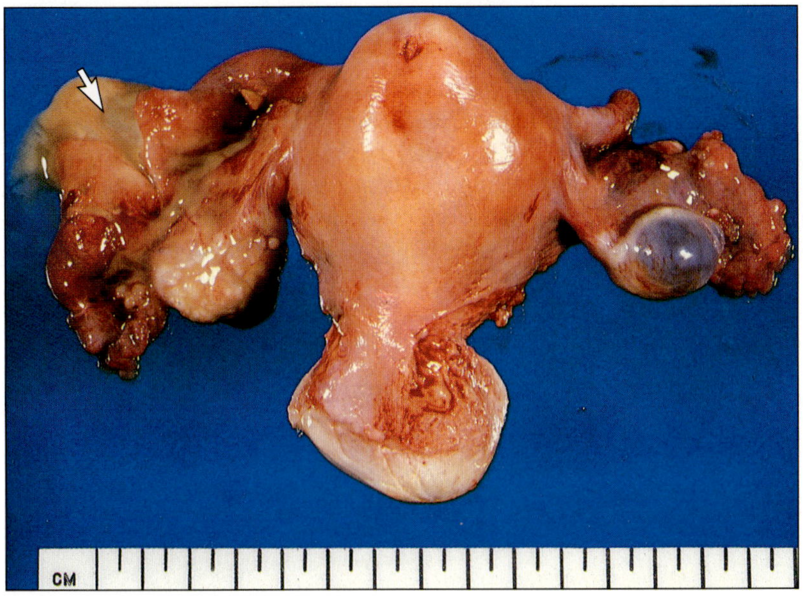

FIGURE 7-20.
Total abdominal hysterectomy and bilateral salpingo-oophorectomy performed for a tubo-ovarian abscess. Grossly purulent exudate is spilling from a ruptured right pyosalpinx (*arrow*). The surgical specimen is from a 39-year-old woman treated in 1978. Modern management of tubal infection emphasizes treatment with broad-spectrum antibiotics. Appropriately selected patients will usually not require surgical intervention. However, laparotomy is indicated when such conservative management fails, or when there is evidence the tubo-ovarian abscess has ruptured, or other diagnoses are suspected (*eg*, appendicitis, sigmoid diverticular abscess). Postmenopausal women should also undergo exploratory laparotomy, given the frequent (44%) association of tubo-ovarian abscess with gynecologic or colorectal malignancies.

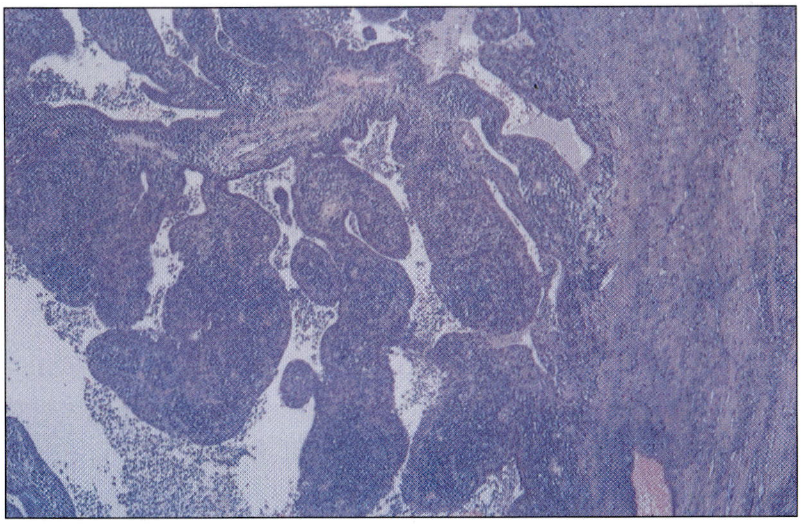

FIGURE 7-21.
Acute salpingitis. Histologic appearance of acute tubal infection, characterized by pus in the tubal lumen and an inflammatory infiltrate in the edematous papillary fronds. The surrounding tubal muscularis (*right*) is also edematous and inflamed. (*Courtesy of* David Dail, MD.)

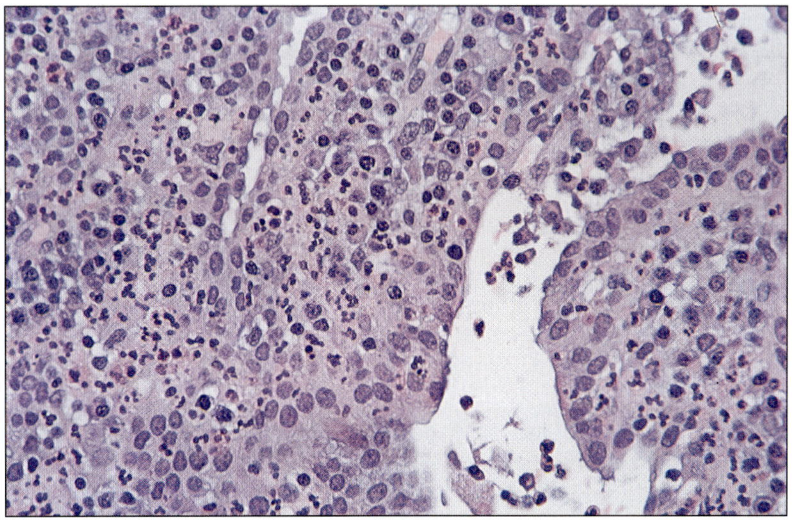

FIGURE 7-22.
Acute salpingitis. Polymorphonucleocytes dominate the inflammatory infiltrate in this high-power photomicrograph of salpingitis. Also note the loss of cilia and the destruction of normal tubal architecture. (*Courtesy of* David Dail, MD.)

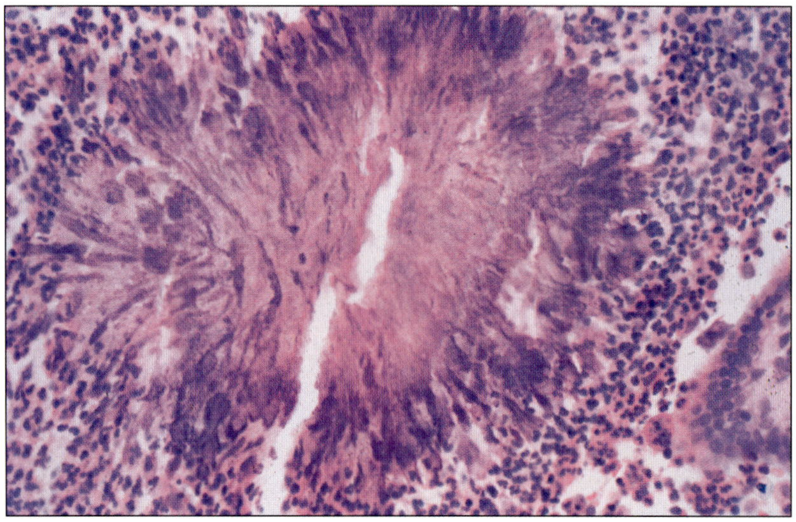

FIGURE 7-23.
Actinomyces "sulfur granule" formed by a colony of actinomyces within the tubal lumen. *Actinomyces israelii* is a gram-positive anaerobic bacterium with a branching filamentous appearance. It is not a pathogen unless normal mucosal barriers are disrupted, as can occur with use of an intrauterine contraceptive device. A chronic severe infection can then result, with the formation of large tubo-ovarian abscesses and extensive "woody" induration of all pelvic tissues. (*Courtesy of* Marit Ek, MD.)

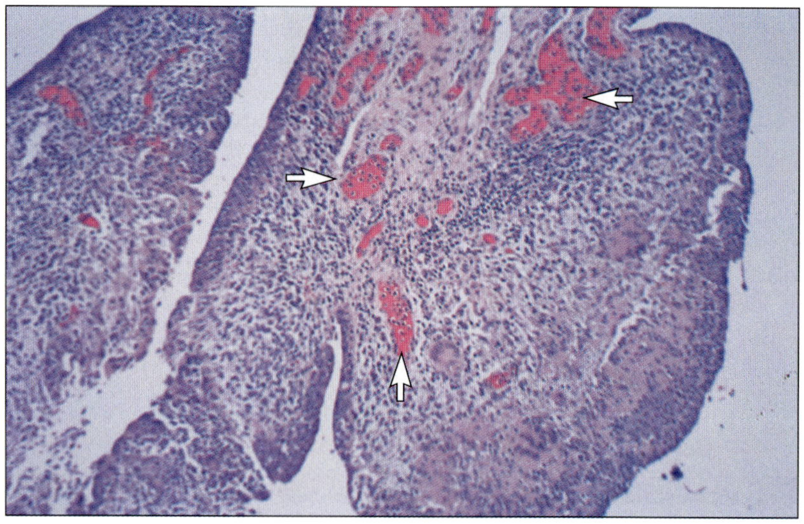

FIGURE 7-24.
Tuberculous salpingitis with Langhans' multinucleated giant cells (*arrows*). Tubal tuberculosis is not sexually transmitted; instead, it results from hematogenous spread in women with systemic tuberculosis. Tuberculosis of the genital tract had become rare in industrialized countries, but with increased immigration and the increased incidence of tuberculosis in patients with AIDS, genital tuberculosis is once again being encountered. Other causes of granulomatous salpingitis are reaction to foreign bodies, including instillation of radiographic contrast media, and sarcoidosis. (*Courtesy of* Marit Ek, MD.)

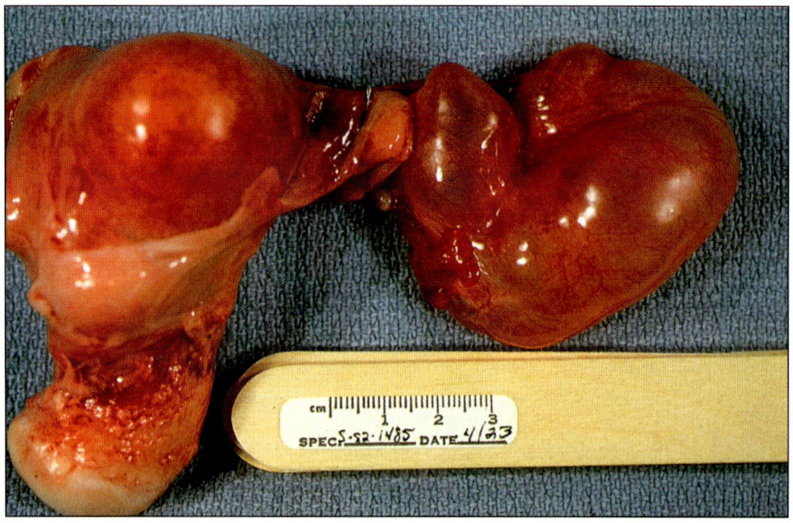

FIGURE 7-25.
Hydrosalpinx. Proximal and distal tubal occlusion following salpingitis may lead to the collection of sterile fluid in the lumen of the fallopian tube. A hydrosalpinx may cause pelvic pain and dyspareunia, or it may be asymptomatic. The surgical specimen shown is from a 65-year-old woman who underwent exploratory surgery and a total abdominal hysterectomy and bilateral salpingo-oophorectomy for a left complex adnexal mass, which was found to be a large but benign hydrosalpinx.

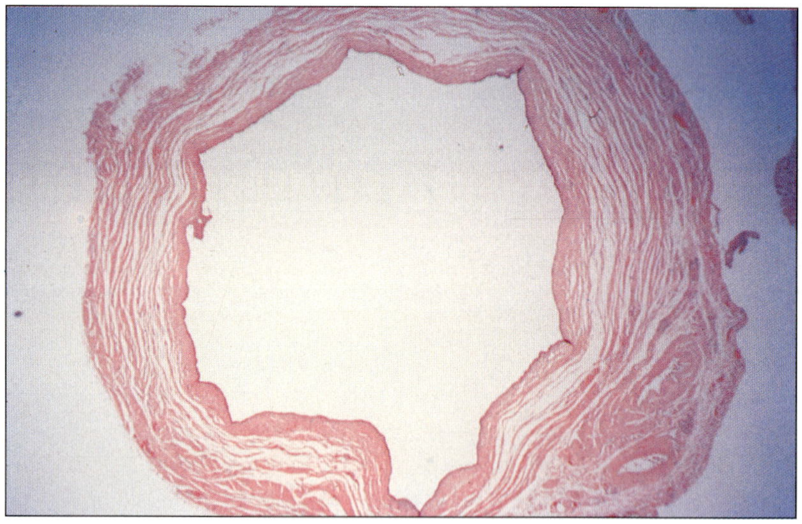

FIGURE 7-26.
Hydrosalpinx. The dilated tubal lumen is lined by simple cuboidal epithelium, with obliteration of the normally complex tubal architecture. Recovery of tubal function is unlikely, and infertility is therefore almost certain. (*Courtesy of* Marit Ek, MD.)

ECTOPIC PREGNANCY

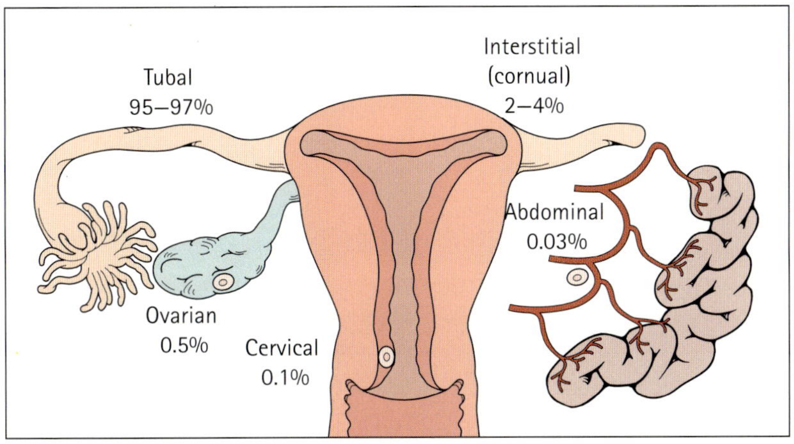

FIGURE 7-27.
Sites of ectopic pregnancies. Approximately 1% to 2% of all conceptions lead to an ectopic pregnancy, in which the developing blastocyst implants at a site other than the endometrial cavity. While over 95% of these errant implantations occur in the fallopian tube, and thus "ectopic" and "tubal" pregnancy are often considered synonyms, other implantation sites are possible (as illustrated). Prior tubal infection, endometriosis, and adhesions from pelvic surgery increase the risk of ectopic implantation as a result of altered structure or function of the fallopian tube.

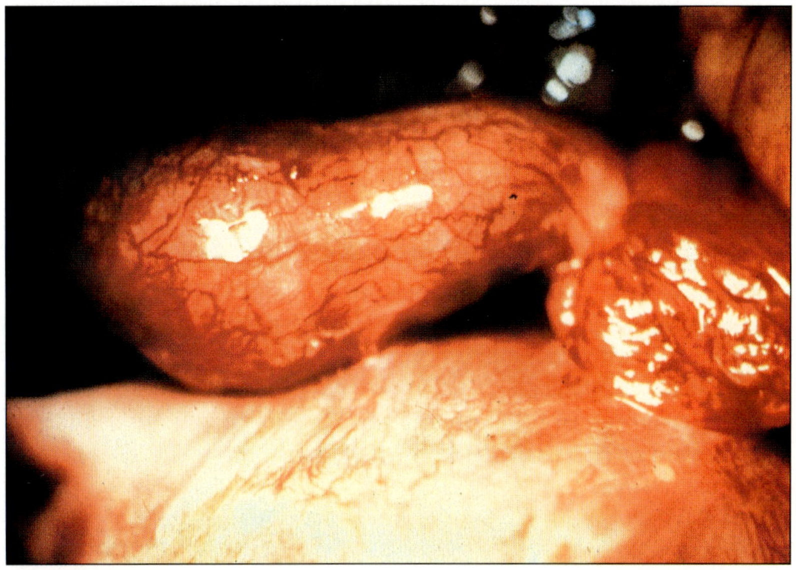

FIGURE 7-28.
Laparoscopic view of a tubal pregnancy. An ectopic gestation is within the ampullary portion of this swollen fallopian tube. Of tubal pregnancies, most occur in the ampulla (75% to 80%) with about 10% to 15% in the isthmus, 5% at the fimbria, and 2% to 4% within the interstitial (or cornual) portion. (*From* Mardh PA, Moller B, Paavonen I, *et al.*: Pelvic inflammatory disease. In *Atlas of Infectious Diseases*. Edited by Mandell G. Philadelphia: Current Medicine; 1996.)

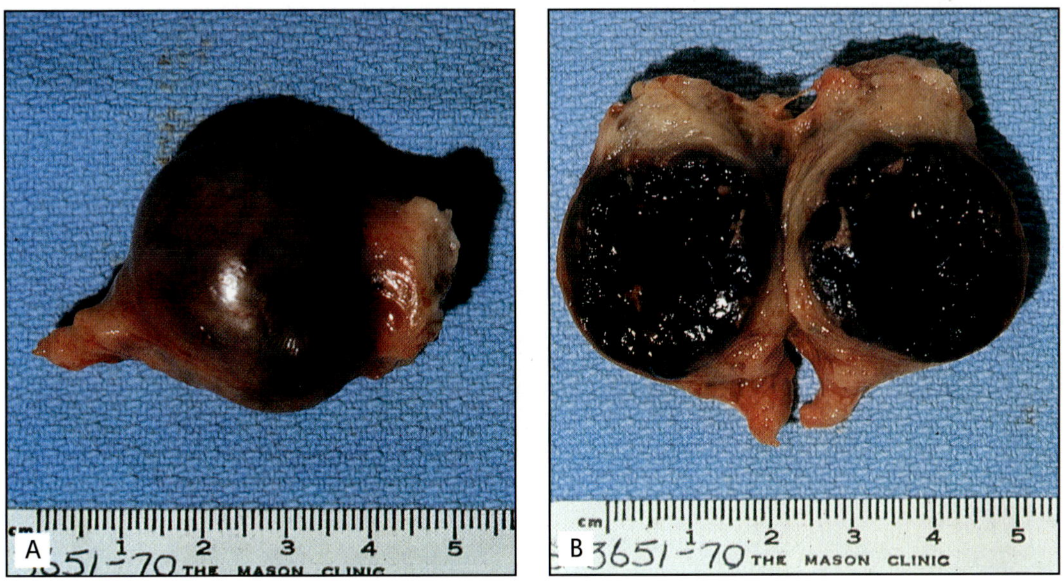

FIGURE 7-29.
Partial salpingectomy specimen with an unruptured 2- to 3-cm tubal pregnancy. The bluish-black discoloration of the intact surgical specimen (**A**) is due to the presence of organized blood clot (**B**) expanding the tubal lumen.

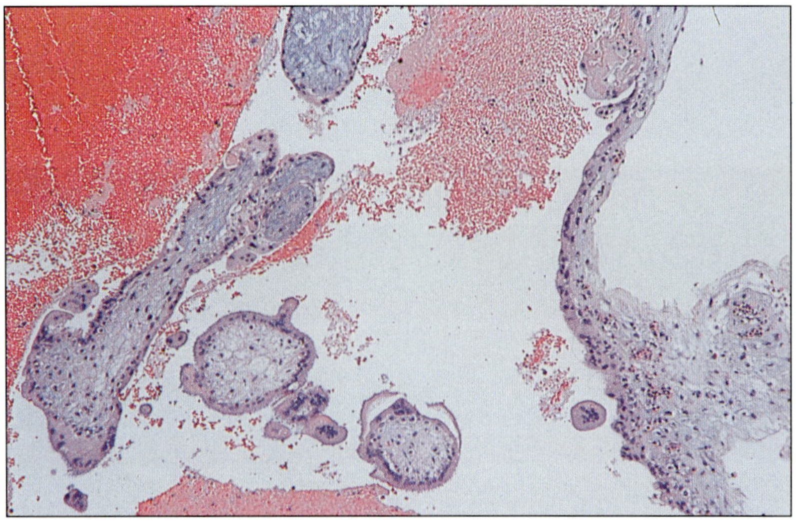

FIGURE 7-30.
Photomicrograph of tubal pregnancy. Chorionic villi are seen in a background of hemorrhage (*left–center*) next to a portion of gestational sac (*right*).

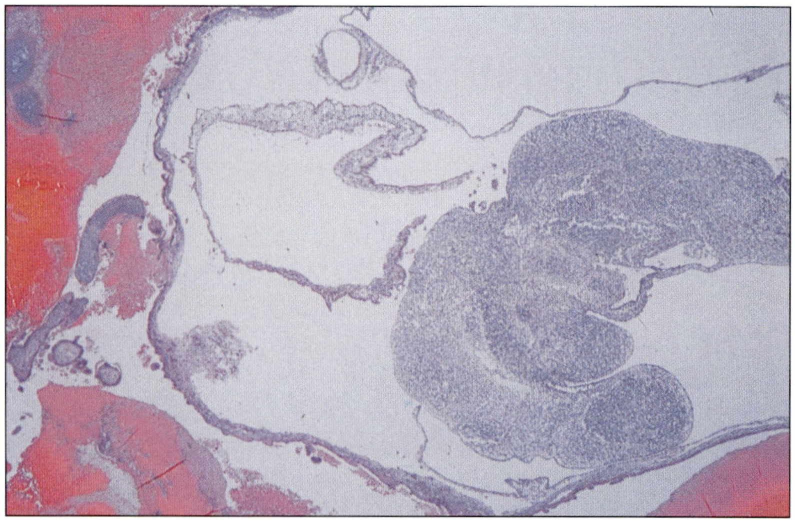

FIGURE 7-31.
Embryo of tubal pregnancy. Up to two thirds of tubal pregnancies contain a grossly or microscopically identifiable embryo. In this cross section of a tubal pregnancy, the early embryo is seen (*right*) inside the gestational sac. Some trophoblastic villi are also seen (*left*). (*Courtesy of* David Dail, MD)

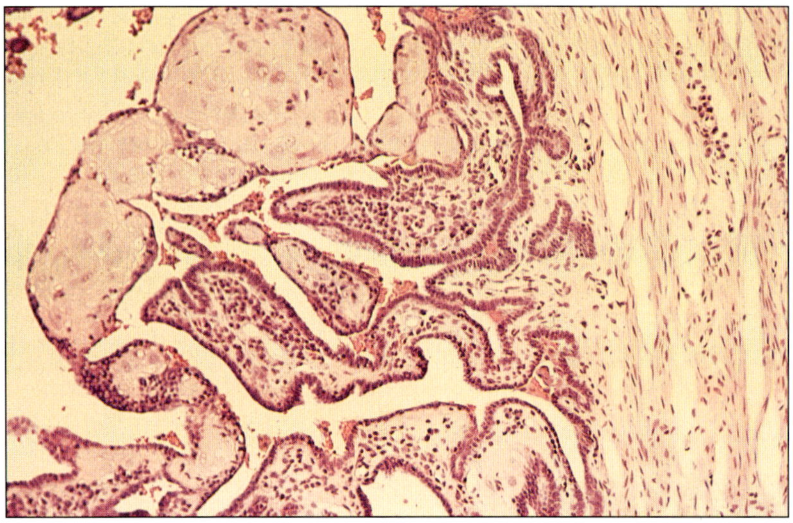

FIGURE 7-32.
Decidual reaction. Decidualization of the tubal epithelium and underlying stroma is a common finding in sections of fallopian tube excised from women with a tubal pregnancy. This reaction also occurs with normal pregnancies and after administration of exogenous progesterone.

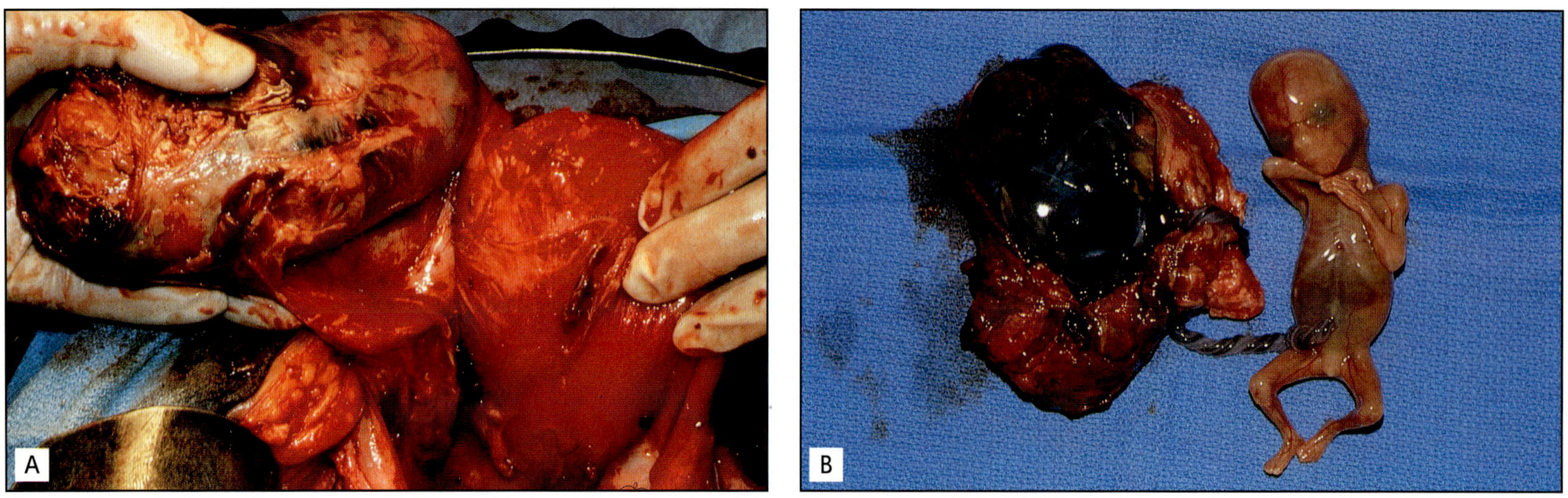

FIGURE 7-33.
Large tubal pregnancy. Intraoperative photograph (**A**) with surgeon holding a massively dilated left fallopian tube, which contained a 14-week fetus (**B**). It is rare, unless implantation occurs in the cornual region, for an ectopic gestation to remain viable into the second trimester. (*Courtesy of* Barbara Goff, MD.)

MALIGNANT NEOPLASMS OF THE FALLOPIAN TUBE

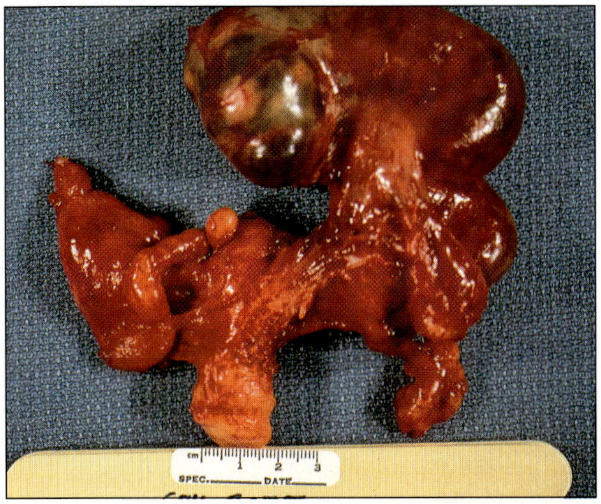

FIGURE 7-34.

Hysterectomy specimen with large malignant tumor of the left fallopian tube. Primary malignancies of the fallopian tube are very rare, comprising less than 0.5% of all female genital tract malignancies. Most women with tubal cancer are post-menopausal, typically in their sixth or seventh decade. The classic signs and symptoms of tubal cancer include vaginal bleeding, clear or serosanguineous vaginal discharge (hydrops tubae profluens), colicky pelvic pain, and a pelvic mass. Many patients, however, similar to women with advanced ovarian cancer, have the insidious onset of abdominal bloating and distention due to ascites, omental metastases, and peritoneal carcinomatosis.

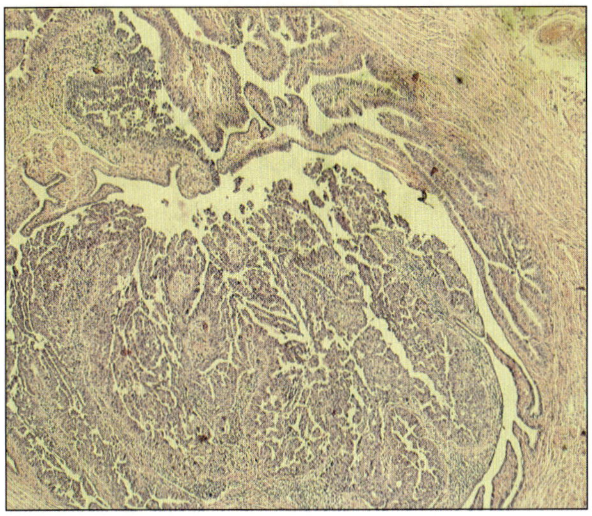

FIGURE 7-35.

Early tubal cancer. The tubal lumen is filled with papillary carcinoma with only minimal invasion of the surrounding muscularis. Such small, good-prognosis lesions comprise only about 10% of most large historical series. Nonetheless, perhaps because patients with fallopian tube cancer will more likely have worrisome clinical symptoms that prompt them to seek medical attention, the overall stage distribution for fallopian tube cancer is better than comparable patients with ovarian cancer. (*From* Muntz HG, *et al.*: Primary adenocarcinoma of the fallopian tube. *Eur J Gynaecol Oncol* 1989, 4:239.)

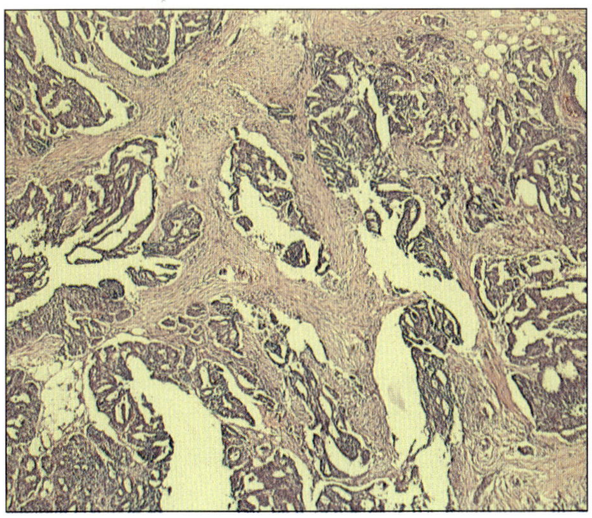

FIGURE 7-36.

Deeply invasive carcinoma of the fallopian tube. Destruction and penetration of the tubal wall, with subsequent peritoneal seeding, is common with fallopian tube cancer. Lymphatic spread is also important. The principal lymphatic drainage appears to be via the para-aortic lymph nodes. Pelvic or para-aortic nodal metastases have been identified in 10% to 30% of patients when careful surgical staging is performed.

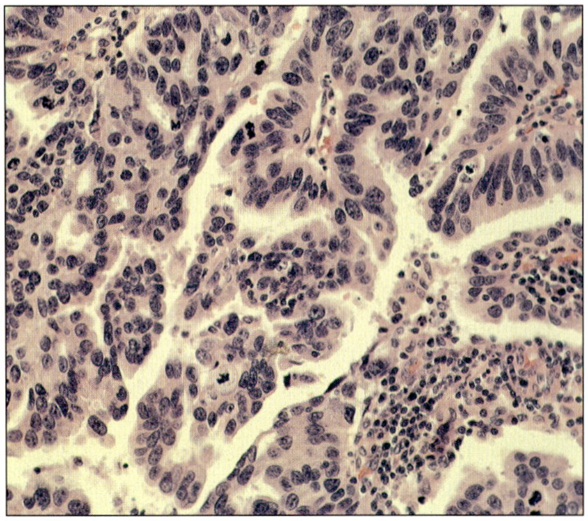

FIGURE 7-37.

Serous papillary carcinoma of the fallopian tube. The majority of tubal cancers are histologically similar to serous adenocarcinomas of the ovary. In this representative photomicrograph, fine branching papillae are covered by malignant epithelium with pleomorphic hyperchromatic enlarged nuclei. Other carcinoma subtypes are uncommon. When they do occur, they also mimic the histologic appearance of the comparable ovarian malignancy (such as endometrioid and clear cell carcinomas).

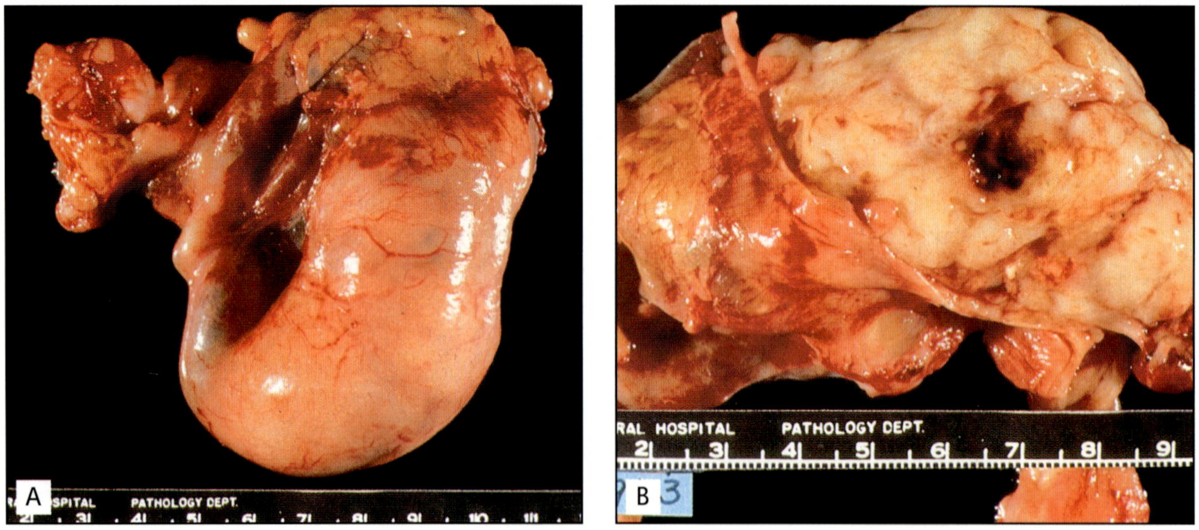

FIGURE 7-38.

Malignant mixed müllerian tumor of the fallopian tube. These unusual tumors of the female genital tract can rarely arise from the fallopian tube. Grossly, they are characterized by a distended tube (**A**), filled with solid, fleshy tumor (**B**), often with areas of central necrosis. (*A, from* Muntz HG, *et al.*: Carcinosarcomas and mixed müllerian tumors of the fallopian tube. *Gynecol Oncol* 1989, 34:109.)

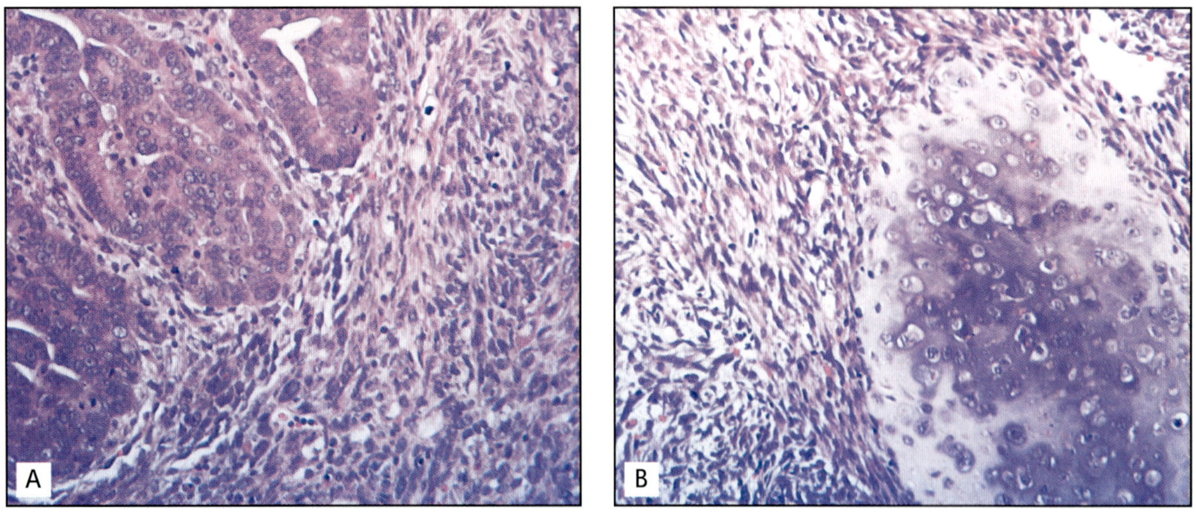

FIGURE 7-39.

A, Malignant mixed müllerian tumors of the fallopian tube contain, by definition, both malignant epithelial (*left*) and malignant mesenchymal elements (*right*). The sarcoma may consist of malignant elements homologous to the tube, such as smooth muscle or stroma. The term "carcinosarcoma" is also used for homologous tumors. **B,** Heterologous sarcomatous components are also encountered, such as the chondrosarcoma pictured.

FIGO STAGING FOR FALLOPIAN TUBE NEOPLASMS

Stage 0	Stage 1	Stage 2	Stage 3	Stage 4
Carcinoma *in situ*	Growth limited to the fallopian tubes	Pelvic extension	Peritoneal or omental implants outside the pelvis and/or positive retroperitoneal or inguinal nodes	Distant metastases

FIGURE 7-40.
International Federation of Gynecology and Obstetrics (FIGO) staging for fallopian tube malignancies. Recognizing the similarity between fallopian tube and ovarian cancers, the current FIGO staging system for fallopian tube cancer closely parallels that of ovarian cancer.

SELECTED BIBLIOGRAPHY

Markman M, Zaino R, Fleming P, Barakat R: Carcinoma of the fallopian tube. In *Principles and Practices of Gynecologic Oncology*, edn 2. Edited by Hoskins WJ, Perez CA, Young RC. New York: Lippincott-Raven; 1997:1025–1038.

Wheeler JE. Diseases of the fallopian tube. In *Blaustein's Pathology of the Female Genital Tract*, edn 4. Edited by Kurman RJ. New York: Springer-Verlag; 1994:529–561.

Wiesenfeld HC, Sweet RL: Progress in the management of tuboovarian abscesses. *Clin Obstet Gynecol* 1993, 36:433–444.

Wiesenfeld HC, Sweet RL: Tuboovarian abscess. In *Atlas of Infectious Diseases*. Edited by Mandell G. Philadelphia: Current Medicine; 1996.

Woodruff JD, Angtuaco TL, Parmley TH: The fallopian tube. In *Atlas of Gynecologic Pathology*. New York: Raven Press; 1993:6.1–6.30.

Epithelial Tumors of the Ovary

CHAPTER 8

Melissa D. Gordon and Karen Ireland

Ovarian neoplasms thought to be derived from surface epithelium are referred to as epithelial or epithelial surface tumors and are separated into five morphologic categories based on cell type: serous, mucinous, endometrioid, clear cell, and transitional (Brenner). As endorsed by the International Federation of Gynecology and Obstetrics (FIGO) and the World Health Organization (WHO), epithelial tumors of the ovary are further subdivided into benign, low malignant potential (borderline or proliferating), and malignant. As a group, the tumors of low malignant potential demonstrate architectural complexity, epithelial stratification and cytologic atypia but lack the destructive stromal invasion seen in frank carcinoma. Additionally, neoplasms in this intermediate category are often associated with extraovarian lesions, referred to as "implants," which, despite widespread involvement or worrisome microscopic features, have a very good prognosis (75% to 90% of patients survive more than 10 years [1–3]). Of the five cell types, serous tumors are the most frequently encountered. Often, more than one cell type is identified within a single tumor. If the second epithelial component comprises at least 10% of the lesion, the term "mixed" epithelial tumor should be used.

Epithelial ovarian tumors are the fifth most commonly occurring tumors in women and are associated with the highest mortality rate of neoplastic disorders of the female genital tract. The following factors are associated with an increased incidence of ovarian neoplasia: low parity, infertility, caucasian race, postmenopausal, and family history of ovarian cancer. Recent investigations suggest that use of oral contraceptives provides a protective effect against the development of invasive ovarian carcinoma [4,5].

Histopathologic grading requires determination of the degree of solid growth within an adequately sampled neoplasm. Grade I tumors have a marked predominance of papillary or glandular growth with less than 5% solid or sheetlike foci. Grade II lesions demonstrate 5% to 50% solid component, whereas tumors categorized as grade III show greater than 50% solid growth. Squamous morules, often accompanying the endometrioid cell type, should not be confused with solid foci within a neoplasm. The degree of cytologic atypia generally parallels the grade. FIGO staging of ovarian epithelial tumors, based on pathologic and surgical findings, takes into account the histologic grading and cell type, as well as assessment of involvement of peritoneal washings and ascites fluid (*see* Fig. 8-1).

FIGO STAGING FOR CARCINOMA OF THE OVARY

Stage I	Growth limited to the ovaries
Stage IA	Growth limited to one ovary; no ascites present containing malignant cells. No tumor on the external surface; capsule intact
Stage IB	Growth limited to both ovaries; no ascites present containing malignant cells. No tumor on the external surfaces; capsule intact
Stage IC*	Tumor classified as either stage IA or IB but with tumor on the surface of one or both ovaries; or with ruptured capsule(s); or with ascites containing malignant cells present or with positive peritoneal washings
Stage II	Growth involving one or both ovaries, with pelvic extension
Stage IIA	Extension and metastases to the uterus and tubes
Stage IIB	Extension to other pelvic tissues
Stage IIC*	Tumor either stage IIA or IIB but with tumor on the surface of one or both ovaries; or with capsule(s) ruptured; or with ascites containing malignant cells present or with positive peritoneal washings
Stage III	Tumor involving one or both ovaries with peritoneal implants outside the pelvis or positive retroperitoneal or inguinal nodes. Superficial liver metastasis equals stage III. Tumor is limited to the true pelvis but with histologically proven malignant extension to small bowel or omentum
Stage IIIA	Tumor grossly limited to the true pelvis with negative nodes but with histologically confirmed microscopic seeding of abdominal peritoneal surfaces
Stage IIIB	Tumor of one or both ovaries with histologically confirmed implants of abdominal peritoneal surfaces none exceeding 2 cm in diameter; nodes are negative
Stage IIIC	Abdominal implants greater than 2 cm in diameter and/or positive retroperitoneal or inguinal nodes
Stage IV	Growth involving one or both ovaries with distant metastases. If pleural effusion is present, there must be positive cytologic findings to allot a case to stage IV. Parenchymal liver metastasis equals Stage IV.

** Notes about the staging: To evaluate the impact on prognosis of the different criteria for allotting cases to stage IC or IIC, it would be of value to know whether the rupture of the capsule was spontaneous or caused by the surgeon and if the source of malignant cells detected was peritoneal washings or ascites.*

FIGURE 8-1.
FIGO staging for carcinoma of the ovary. (*From* International Federation of Gynecology and Obstetrics (FIGO) [6].)

SEROUS TUMORS

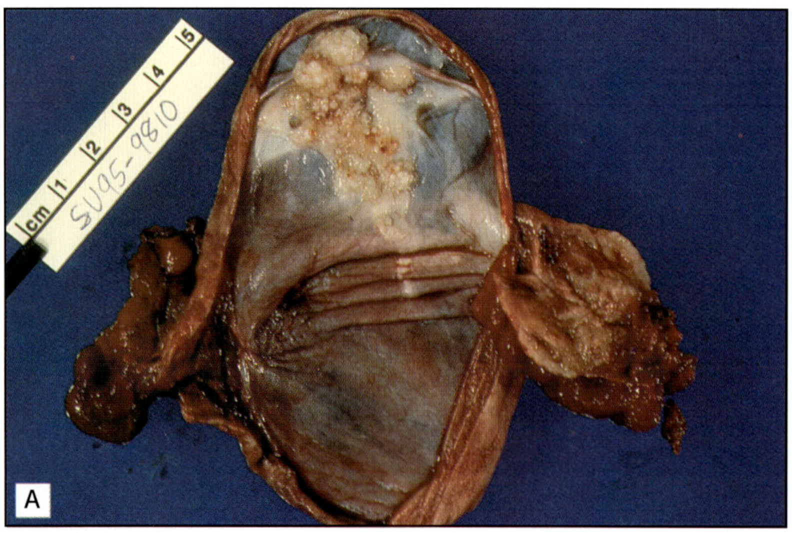

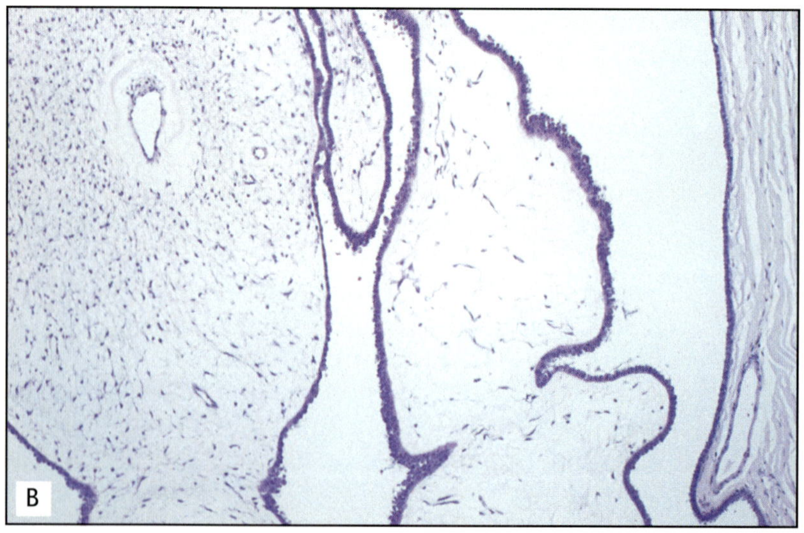

FIGURE 8-2.
Benign serous tumors. Nearly 25% of all benign ovarian neoplasms are serous in nature. These tumors may be uni- or multiloculated and are bilateral in 15% to 20% of patients. Papillary structures frequently occur and often are grossly visible as excrescences on the inner and outer surfaces of the cysts. **A**, Open serous ovarian neoplasm. Microscopically, the papillae consist of loose myxoid connective tissue (**B**) with a single layer of columnar lining epithelium that closely resembles fallopian tube mucosa, including

(*Continued on next page*)

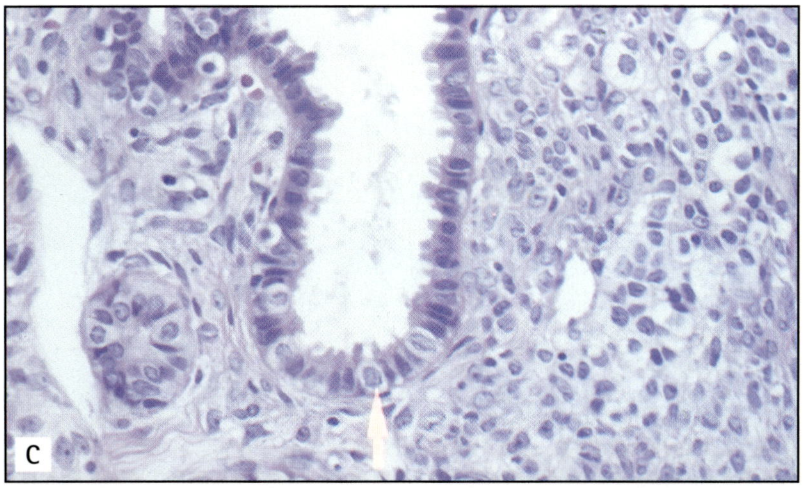

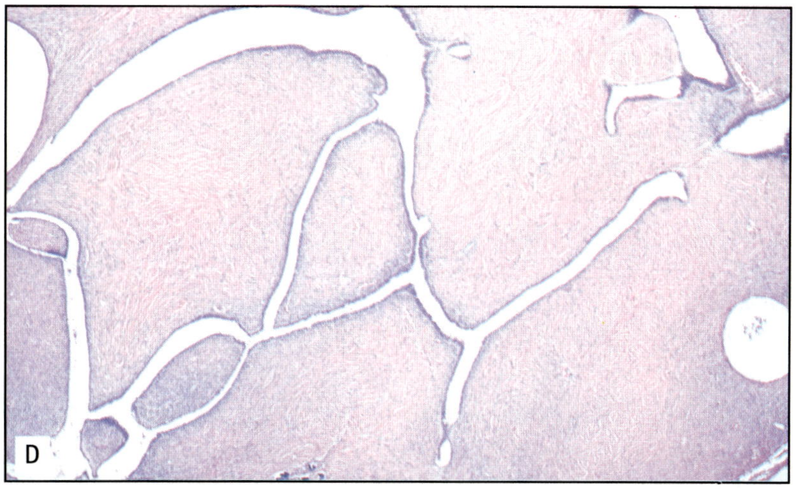

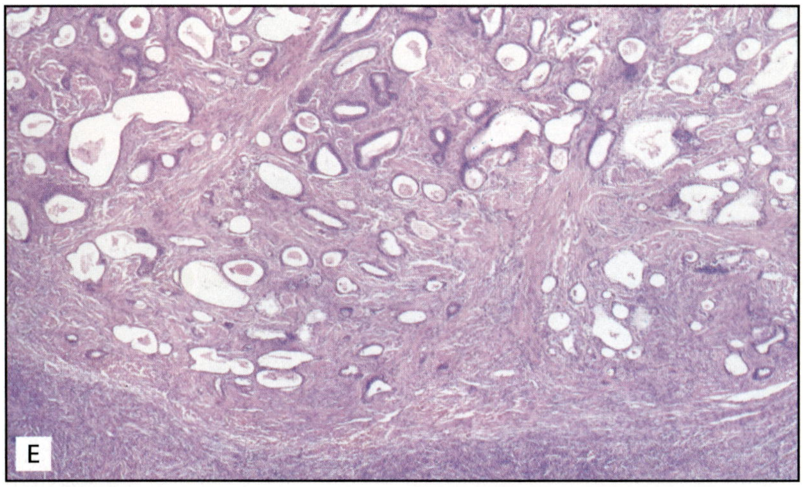

FIGURE 8–2 *(Continued)*

ciliated and peg cells (**C**, *arrow* denotes a peg cell). Moreover, cuboidal cells are often encountered, especially in large cysts where the lining is attenuated. Serous adenofibroma describes lesions which, in addition to the epithelial features above, have an abundant amount of dense fibrous stroma (**D** and **E**). (*B* to *E*, photomicrographs, H & E stain; Original magnification, *B* × 100, *C* × 400, *D* and *E* × 40.)

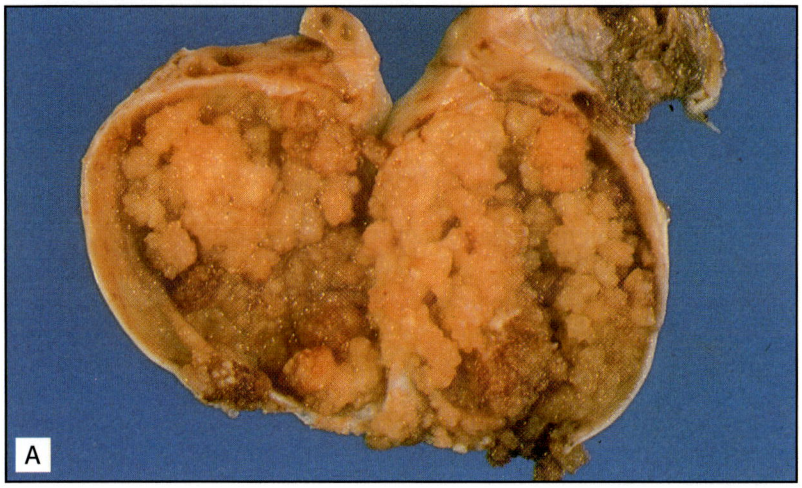

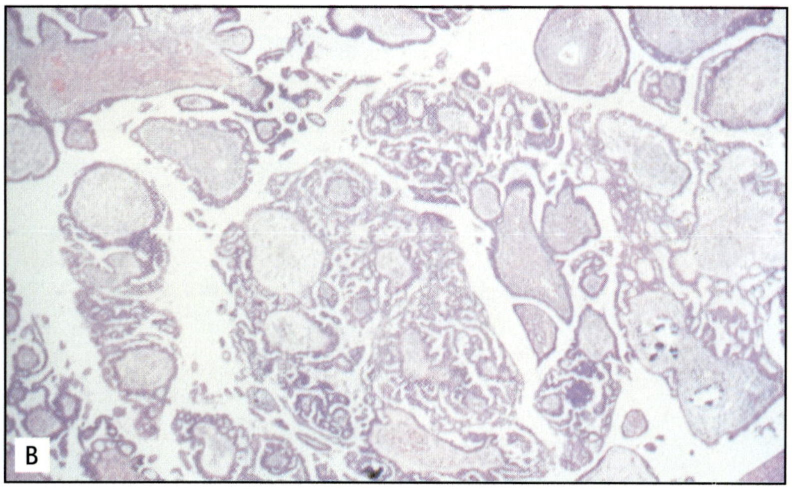

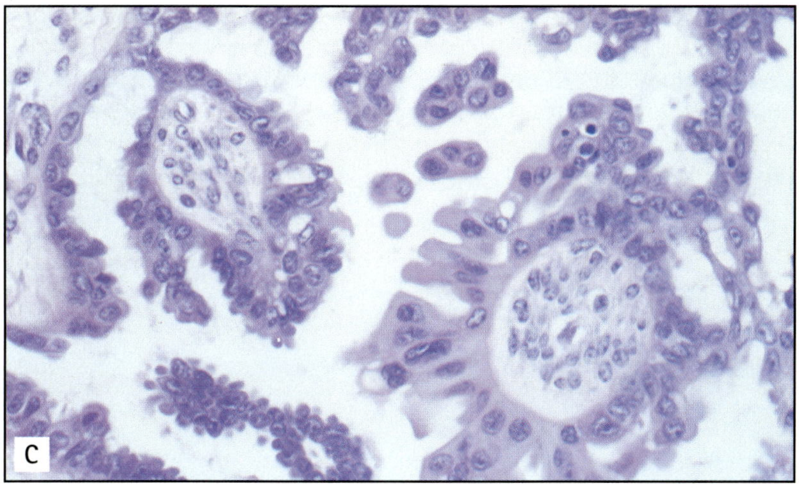

FIGURE 8–3.

Low malignant potential (LMP) serous tumors. Serous tumors of low malignant potential account for approximately 15% of ovarian serous neoplasms and generally occur in postmenopausal women. Usually multicystic, these tumors tend to have numerous friable papillary projections not only protruding into the cystic spaces but also present on the external surface. Macroscopic borderline tumor (**A**). Microscopically, there is complex arborizing papillary architecture (**B**), as well as epithelial stratification and cellular budding (**C**). Cytologically, the tumor cells may resemble those of benign serous tumors or show mild pleomorphism with prominent nucleoli. Fifty percent of LMP serous tumors have psammoma bodies.

(*Continued on next page*)

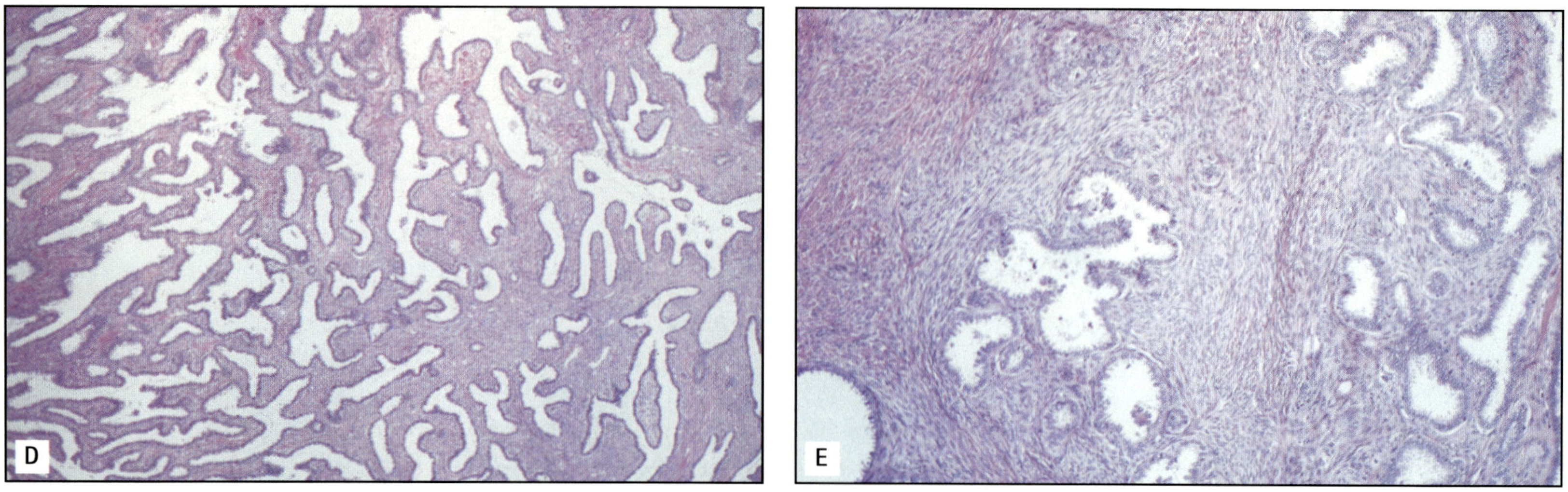

FIGURE 8-3. *(Continued)* Although rare, adenofibromatous serous tumors showing similar architectural and cytologic complexity do exist and are referred to as proliferating adenofibromas (**D** and **E**). The vast majority of these neoplasms behave in a benign fashion. (*B to* E, photomicrographs, H & E stain; Original magnification, *A* × 40, *C* × 400, *D* × 40, *E* × 100.)

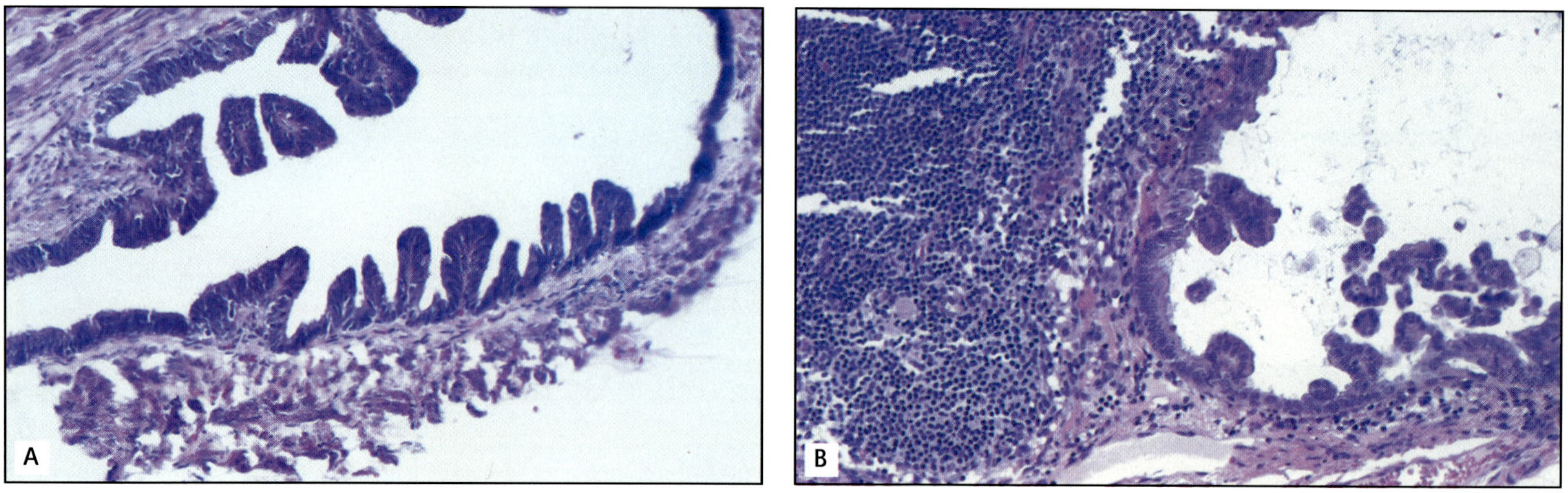

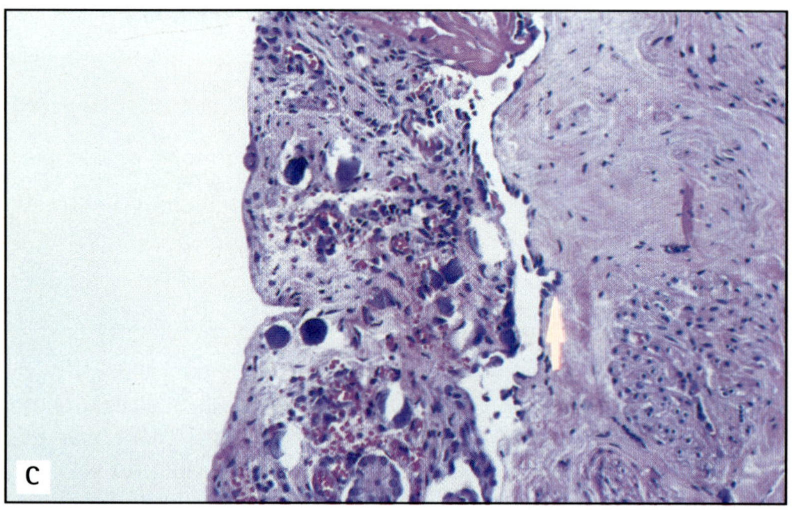

FIGURE 8-4.
Noninvasive implants occurring with low malignant potential (LMP) serous tumors. Twenty to forty percent of patients with LMP serous tumors have extraovarian serous proliferations that typically appear histologically similar to the primary ovarian neoplasm. Two types of implants have been described. Noninvasive implants are the most frequently encountered and are subdivided into epithelial and desmoplastic [1]. **A** and **B**, The epithelial subtype consists of smoothly contoured foci composed of serous epithelium showing mild to moderate cytologic atypia. (*A*) shows a peritoneal implant; (*B*) is a pelvic lymph node implant. The underlying tissue does not demonstrate a desmoplastic reaction. **C**, The second subtype is termed "desmoplastic" owing to the fibroblastic stromal reaction that is limited to the surface peritoneum or fibrous omental septa containing the noninvasive implant (*arrow* denotes surface mesothelial lining, to the right of the desmoplastic implant). Psammoma bodies are common in either type. (Photomicrographs, H & E stain; Original magnification, × 200.)

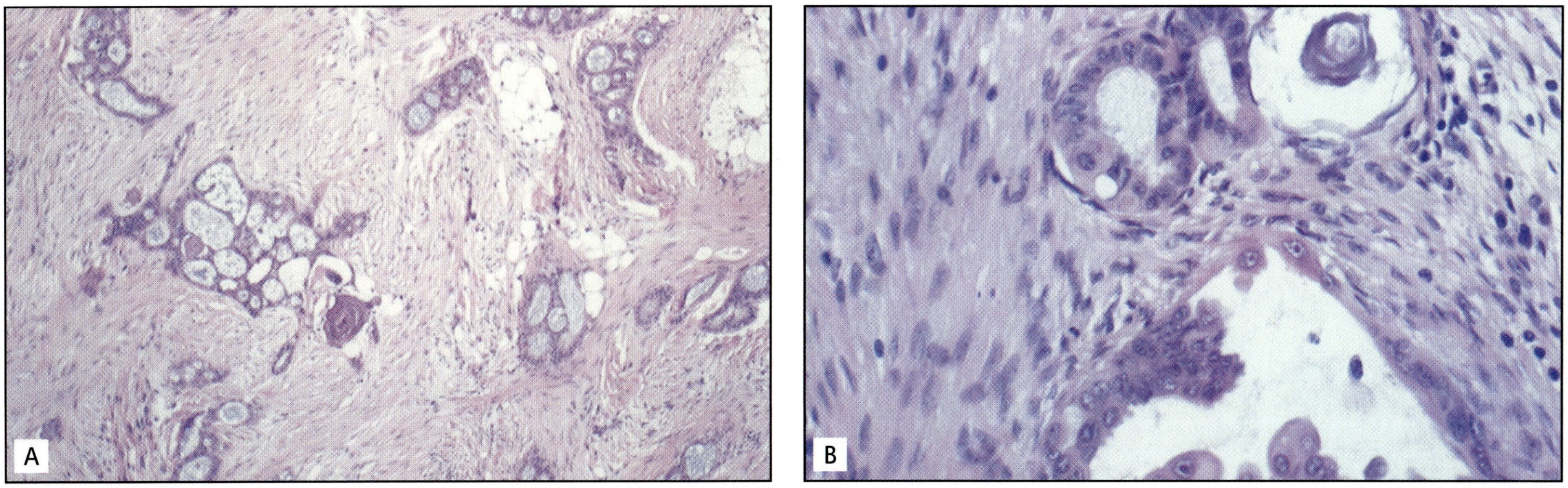

FIGURE 8-5.

Invasive implants found with low malignant potential (LMP) serous tumors. Invasive implants are much less common and comprise the second type of implant found in serous tumors of LMP. **A**, A marked and diffuse desmoplastic stromal response is mounted against these irregular, jagged glandular proliferations. **B**, Unlike noninvasive implants, marked cytologic atypia is often noted. Because patients may have both patterns of implants, it is recommended that the lesions be classified according to the most infiltrative type. Controversy exists as to the prognostic significance of the histologic appearance of peritoneal implants [1,2,7–9]. (Photomicrographs, H & E stain; Original magnification, $A \times 100$, $B \times 400$.)

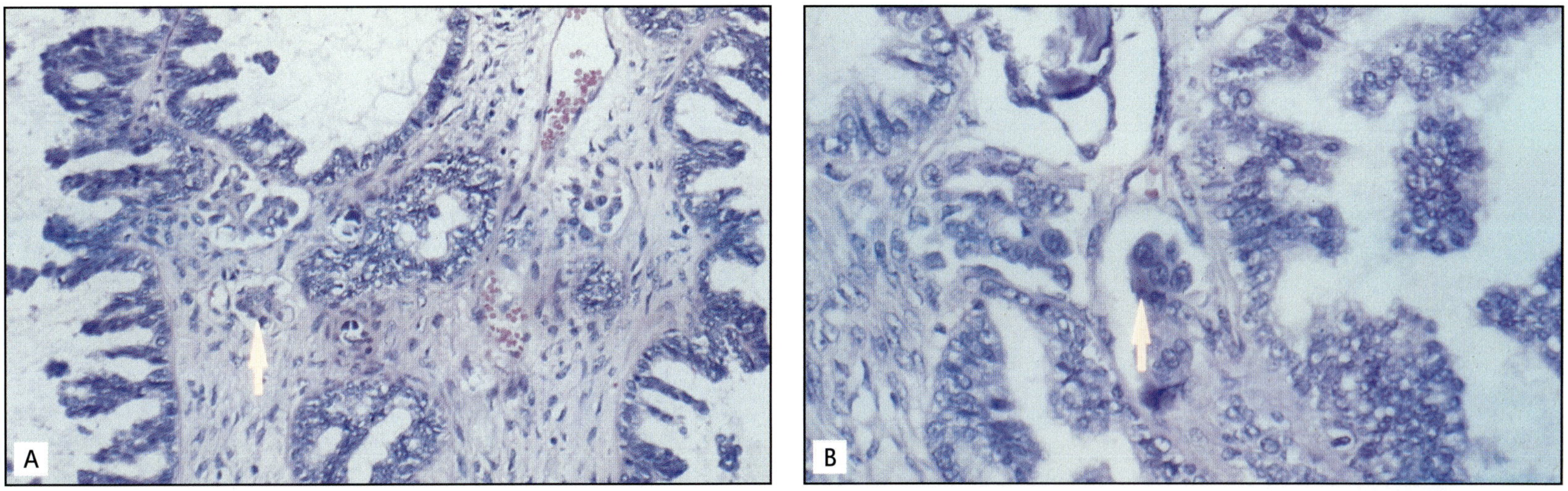

FIGURE 8-6.

Stromal microinvasion. Only recently has microinvasion in serous tumors of low malignant potential (LMP) been recognized. From the few cases investigated, it appears that tumors with stromal microinvasion behave in a similar manner as LMP serous tumors of the same stage [10–12]. In addition to the usual features seen in serous tumors of LMP, tumors with microinvasion typically demonstrate a population of cells with abundant eosinophilic cytoplasm infiltrating the stromal stalk of the papillae (**A** and **B**; *arrows* on invasive foci). A desmoplastic stromal response may or may not be present. Bell and Scully [10] define foci of microinvasion as being no greater than 3mm in maximum dimension. (Photomicrographs, H & E stain; Original magnification, $A \times 200$, $B \times 400$.)

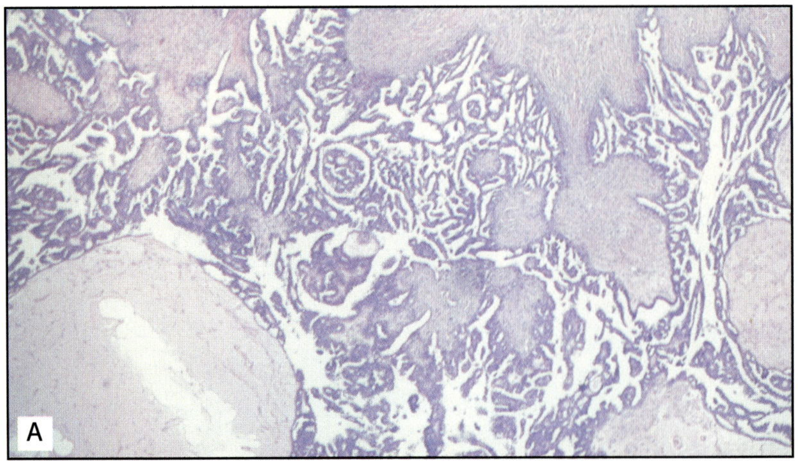

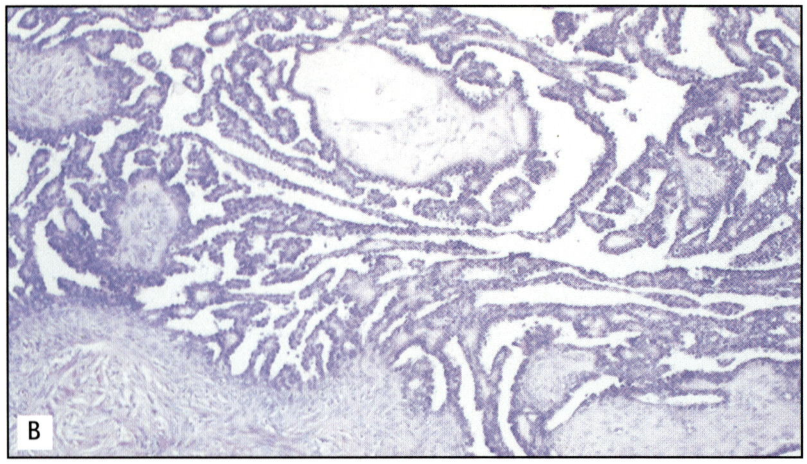

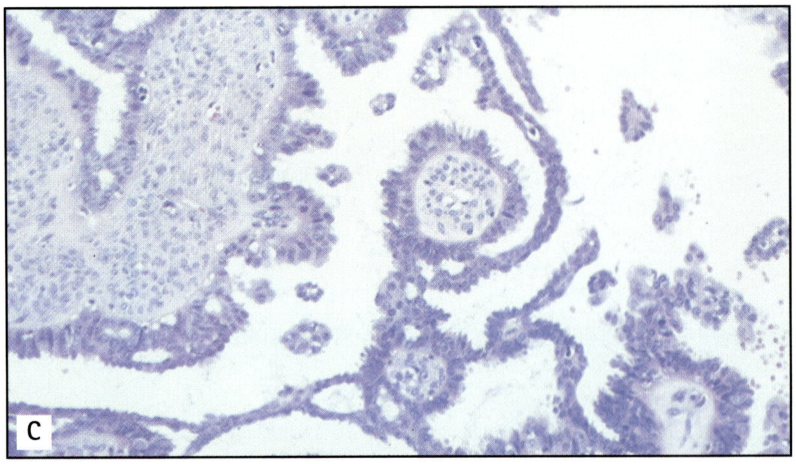

FIGURE 8–7.

Micropapillary type of serous tumors. Recent interest has been shown in investigating the significance of certain unusual patterns in serous tumors of low malignant potential (LMP). Of particular controversy is the so-called micropapillary type, which has a filigree pattern of complex micropapillae arising from larger papillary structures (**A** and **B**). The cytologic features are identical to those described in serous tumors of LMP, including cellular budding (**C**). Although some authors argue that neoplasms exhibiting this pattern have a worse prognosis stage for stage than usual serous tumors of LMP [13], others have found no difference in patient outcome [14]. Additional studies will be necessary to resolve this issue. (Photomicrographs, H & E stain; Original magnification, *A* × 40, *B* × 100, *C* × 200.)

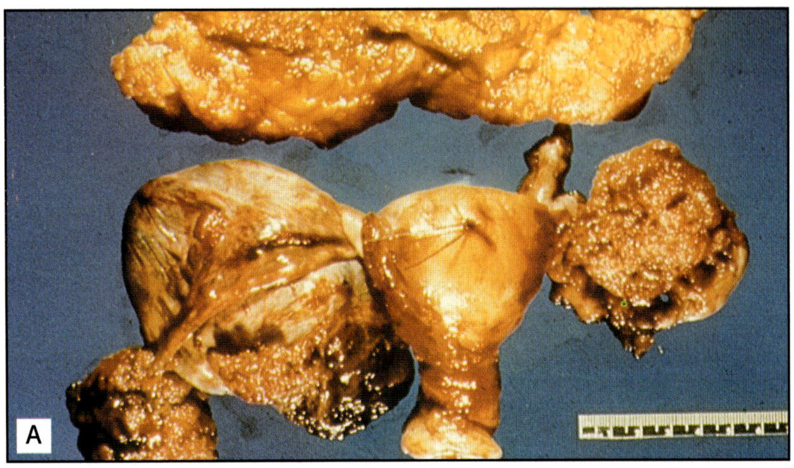

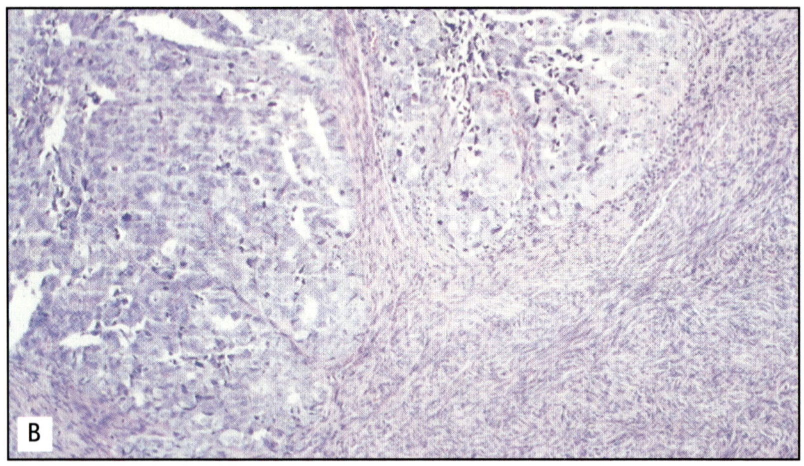

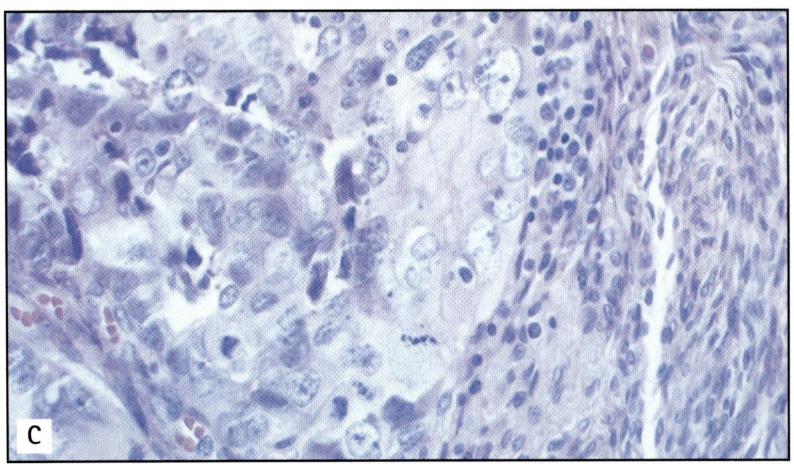

FIGURE 8–8.

Histologic criteria for stromal invasion. Separation of serous tumors of low malignant potential (LMP) from invasive serous carcinoma is characterized by destructive stromal invasion, as defined by the World Health Organization and the International Federation of Gynecology and Obstetrics. Morphologic patterns accepted for stromal invasion in serous tumors [15] include 1) irregularly shaped glands in an edematous stroma; 2) irregular small projections of cells infiltrating the stroma; 3) back-to-back glands without intervening stroma; 4) randomly distributed clusters of cells surrounded by a clear space; 5) small clusters or individual cells infiltrating the stroma.

Two thirds of serous carcinomas are bilateral (**A**) and occur typically between the ages of 45 and 65. The neoplasms range histologically from well-differentiated tumors with numerous papillary structures with mild cellular atypia to poorly differentiated tumors forming solid sheets of markedly pleomorphic cells (**B** and **C**). (*B* and *C*, Photomicrographs, H & E stain; Original magnification, *B* × 200, *C* × 400.)

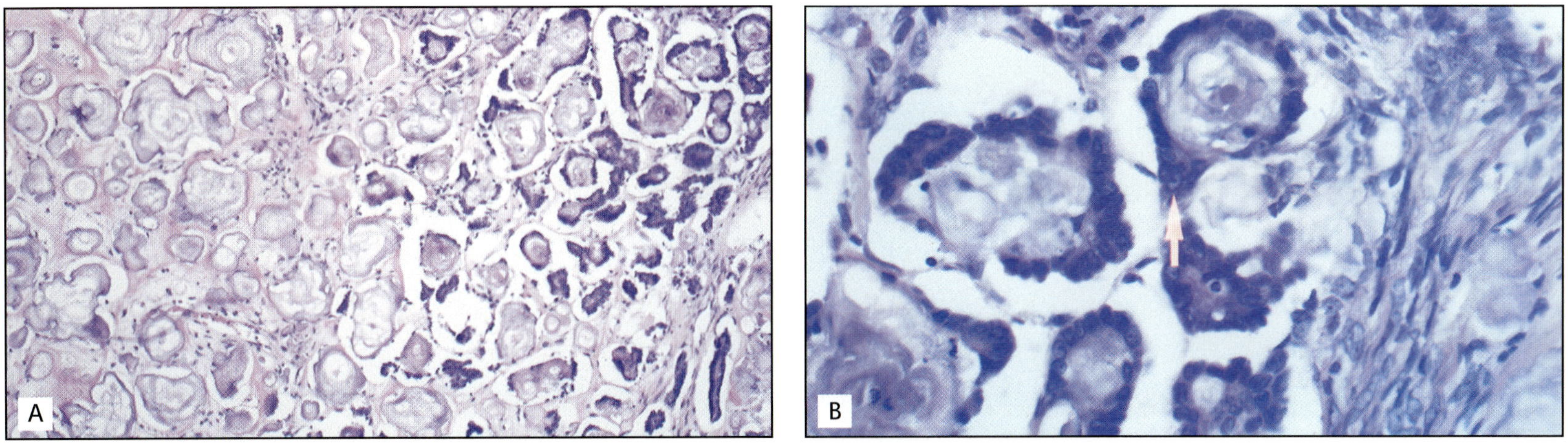

FIGURE 8-9.

Serous psammocarcinoma. Serous psammocarcinoma is a rare ovarian neoplasm characterized by a predominance of psammoma bodies, often coalescing to form lobulated calcified masses. Note the numerous round laminated basophilic structures (psammoma bodies) (**A**). Small clusters and papillae of mildly atypical epithelial cells are present (**B**) but make up less than 25% of the lesion. Although, classified as a carcinoma due to the stromal invasion, these neoplasms have a natural history more akin to serous tumors of low malignant potential [16]. (Photomicrographs, H & E stain; Original magnification, *A* × 100, *B* × 400.)

MUCINOUS TUMORS

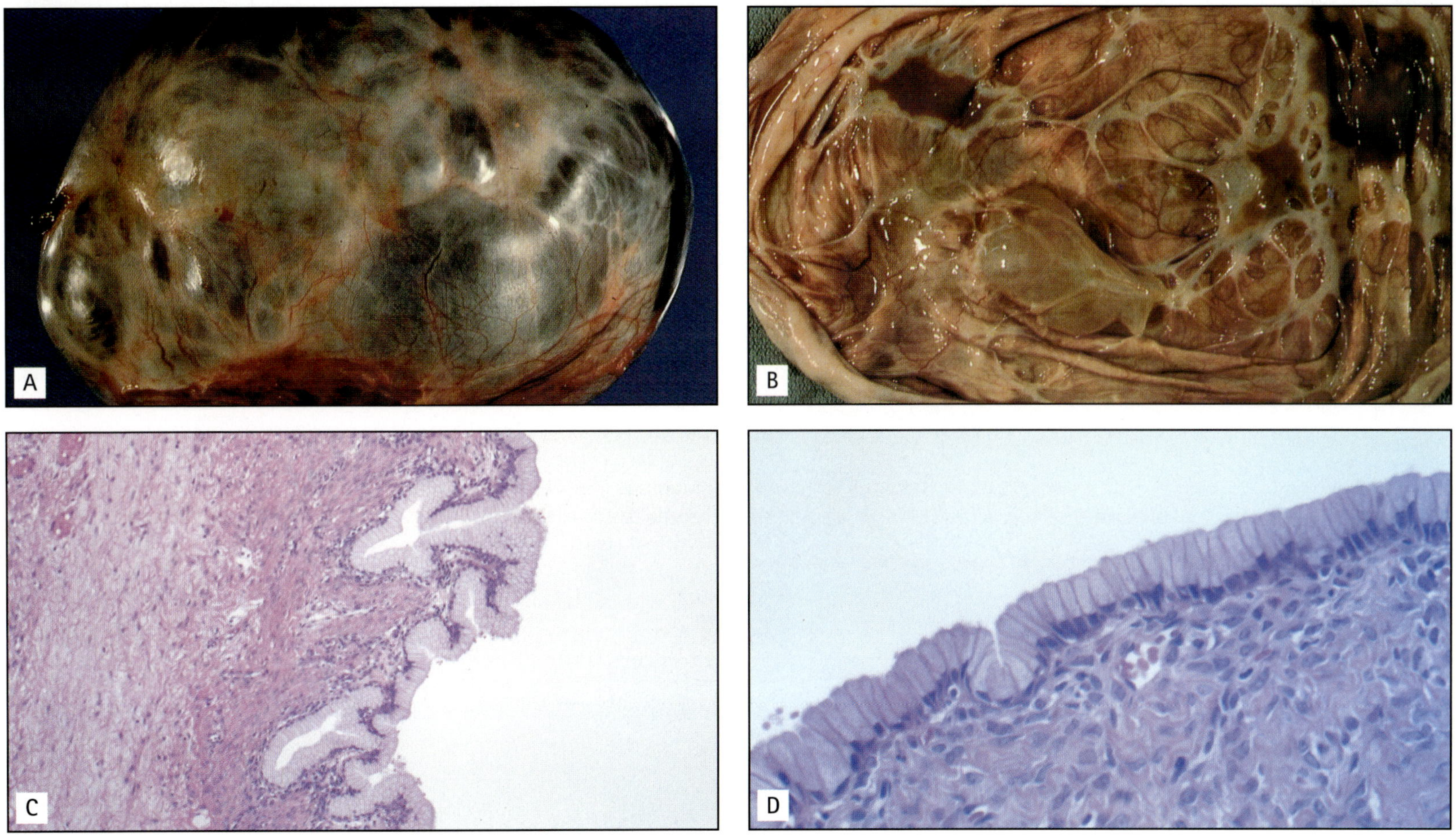

FIGURE 8-10.

Benign mucinous cysts. The most common mucinous ovarian neoplasms are benign mucinous cysts, constituting approximately 25% of all benign ovarian tumors. Usually multiloculated, these tumors contain thick gelatinous material within the cysts (**A** and **B**). The single layered lining epithelium may be of intestinal or endocervical type. The intestinal type (**C** and **D**) is composed of mucinous columnar cells with basally oriented nuclei intermixed with goblet cells and occasional Paneth cells. Approximately 50% of these lesions have a predominance of epithelia that are uniform tall columnar mucinous cells, the so-called endocervical type. While coarse papillae may be present, complex branching, nuclear atypia and multilayering of the lining epithelium are features not seen in benign mucinous tumors. If such findings are encountered, one should consider a diagnosis of a tumor of low malignant potential. (*C* and *D*, photomicrographs, H & E stain; Original magnification, *C* × 200, *D* × 400)

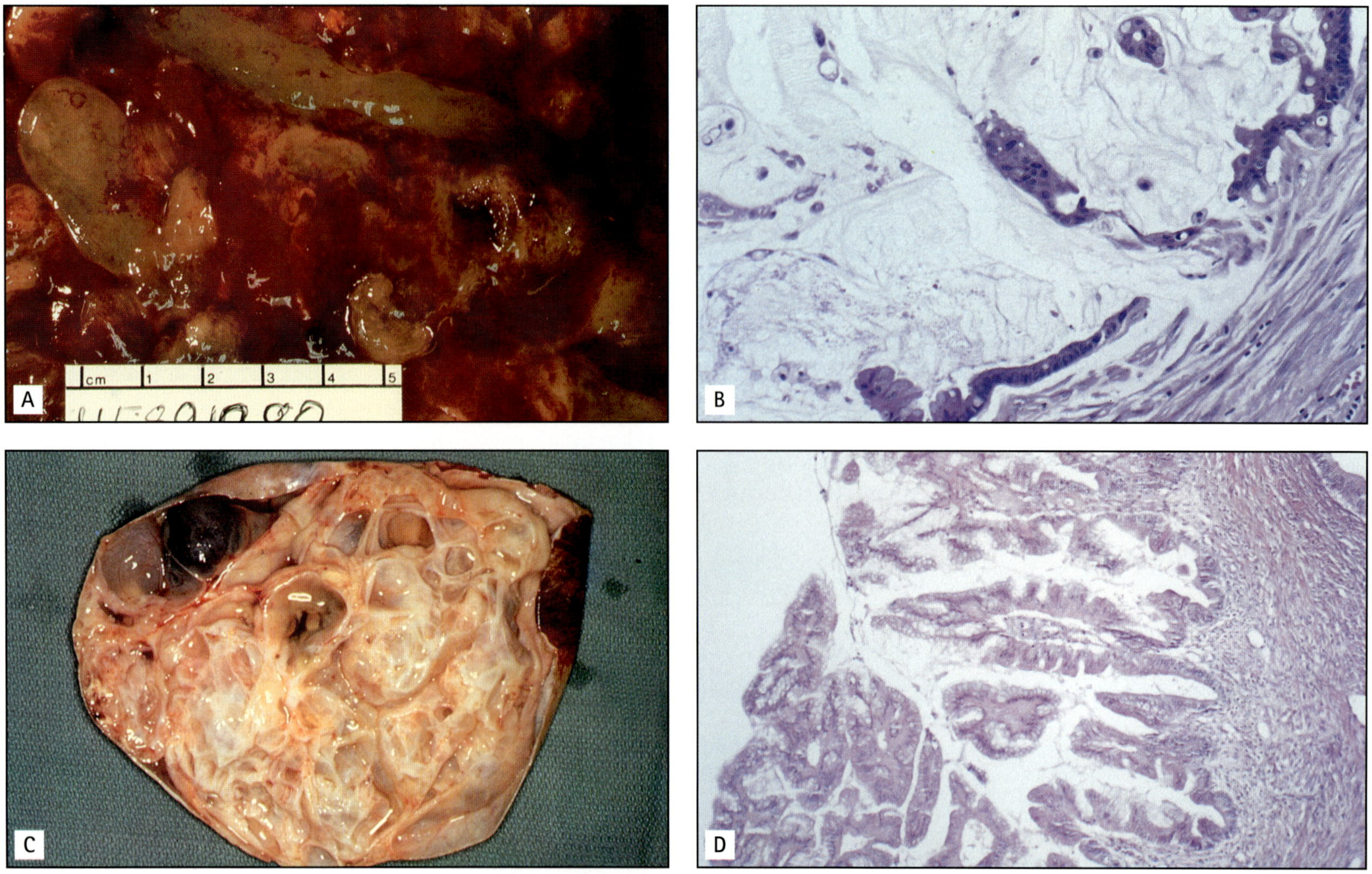

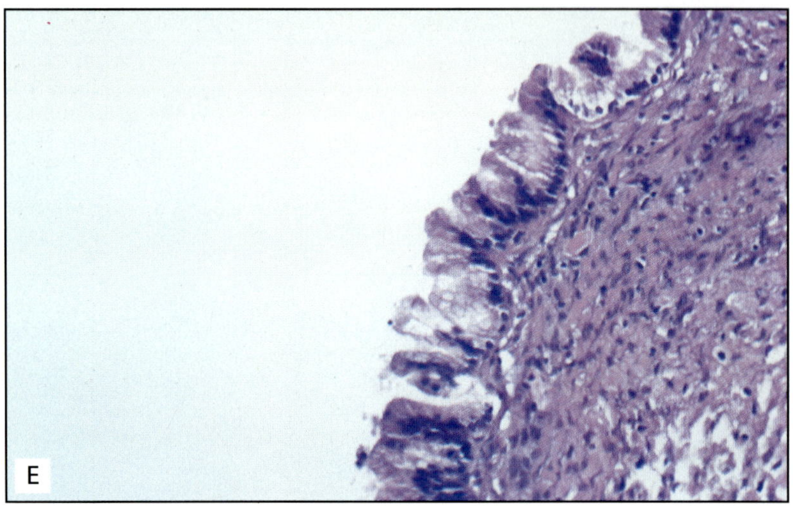

FIGURE 8-11.

Endocervical versus intestinal type of low malignant potential (LMP) mucinous tumors. The importance of subclassifying mucinous tumors of LMP into endocervical (müllerian) and intestinal types has recently been recognized [17]. The biologic differences between these two types primarily involve the pattern of peritoneal implants. Peritoneal implants of the endocervical type take the form of well circumscribed nodules of mucinous or glandular elements within a fibrous stroma. **A**, The intestinal type, however, often forms pools of mucin in association with its implants termed "pseudomyxoma peritonei" [18,19]. This entity, which has a morbid prognosis, is characterized histologically by cellular clumps of epithelium floating within extravasated mucin (**B**). The intestinal type of LMP mucinous tumors is by far the most frequently occurring variant and presents as a large multiloculated ovarian mass filled with tenacious mucinous material (**C**). Histologically, short papillae are lined by often multilayered mucinous columnar and goblet cells (**D** and **E**).

(*Continued on next page*)

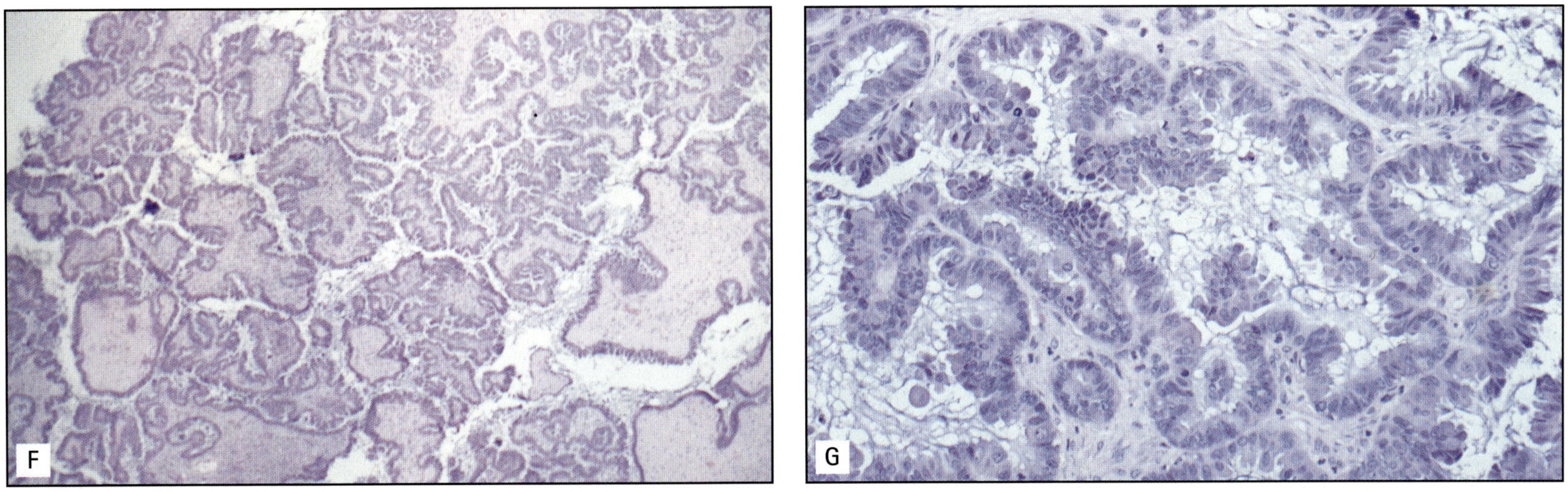

FIGURE 8-11. *(Continued)*
Cellular budding and complex arborization are typically absent. In contrast, the endocervical type shows intricate branching of papillary structures (**F**), which are lined by tall columnar cells resembling endocervical epithelium. Tufting and detached cell fragments are common (**G**). Importantly, by International Federation of Gynecology and Obstetrics and World Health Organization criteria, stromal invasion must be absent in order to place a mucinous neoplasm into this category. (*B, D, E* to *G*, photomicrographs, H & E stain; Original magnification, *B* × 400, *D* × 150, *E* × 200, *F* × 40, *G* × 200.)

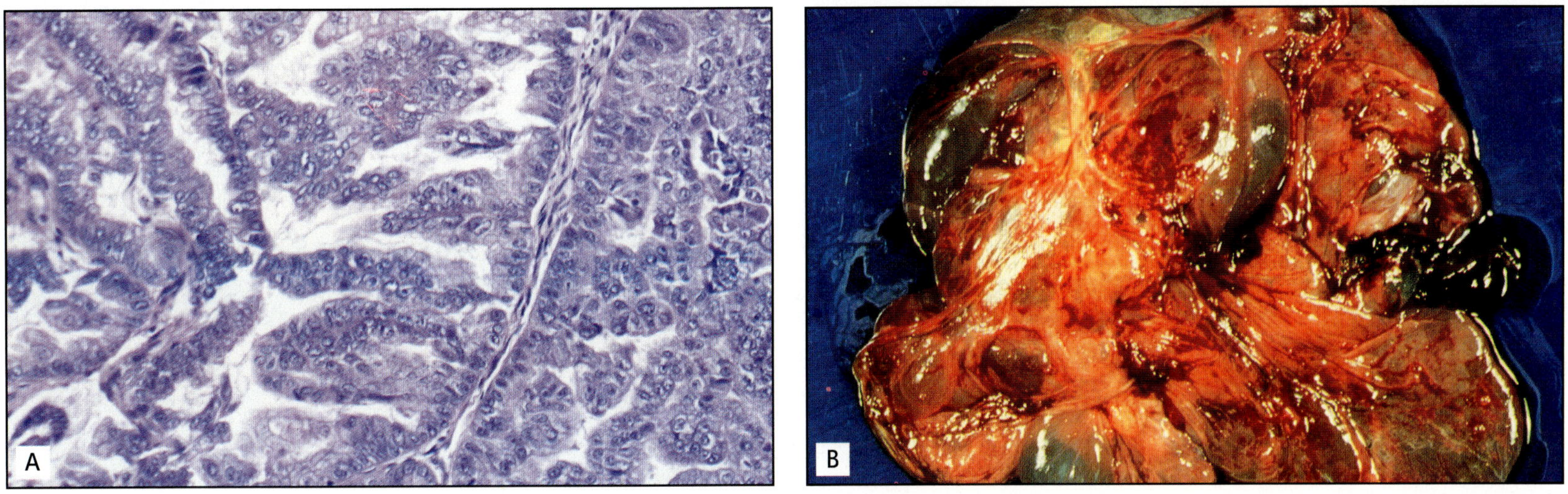

FIGURE 8-12.
Invasive mucinous adenocarcinoma. The findings of irregular gland contours and atypical cellular budding with a desmoplastic stromal response may be the only features present in an early invasive mucinous adenocarcinoma. Frankly invasive tumors (**A**) show a moderate to marked degree of nuclear atypia, architectural complexity (cribriforming, branching, and tufting of the epithelial elements), and necrosis. Noteworthy is the frequent occurrence of histologically benign mucinous foci within these tumors, emphasizing the importance of sampling. **B**, Grossly these tumors have cystic and solid areas. Bilateral tumors occur in 8% to 10% of cases. Distinction from a metastatic colon primary may be difficult on a histologic basis alone; therefore clinicopathologic correlation is necessary in these situations. (*A*, photomicrograph, H & E stain, × 400.)

ENDOMETRIOID TUMORS

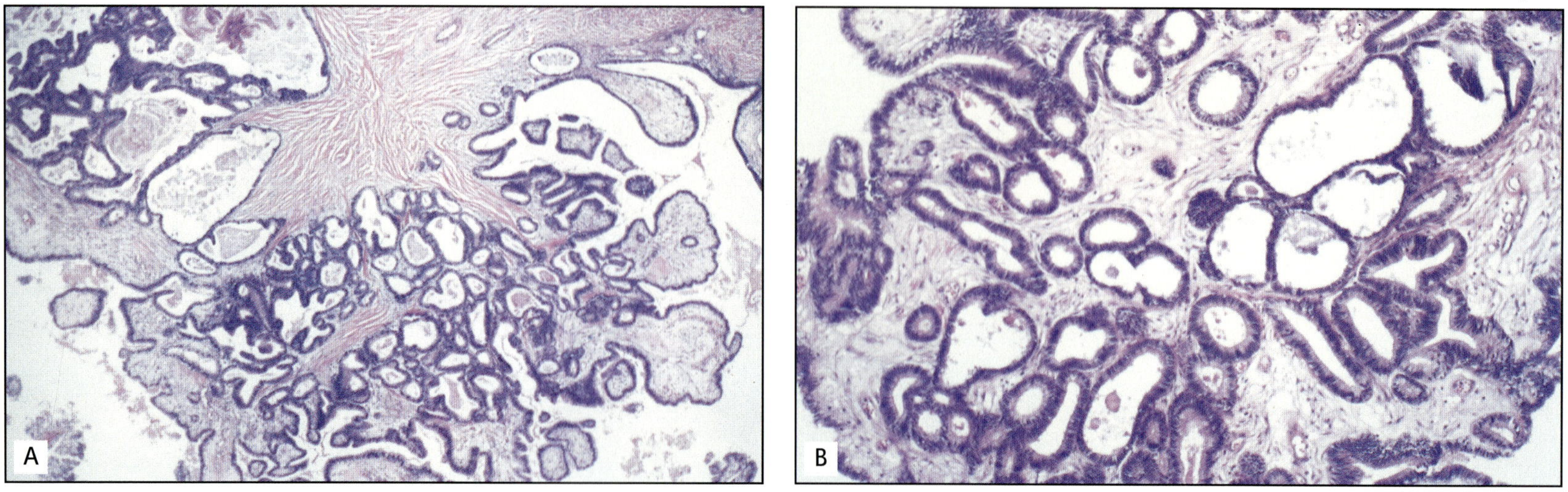

FIGURE 8–13.

Intermediate endometrioid tumors. Unlike serous and mucinous tumors of low malignant potential (LMP) there is a lack of uniformly accepted criteria for intermediate endometrioid tumors [20,21]. It is agreed, however, that these lesions behave in a benign fashion, with no reports of metastases, and that they occur in postmenopausal women whose main complaints are vaginal bleeding, abdominal enlargement, and pain. The majority of these lesions are adenofibromatous in nature possessing prominent stroma "punctuated" with round or tubular branching glands or dilated cysts of varying size (**A**) lined by pseudostratified or stratified columnar epithelial cells usually with minimal atypia. Although typically the glands and tubules are distributed in a dense fibrous stroma, occasional endometrioid tumors show complex architecture with glandular branching and budding and lack an associated fibrous stroma (**B**). Terms such as low malignant potential, atypical, or proliferating endometrioid tumor have been used to describe these intermediate lesions. (Photomicrographs, H & E stain, *A* × 40, *B* × 100.)

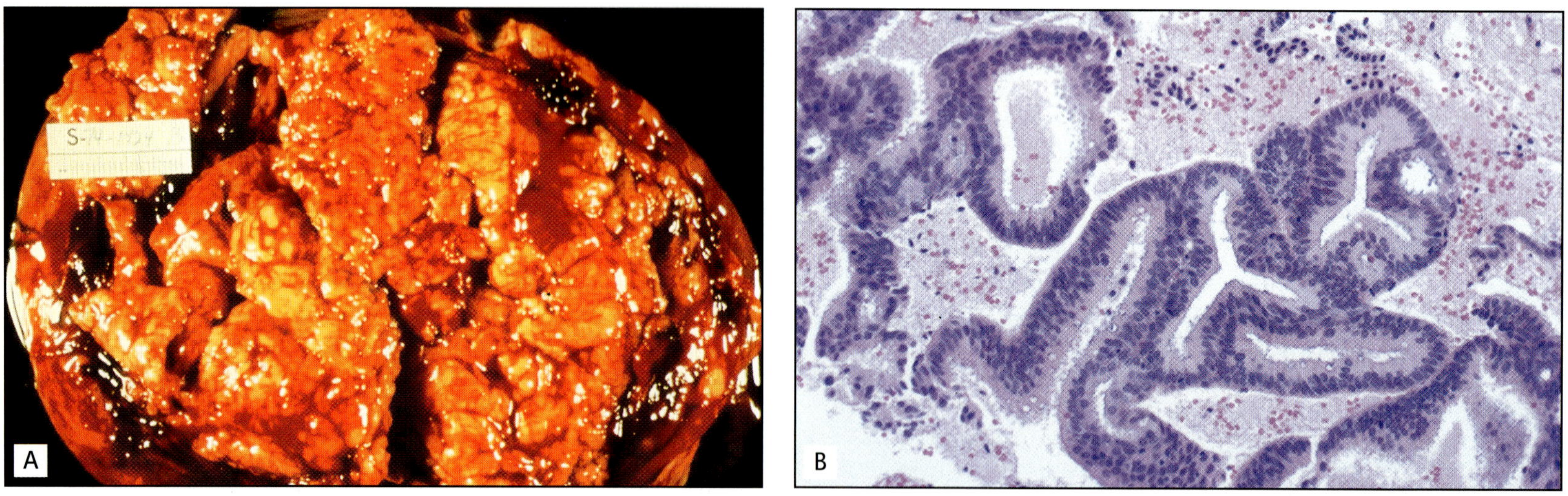

FIGURE 8–14.

Malignant endometrioid tumors. Malignant endometrioid tumors can be cystic or solid (**A**). Endometrioid carcinomas exhibit stromal invasion as evidenced by infiltrative, irregular, jagged glands set within a desmoplastic stroma. **B**, A low-grade tumor is seen, which is characterized by back to back glands (no intervening stroma) lined by pseudostratified columnar cells with mild atypia. High-grade endometrioid carcinomas, in addition to having a predominantly solid growth pattern, demonstrate a lack of polarity of the lining epithelial cells, which are hyperchromatic and pleomorphic. Numerous apoptotic bodies and necrosis are present as well. (Photomicrograph, H & E stain, × 400.)

CLEAR CELL TUMORS

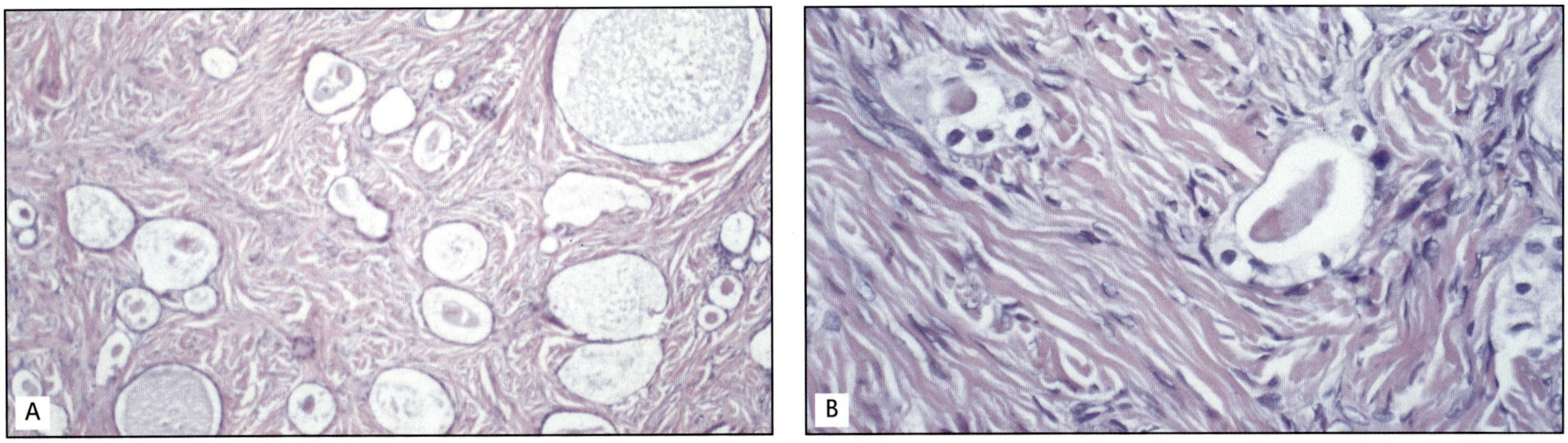

FIGURE 8-15.

Clear cell adenofibroma. Clear cell adenofibroma, also known as parvilocular cystadenoma, is considered by some authors to represent a tumor of low malignant potential for the following reasons: 1) many of these lesions show at least focal significant cytologic atypia, and 2) this pattern has been found in frankly malignant clear cell carcinomas (thus these tumors require thorough sampling). Needless to say, the vast majority of these tumors behave in a benign fashion [22,23]. Grossly, these unilateral lesions have abundant stroma with numerous small cystic spaces filled with watery fluid. The cysts embedded within the fibrous stroma (**A**) are lined by two distinct cell types, clear cells (**B**) and hobnail cells, both of which are glycogen-rich. The nuclei are generally hyperchromatic and show varying degrees of atypia and epithelial tufting. The epithelial-stromal interface is smooth with no evidence of invasion. The existence of truly benign clear cell tumors remains controversial in our opinion. (Photomicrographs, H & E stain, *A* × 100, *B* × 400.)

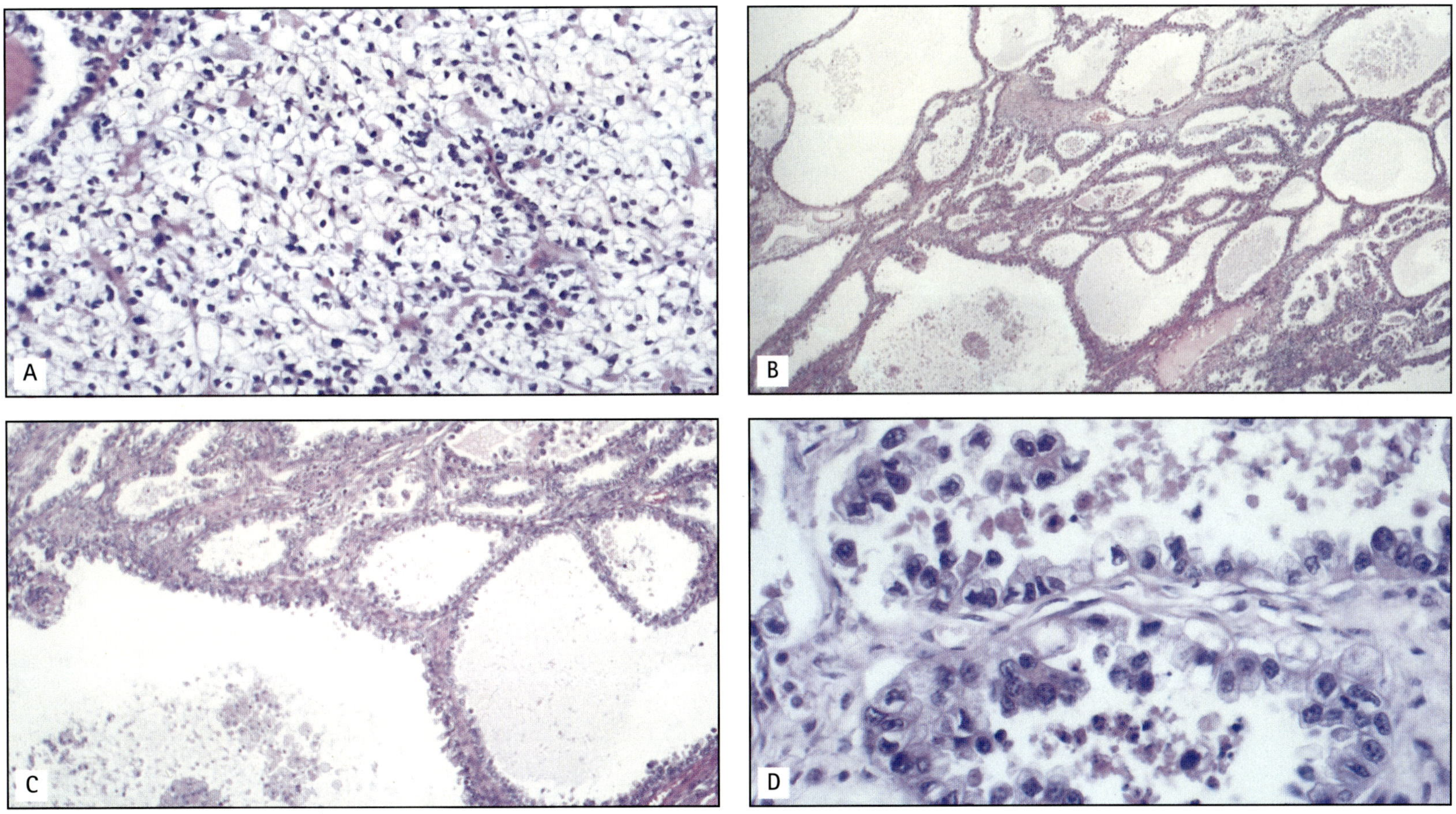

FIGURE 8-16.

Clear cell carcinoma. Clear cell carcinoma accounts for approximately 6% of all ovarian epithelial tumors with as many as two thirds of the affected women being nulliparous. A variety of architectural patterns are recognized: solid (**A**), tubulocystic (**B** and **C**), and papillary. Designation as clear cell carcinoma relies most heavily on the presence of cells with abundant clear cytoplasm (containing glycogen), hobnail cells with eosinophilic cytoplasm, or columnar cells with cytoplasmic vacuoles (**D**). Also note the irregular and hyperchromatic nuclei. A poorer survival rate has been reported in patients with clear cell carcinoma as compared with other epithelial ovarian neoplasms. Additionally, histologic grading of tumors with this cell type does not correlate with prognosis [24]. (*A* to *D*, photomicrographs, H & E stain; Magnification, *A* × 200, *B* × 40, *C* × 200, *D* × 400.)

BRENNER TUMORS

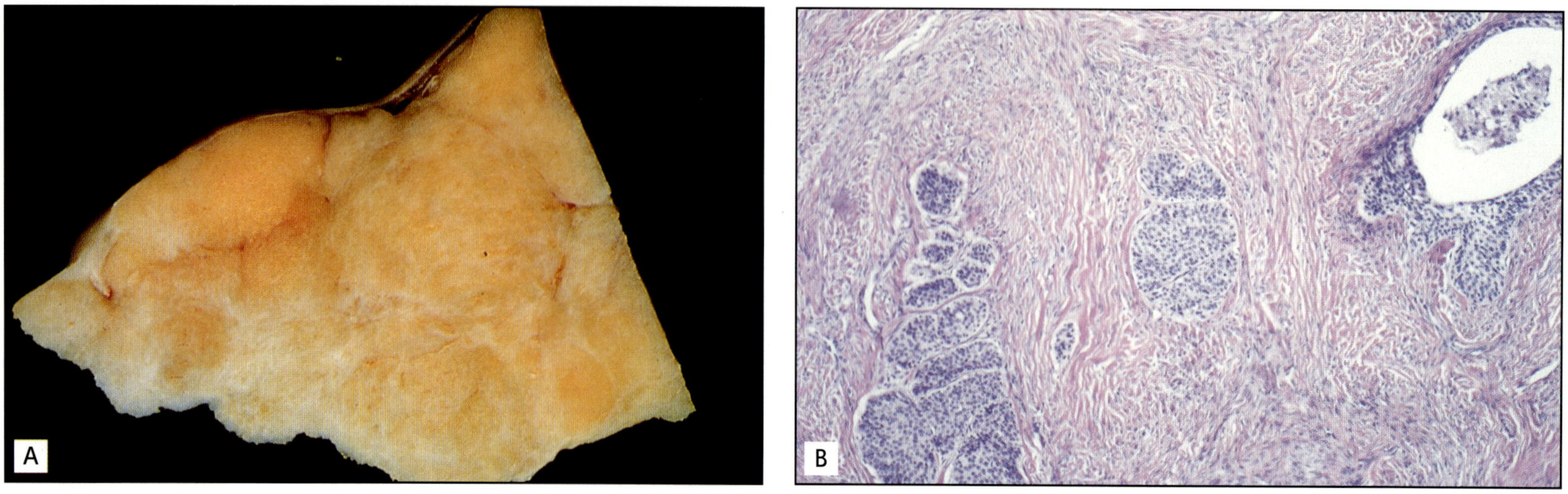

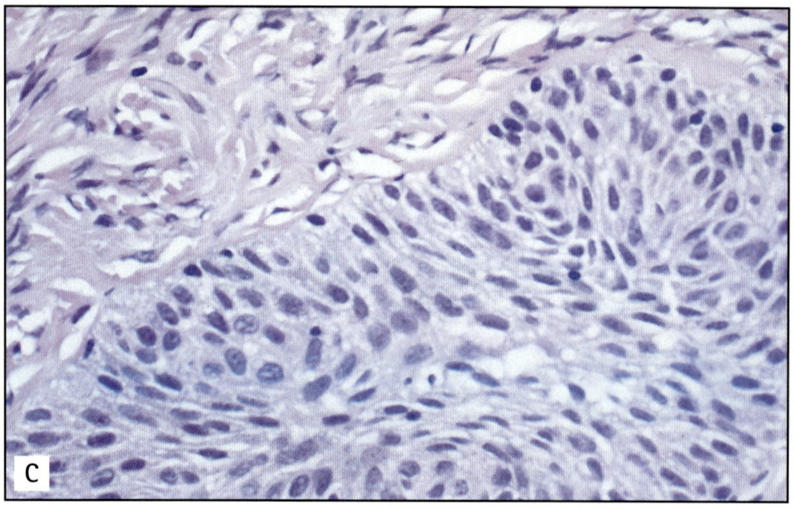

FIGURE 8-17.

Benign Brenner tumor. Benign Brenner tumors are typically identified incidentally in peri- and postmenopausal women. These are well circumscribed, yellow solid tumors (**A**). Sharply demarcated epithelial nests composed of uniform, small transitional cells are characteristic of this uncommon entity. The cellular nests are often cystic(**B**), with resultant flattening of the epithelial cells. The surrounding stroma consists of bland spindle cells with varying degrees of hyalinization and dystrophic calcification. The nests are composed of transitional cells that tend to be round to oval, with small nucleoli and identifiable nuclear grooves, imparting a coffee bean appearance (**C**). Nuclear atypia and mitoses are absent or rare. (*B* and *C*, photomicrographs, H & E stain; Magnification, *B* × 100, *C* × 400.)

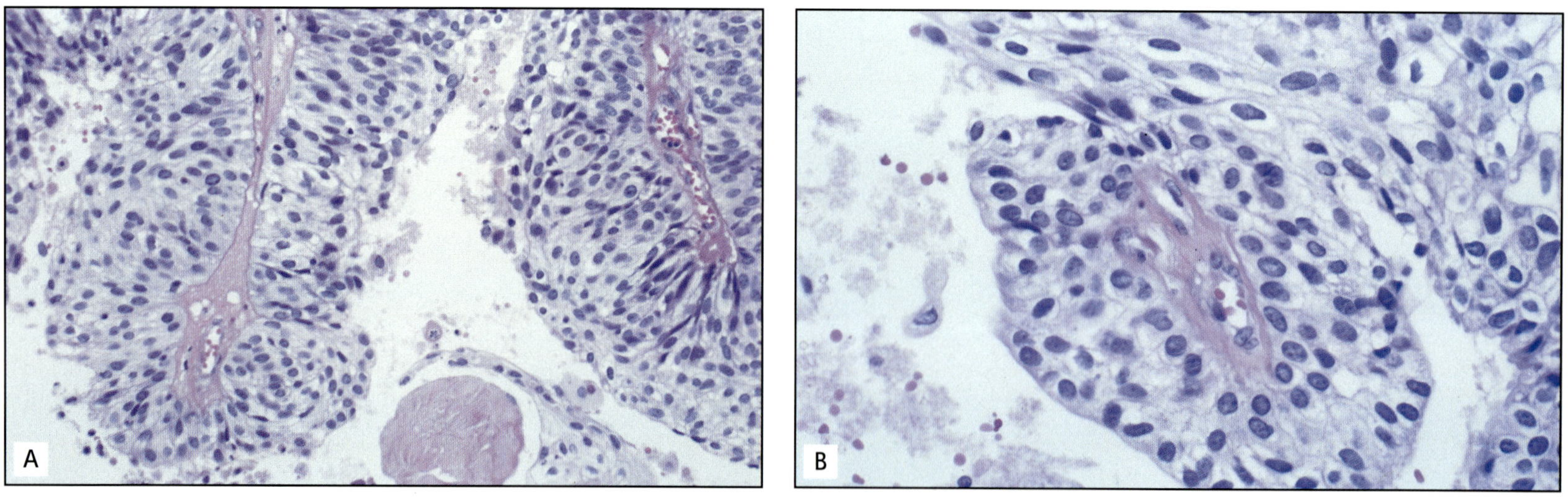

FIGURE 8-18.

Borderline Brenner tumor. Occurring in an older age group than the benign Brenner tumor, the proliferating (or borderline) Brenner tumor tends to present as a mass lesion with concomitant symptoms. Relatively small and uniform nuclei are arranged on a fibrovascular stalk (**A**), paralleling the histologic characteristics of a grade I transitional cell carcinoma of the urinary bladder Exophytic (papillary) as well as endophytic (downward) growth can be present. By definition, stromal invasion is absent. Individual tumor cells have identical features to those described for benign Brenner tumors (**B**). Nearly all examples of this entity possess a benign transitional cell tumor. Only rare recurrences have been recorded after a conservative surgical approach [25]. (Photomicrographs, H & E stain; Magnification, *A* × 200, *B* × 400.)

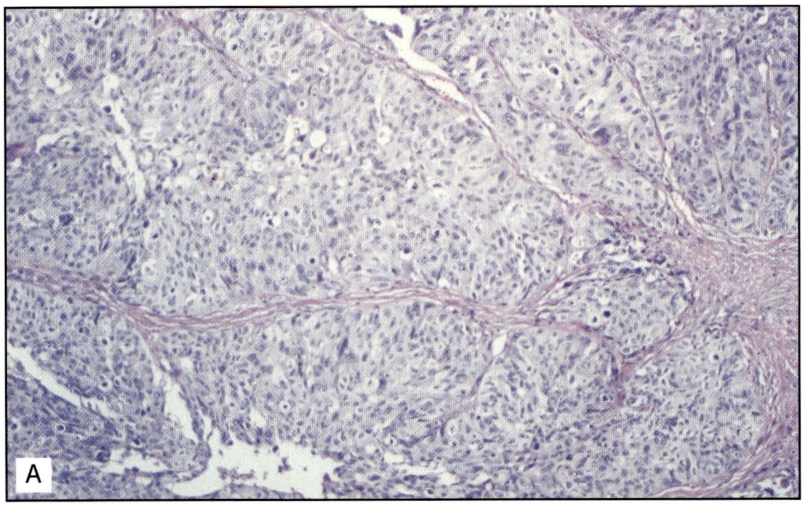

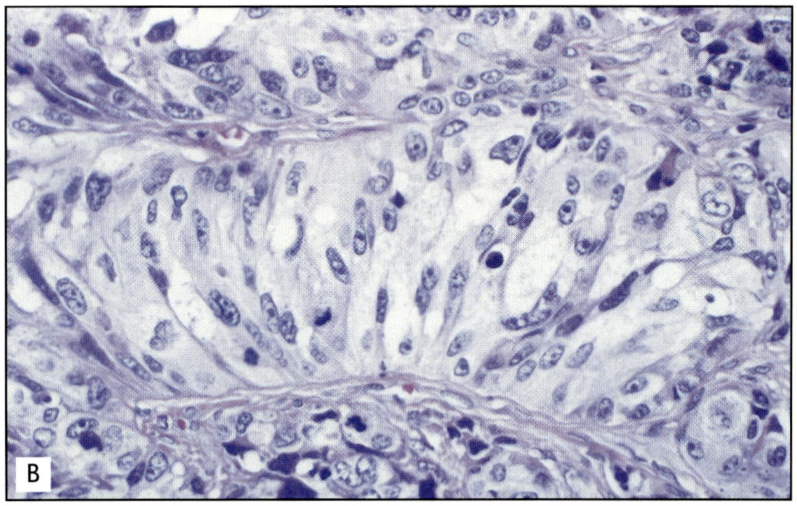

FIGURE 8-19.

Malignant Brenner tumor. Malignant Brenner tumors are invasive transitional cell carcinomas, usually of high grade, and by definition are associated with either a benign or proliferating Brenner component. Typically, there is an invasive solid growth pattern with accompanying cysts and papillae (**A**). The cellular nests often undergo central necrosis. The neoplastic cells demonstrate moderate to marked pleomorphism, prominent eosinophilic nucleoli and numerous atypical mitoses (**B**). It is important to distinguish this entity from a primary transitional cell carcinoma of the ovary because of the significant differences in their clinical courses [26]. (Photomicrographs, H & E stain; Magnification, *A* × 200, *B* × 400.)

TRANSITIONAL CELL CARCINOMA

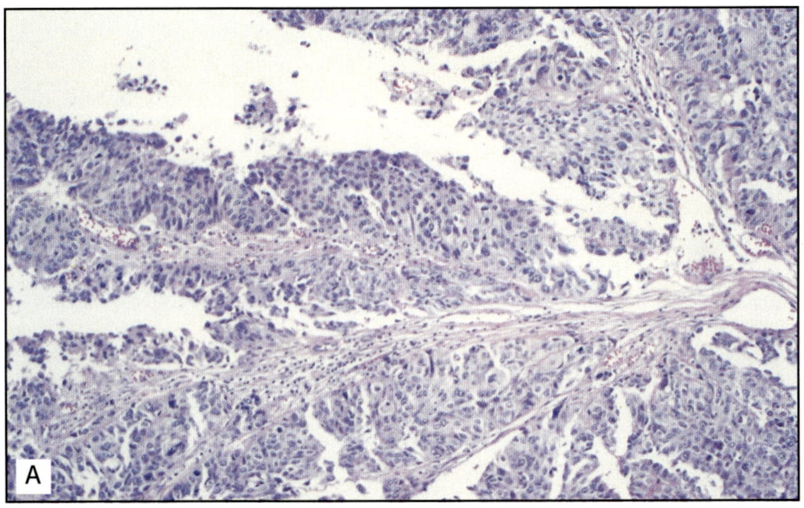

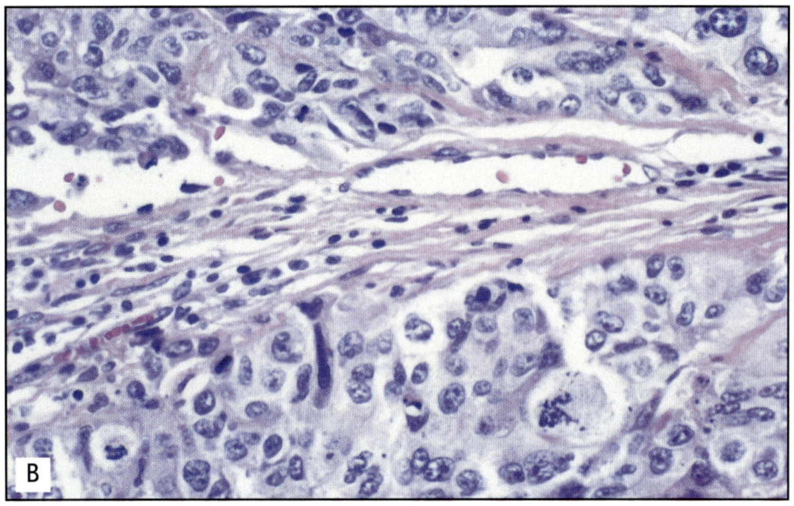

FIGURE 8-20.

Ovarian transitional cell carcinoma (TCC). Resembling transitional cell carcinoma of the urinary bladder histologically, primary TCC of the ovary is rare accounting for only 1% of ovarian carcinomas. Patients are typically postmenopausal and present with abdominal distention and pain. Thick papillary fronds, with fibrovascular cores, projecting into cystic spaces are typical of the histologic appearance (**A**); however, grade III lesions demonstrate more solid areas. The lining cells have moderate amounts of cytoplasm, distinct cytoplasmic borders, and varying degrees of nuclear atypia (**B**). Unlike a malignant Brenner tumor, a primary TCC of the ovary lacks a benign or proliferating Brenner component. The importance of distinguishing a primary TCC from a malignant Brenner tumor lies in the fact that the former is more sensitive to chemotherapy than other poorly differentiated ovarian carcinomas [27,28].

REFERENCES

1. Bell DA, Weinstock MA, Scully RE: Peritoneal implants of ovarian serous borderline tumors: Histologic features and prognosis. *Cancer* 1988, 62:2212–2222.
2. Gershenson DM, Silva EM: Serous ovarian tumors of low malignant potential with peritoneal implants. *Cancer* 1990, 65:578–585.
3. Kurman RJ, Trimble CL: The behavior of serous tumors of low malignant potential: are they ever malignant? *Int J Gynecol Pathol* 1993, 12:120–127.
4. Hartage P, Schiffman MH, Hoover R, *et al.*: A case-control study of epithelial ovarian cancer. *Am J Obstet Gynecol* 1989, 161:10–16.
5. Booth M, Beral V, Smith P: Risk factors for ovarian cancer: a case-control study. *Br J Cancer* 1989, 60:592–598.
6. International Federation of Gynecology and Obstetrics: Annual report on the results of treatment in gynecological cancer. *Int J Gynecol Obstet* 1989, 28:189–190.
7. McCaughey WTE, Kirk ME, Lester W, *et al.*: Peritoneal lesions associated with proliferative serous tumors of the ovary. *Histopathology* 1984, 8:195–208.
8. Bostwick DG, Tazelaar HD, Ballon SC, *et al.*: Ovarian epithelial tumors of borderline malignancy: a clinical and pathologic study of 109 cases. *Cancer* 1986, 52:2052–2065.
9. Micheal H, Roth L: Invasive and noninvasive implants in ovarian serous tumors of low malignant potential. *Cancer* 1986, 57:1240–1247.
10. Bell DA, Scully RE: Ovarian serous borderline tumors with stromal microinvasion: a report of 21 cases. *Hum Pathol* 1990, 21:397–403.
11. Tavassoli HD: Serous tumor of low malignant potential with early stromal invasion (serous LMP with microinvasion). *Mod Pathol* 1988, 1:407–414.
12. Nayar R, Siriaunkgul S, Robbins KM, *et al.*: Microinvasion in low malignant potential tumors of the ovary. *Hum Pathol* 1996, 27(6):521–527.
13. Burks RT, Sherman ME, Kurman, RJ: Micropapillary serous carcinoma of the ovary: a distinctive low-grade carcinoma related to serous borderline tumors. *Am J Surg Pathol* 1996, 20(11):1319–1330.
14. Eichhorn JH, Bell DA, Young RH, Scully RE: Ovarian serous borderline tumors of solid, micropapillary and cribriform types: a study of 42 cases. *Mod Pathol* 1997, 10:99A.
15. Katzenstein A-LA, Mazur MT, Morgan TE, *et al.*: Proliferative serous tumors of the ovary: histologic features and prognosis. *Am J Surg Pathol* 1978, 2:339–355.
16. Gilks CB, Bell DA, Scully RE: Serous psammocarcinoma of the ovary and peritoneum. *Int J Gynecol Pathol* 1990, 9:110–121.
17. Rutgers, JL, Scully RE: Ovarian mixed-epithelial papillary cystadenomas of borderline malignancy of müllerian type: a clinicopathologic analysis. *Cancer* 1988, 61:546–554.
18. Kahn MA, Demopoulos RI: Mucinous ovarian tumors with pseudomyxoma peritonei: a clinicopathologic study. *Int J Gynecol Pathol* 1992, 11:15–23.
19. Prayson RA, Hart WR, Hood DL, *et al.*: Pseudomyxoma peritonei: a clinicopathologic study of 16 cases. *Mod Pathol* 1992, 5:68A.
20. Bell DA, Scully RE: Atypical and borderline endometrioid adenofibromas of the ovary: a report of 27 cases. *Am J Surg Pathol* 1985, 9:205–214.
21. Snyder RR, Norris HJ, Tavassoli F: Endometrioid proliferative and low malignant potential tumors of the ovary: a clinicopathologic study of 46 cases. *Am J Surg Pathol* 1988, 12:661–671.
22. Bell DA, Scully RE: Benign and borderline clear cell adenofibromas of the ovary. *Cancer* 1985, 56:2922–2931.
23. Roth LM, Langely FA, Fox H, *et al.*: Ovarian clear cell adenofibromas: benign, of low malignant potential and associated with invasive clear cell carcinoma. *Cancer* 1984, 53:1156–1163.
24. Jenison EL, Montag AG, Grifffiths CT, *et al.*: Clear cell adenocarcinoma of the ovary: a clinical analysis and comparison with serous carcinoma. *Gynecol Oncol* 1989; 32:65–71.
25. Roth LM, Dallenbach-Hellwag G, Czernobilsky B: Ovarian Brenner tumors: metaplastic, proliferating and low malignant potential. *Cancer* 1985, 56:582–591.
26. Austin RM, Norris HJ: Malignant Brenner tumor and transitional cell carcioma of the ovary: a comparison. *Int J Gynecol Pathol* 1987, 6:29–39.
27. Robey SS, Silva EG, Gershenson DM, *et al.*: Transitional cell carcinoma in high-grade high stage ovarian carcinoma. An indication of favorable response to chemotherapy. *Cancer* 1989, 63:839–847.
28. Silva EG, Robey-Cafferty SS, Smith TL, *et al.*: Ovarian carcinomas with transitional cell carcinoma pattern. *Am J Clin Pathol* 1990, 93:457–465.

CHAPTER 9

Germ Cell Tumors of the Ovary

Cornelia Liu Trimble and Barbara Goff

Germ cell tumors are derived from primordial germ cells of the ovary. Germ cell tumors are the second most common ovarian neoplasms, after epithelial tumors. Germ cell tumors make up 15% to 20% of all ovarian neoplasms. Although they may occur at all ages, they are more common in younger patients. The most common germ cell neoplasm is the benign cystic teratoma. Only 2% to 3% of germ cell tumors are malignant. The younger the patient, however, the more likely that the germ cell tumor is malignant. In order of decreasing frequency, malignant ovarian germ cell tumors are dysgerminoma, endodermal sinus tumor, immature teratoma, embryonal carcinoma, choriocarcinoma, and poplyembryoma. Gonadoblastomas are included among germ cell tumors because of their propensity to give rise to germ cell tumors. On average, 60% to 75% of malignant germ cell tumors are stage I at diagnosis, and cure rates of over 90% have been achieved with surgery and combination chemotherapy.

Sex cord stromal tumors of the ovary are the third most commom ovarian neoplasm and account for approximately 5% of all ovarian malignancies. These tumors are derived from the ovarian stroma, and many can synthesize estrogen and progesterone, as well as androgens. Because the embryonic gonad is sexually bipotential, these gonadal stromal tumors can differentiate histologically and hormonally toward male or female gonadal cells. Sex cord stromal tumors are usually composed of either "female" cells (granulosa and theca cells), or "male" cells (Sertoli and Leydig cells). The gynandroblastoma contains elements of both male and female cells. Clinically, the majority of these tumors behave in a low-grade fashion, and many are curable with surgery alone.

Metastatic tumors account for approximately 5% of ovarian malignancies. The most common sources of metastases to the ovary are malignancies of the female genital tract, the breast, and the gastrointestinal tract. In 75% of cases, metastatic disease involves both ovaries.

PATHOGENESIS AND CLASSIFICATION

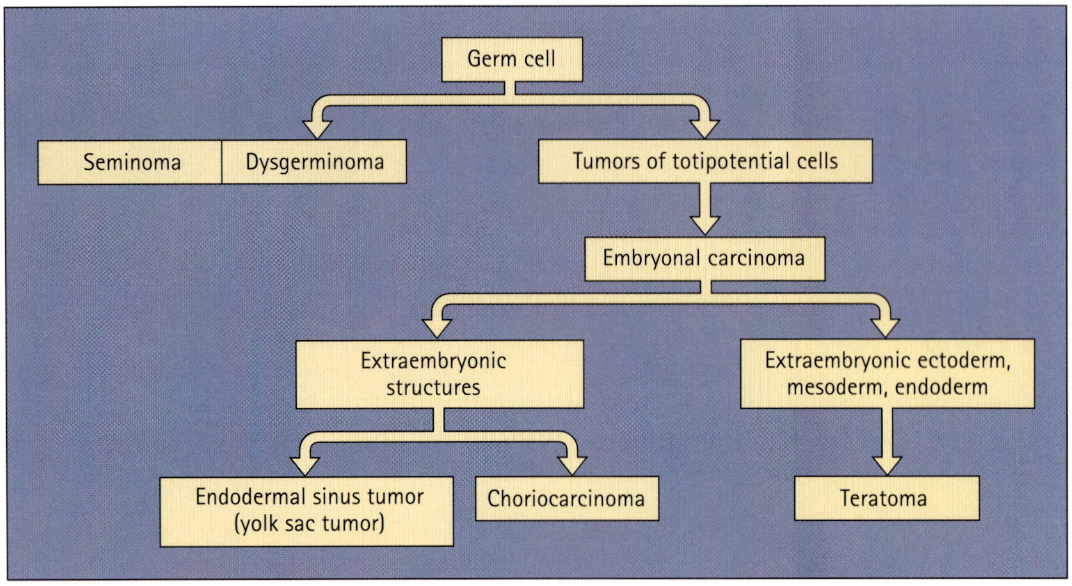

FIGURE 9-1.
Pathogenesis. Germ cell tumors are believed to arise from primordial germ cells of the embryonic gonad. A putative histogenesis has been proposed by Teilum. Those tumors arising from cells without potential for differentiation are classified as dysgerminomas. Embryonal carcinomas, on the other hand, represent those tumors arising from multipotential cells capable of differentiation. Tumors consisting of embryonal elements are grouped as teratomas. Those arising from extraembryonal elements are subdivided into those arising from trophoblastic precursors, *ie*, choriocarcinomas, or from the endoderm, *ie*, yolk sac tumors.

CLASSIFICATION OF GERM CELL TUMORS

- Dysgerminoma
- Yolk sac tumor
- Teratoma
  - Mature cystic teratoma
  - Malignant transformation of mature elements of teratoma
  - Immature teratoma
  - Monodermal teratoma
- Choriocarcinoma
- Embryonal carcinoma
- Polyembryoma
- Mixed germ cell tumor
- Germ cell/sex cord–stromal tumor
- Gonadoblastoma

FIGURE 9-2.
Classification of germ cell tumors. The categorization of ovarian germ cell tumors proposed by the World Health Organization (WHO) in 1973 is the one most widely accepted. Dysgerminomas appear to be the most common, comprising 48% of germ cell tumors, followed by yolk sac tumors (22%), immature teratomas (18%), mixed germ cell tumors (8%), and embryonal carcinomas (4%).

DIAGNOSTIC TESTS

GERM CELL TUMOR MARKERS

Tumor	Marker
Endodermal sinus tumor	AFP
Embryonal carcinoma	AFP, hCG
Choriocarcinoma	hCG
Dysgerminoma	LDH
Immature teratoma	None

FIGURE 9-3.
Tumor markers. Several biologic markers can be identified either within tumor cells or circulating in the patient's serum. These markers can be helpful in diagnosing tumor types and in documenting and evaluating response to therapy in cases of malignancy. Any tumor with yolk sac elements will express α-fetoprotein (AFP). After removal of yolk sac elements, serum AFP levels normalize within 4 to 6 weeks. Human chorionic gonadotropin (hCG) is produced normally by placental synctiotrophoblast and intermediate trophoblast. It is produced by tumors with trophoblastic cells, such as choriocarcinomas, and can be measured in the serum. Less specific markers include alkaline phosphatase and lactate dehydrogenase (LDH) isoenzymes. Alkaline phosphatase may be identified in the plasma membrane of germ cells and thus may be useful in differentiating germ cell tumors such as dysgerminomas from non–germ cell tumors such as malignant lymphoma. LDH isoenzymes, which are normally produced by the liver and the central nervous system, may be found in dysgerminomas and in yolk sac tumors.

DYSGERMINOMA

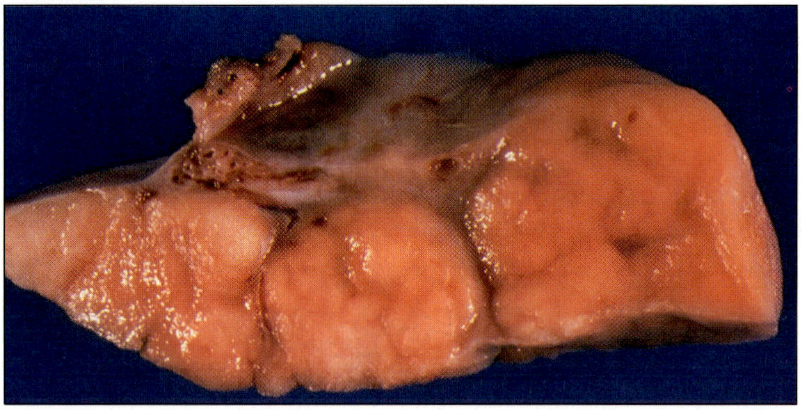

FIGURE 9-4.
Dysgerminoma. Dysgerminoma is histologically identical to seminoma of the testis. The tumor is solid, with a smooth, lobulated surface. The cut surface is tan, often with central necrosis and hemorrhage. In those specimens with cystic degeneration without a history of torsion, the possibility of mixed germ cell tumor should be entertained. Dysgerminoma is the most common malignant germ cell tumor. Most present with abdominal enlargement. In those in whom the tumors grow rapidly, torsion and subsequent hemoperitoneum may ensue. Although dysgerminoma is not assoicated with endocrine manifestations in the great majority of cases, young patients may present with precocious puberty. The median age at diagnosis is 20 years, with 80% occurring in those under 30 years. About two thirds of women are diagnosed with stage I disease. Dysgerminomas are usually unilateral, but bilateral tumors occur in 10% to 15% of women. About 5% of dysgerminomas are found in girls with chromosomal abnormalities such as 46,XY or 45,X/46,XY mosaicism. Prepubertal patients with dysgerminomas should undergo karyotyping. If gonadal dysgenesis is diagnosed, both ovaries should removed.

Dysgerminoma tends to spread via lymphatics. With tumor rupture, or extracapsular disease, tumor may also spread locally by direct extension. The great majority, 70%, of patients are diagnosed with stage IA disease. Primary treatment is surgical. If the tumor is grossly stage I, a unilateral oophorectomy is performed. Staging must be performed, including pelvic and para-aurtic node dissection, omental biopsy, and washings. Ten-year survival for those with stage IA disease has been reported at greater than 90%. For patients with more advanced stages prognosis is still quite good because this tumor is extremely radiosensitive and chemosensitive. With the use of adjuvant radiotherapy, or BEP (bleomycin, etoposide, cisplatin) combination chemotherapy, cures are often achieved even with metastic disease.

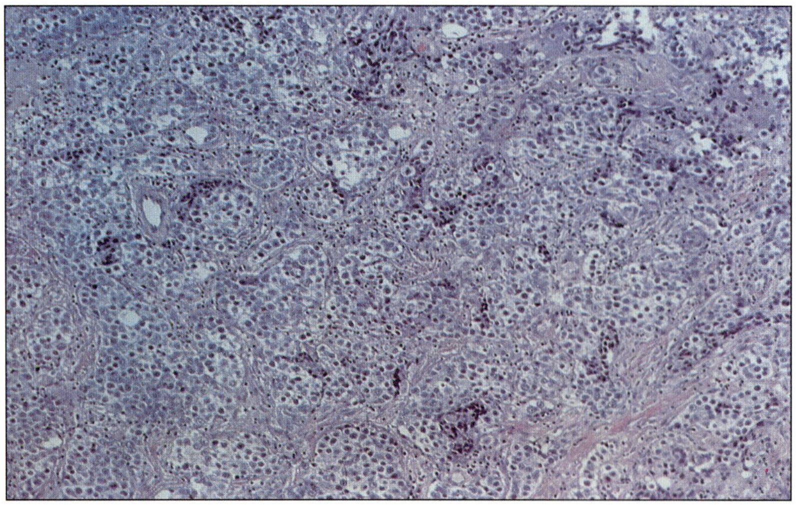

FIGURE 9-5.
Dysgerminoma—microscopic appearance. Histologically, the tumor is composed of three cell types: nests of germ cells, intervening fibrous septations, and lymphocytic infiltrates. The germ cells are round, measuring up to 25 μm in diameter. The cytoplasm contains glycogen, which may be demonstrated using periodic acid–Schiff (PAS) stain. Lipid can be identified using fat stains. Dysgerminoma cells in general are negative for cytokeratin, carcinoembryonic antigen (CEA), α-fetoprotein (AFP), and human chorionic gonadotropin (hCG). However, they show membrane-bound positivity for placental alkaline phosphotase (PLAP). Cell membranes are distinct. Nuclei are large, and display a vesicular chromatin pattern, often with prominent eosinophilic nucleoli. Mitotic activity is almost invariably present.

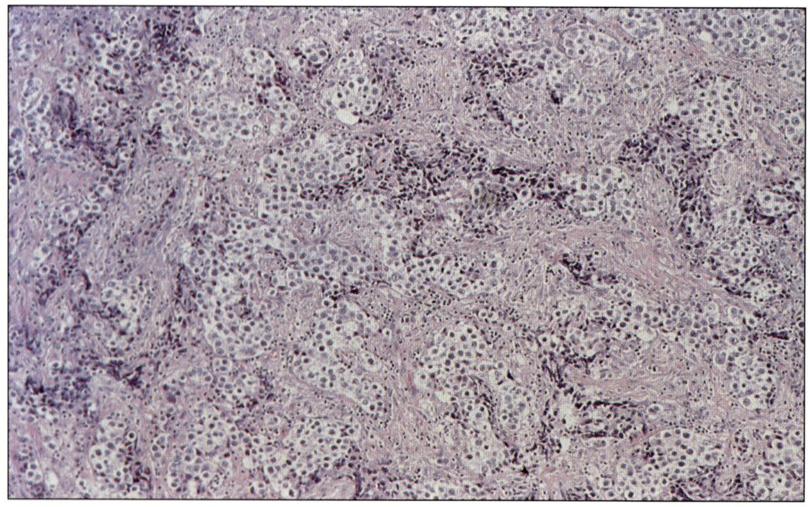

FIGURE 9-6.
Dysgerminoma. The stroma surrounding nests of germ cells is infiltrated by lymphocytes. Most of these cells are T cells and macrophages. Lymphoid follicles and granulomatous reactions may be identified. Although areas of necrosis and hemorrhage may represent the sequelae of torsion, the presence of calcifications may represent burnt-out gonadoblastoma. Some tumors may contain collections of syncytiotrophoblast giant cells. These may in turn produce hCG. The presence of these cells does not convey a worse prognosis.

YOLK SAC TUMOR (ENDODERMAL SINUS TUMOR)

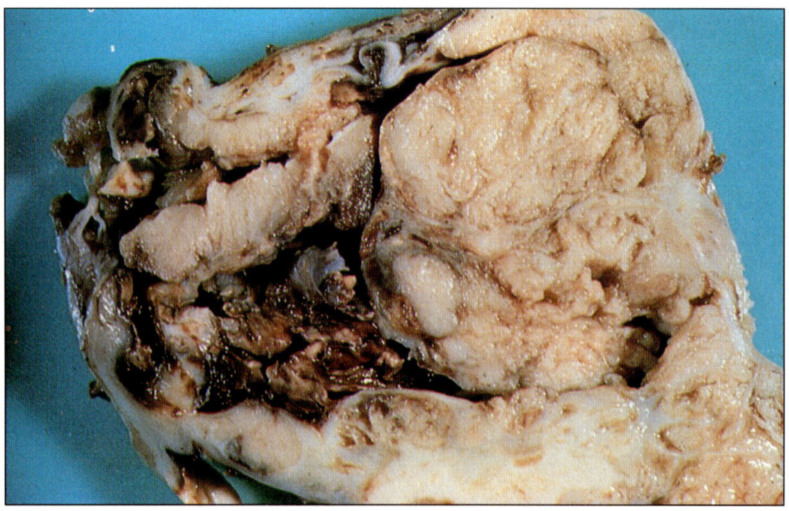

FIGURE 9-7.
Yolk sac tumor. Yolk sac tumor is the second most common germ cell tumor of the ovary. It is thought to arise from the multipotential cells of the embryonal carcinoma which differentiate toward vitelline structures. This tumor has also been known as endodermal sinus tumor. It comprises approximately 20% of all ovarian germ cell malignancies. Yolk sac elements are frequently found in mixed germ cell tumors. The median age at diagnosis is 19 years. Because this tumor typically grows rapidly, patients often present with acute abdominal symptoms. It is usually not associated with endocrine symptoms; the presence of these should lead to the consideration of a mixed tumor. Serum α-fetoprotein (AFP) levels are elevated, and can be used to assess the efficacy of treatment. Most patients (70%) have stage I disease at diagnosis. Because of its rapid growth, this tumor is typically large at the time of diagnosis, ranging up to 30 cm in greatest dimension. The surface is smooth, and may be lobulated. The cut surface is pink to grayish-yellow with areas of cystic, mucinous change, as well as areas of necrosis and hemorrhage.

Yolk sac tumors spread by direct extension, and by lymphatics, to the pelvic and para-aortic lymph nodes. Hematogenous spread occurs later in the course of the disease to the liver and lungs. Local recurrences are common. The prognostic factor most affecting survival is stage at diagnosis. Neither the patient's age nor preoperative AFP level affects prognosis. Postoperative adjuvant multiagent chemotherapy with BEP (bleomycin, etoposide, cisplatin) renders a complete cure at rates higher than 80%. All patients, even those with early-stage disease, should receive adjuvant chemotherapy. Serum AFP levels may be used to assess response to therapy, and for early detection of metastases.

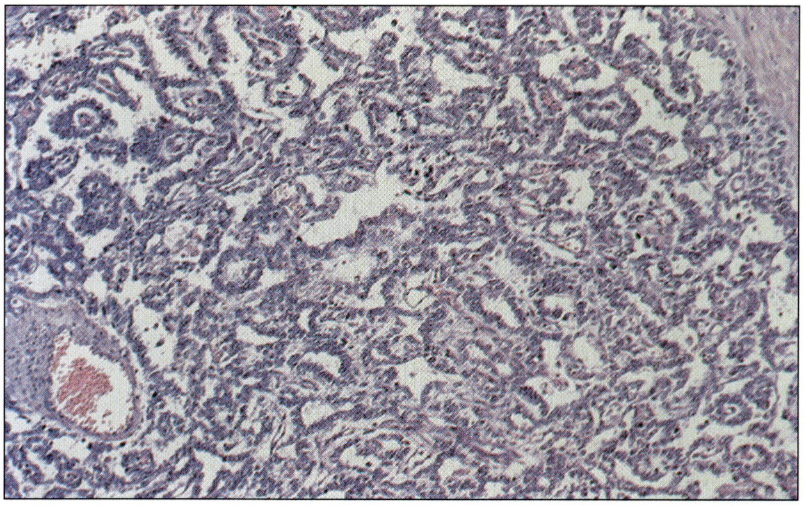

FIGURE 9-8.
Yolk sac tumor—microscopic appearance. Yolk sac tumors display a wide range of histologic patterns, often in a single lesion. These may include microcystic, macrocystic, endodermal sinus, solid, glandular-alveolar, papillary, polyvesicular-vitelline, myxomatous, hepatoid, and glandular patterns. Although these patterns differ very much from each other, most yolk sac tumors share certain histopathologic features. These include a loose reticular meshwork lined by flattened endodermal cells. Hyaline bodies which stain with periodic acid–Schiff, and contain α-fetoprotein and α-antitrypsin, are common. Mitotic activity is usually quite brisk.

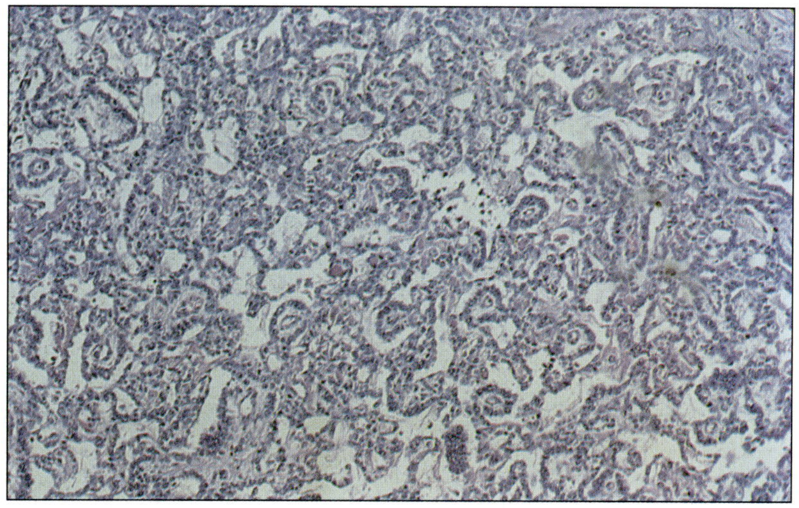

FIGURE 9-9.
Yolk sac tumor. The endodermal sinus pattern is most easily recognized by the identification of Schiller-Duval bodies. These structures are rounded, papillary configurations around a central vessel. The papillary appearance on cross section is due to malignant endodermal cells with large, pleomorphic nuclei, often with prominent nucleoli. The perivascular formation bears some resemblance to immature renal glomeruli.

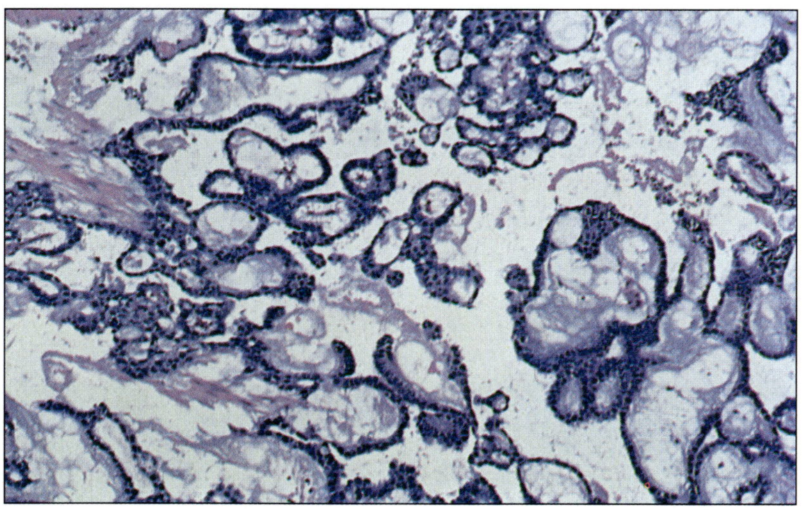

FIGURE 9-10.
Yolk sac tumor. Other histologic patterns of yolk sac tumor are less common. All, however, are characterized by a loose meshwork of sinuses lined by endodermal cells with large, pleomorphic nuclei. The polyvesicular-vitelline pattern is composed of cystic spaces lined by epithelial cells with clear cytoplasm. The stroma which contains the cystic spaces is densely cellular, often with a streaming appearance. The microcystic and myxomatous patterns are composed of loose meshworks of small cystic spaces in a more regular, or honeycomb, pattern. The cystic spaces are lined by flat mesothelial cells with large hyperchromatic nuclei. Hyaline material is found both within and without the cells.

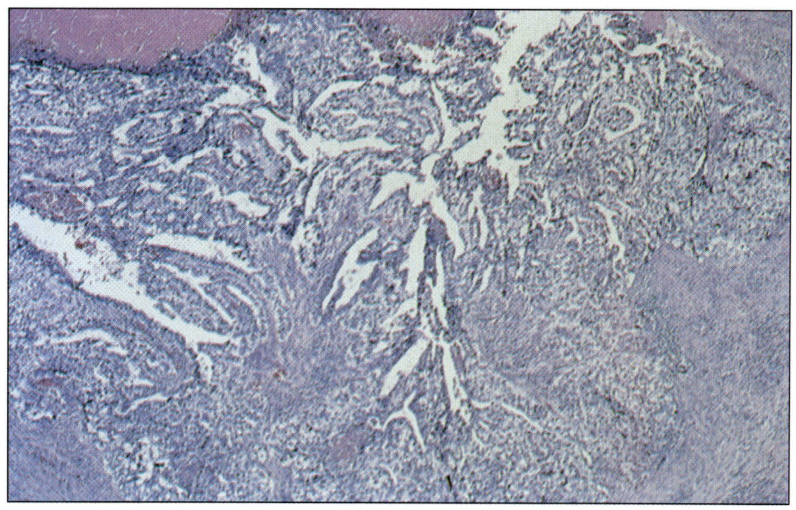

FIGURE 9-11.
Yolk sac tumor. The papillary pattern of yolk sac tumor is composed of hyaline cores lined with endodermal tumor cells. The hepatoid pattern is largely solid, and is composed of large polygonal or rounded cells with eosinophilic, granular cytoplasm. The intestinal, or glandular, pattern is characterized by aggregates of immature endodermal glands, some with goblet cells.

DIFFERENTIAL DIAGNOSIS OF YOLK SAC TUMOR

	Cytokeratin	Vimentin	AFP
Yolk sac tumor	+	-	+
Clear cell tumor	+	+	-
Dysgerminoma	-	+	-
Granulosa cell tumor	-	±	-

+ positive; - negative; ± ?

FIGURE 9-12.
Yolk sac tumor—differential diagnosis. The differential diagnosis for yolk sac tumor includes clear cell epithelial tumors of the ovary, dysgerminoma, embryonal carcinoma, various vascular tumors, and juvenile granulosa cell tumor. Clear cell epithelial tumor of the ovary may be distinguished from yolk sac tumor by its hobnail cells, and absence of perivascular formations and endodermal sinuses. Clear cell tumors of the ovary tend to occur in older patients. Dysgerminoma may be distinguished from the solid pattern of yolk sac tumor by staining for cytokeratin. Yolk sac tumor cells will stain with cytokeratin, whereas dysgerminoma cells, in general, do not. Yolk sac tumors will also stain with α-fetoprotein (AFP). Nests of dysgerminoma cells, furthermore, are typically accompanied by fibrous stroma and lymphocytic infiltrates. Embryonal carcinoma may be distinguished from yolk sac tumors by its larger tumor cells and more granular cytoplasm. Nucleoli are more prominent, and it will not display the multitude of typical patterns of yolk sac tumor. Vascular tumors will stain with both vimentin and with factor VII, whereas yolk sac tumors will not. Finally, the juvenile granulosa cell tumor will not stain with AFP.

TERATOMA

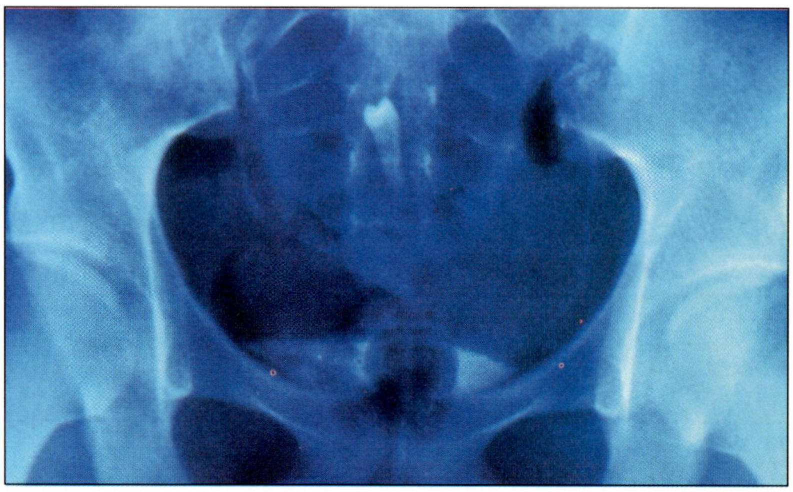

FIGURE 9-13.
Teratoma. Approximately one fourth of all ovarian neoplasms are benign cystic teratomas. These tumors occur most commonly in women of reproductive age. Many patients are asymptomatic. However, torsion or rupture may cause peritonitis and acute abdominal pain. Radiologic examination of the abdomen may reveal bone, cartilage, or teeth, as in this radiograph. Approximately 15% of these lesions are bilateral.

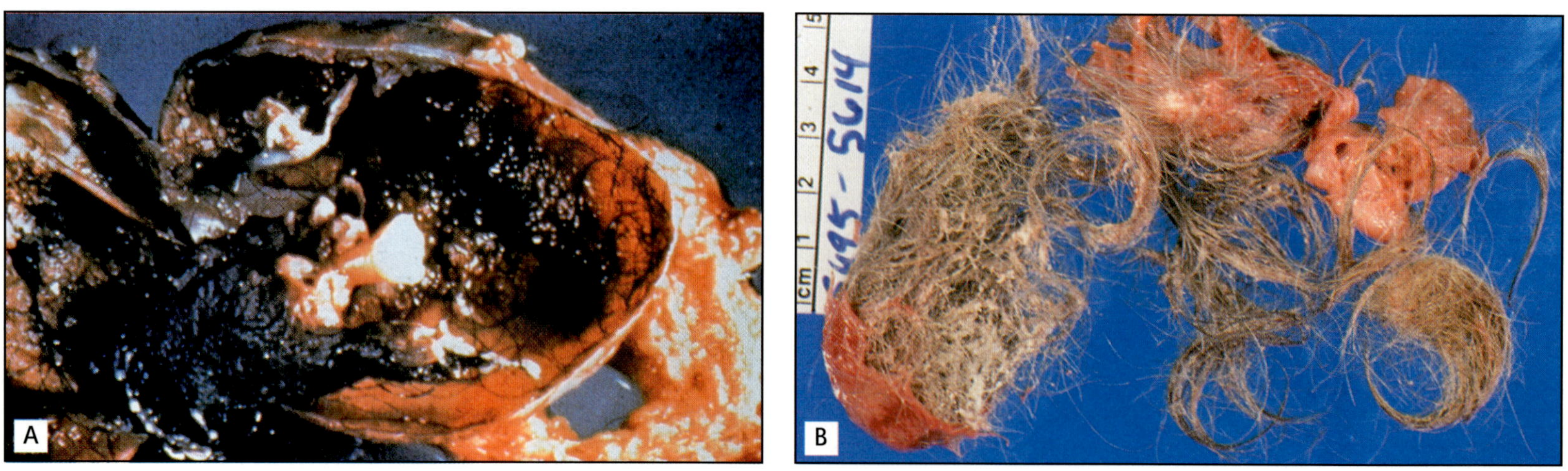

FIGURE 9-14.
Mature cystic teratoma—gross appearance. Mature cystic teratomas range in size from microscopic to very large. **A**, Intact, the tumor is globular with a glistening capsule. On palpation, immediately after surgical removal, the tumor will be fluctuant, with focal firm areas. As the tumor cools to room temperature, the sebum found in association with epithelial areas of the lesion will solidify. **B**, When opened, mature teratomas are often unilocular, filled with hair and sebum. Occasionally, calcified areas of formed teeth will be identified. The cyst wall is focally thickened and relatively smooth. At one pole, a nodule, Rokitansky's protuberance, can be identified. Adequate sampling of solid areas is prudent, because immature elements, if any, will be found in these areas.

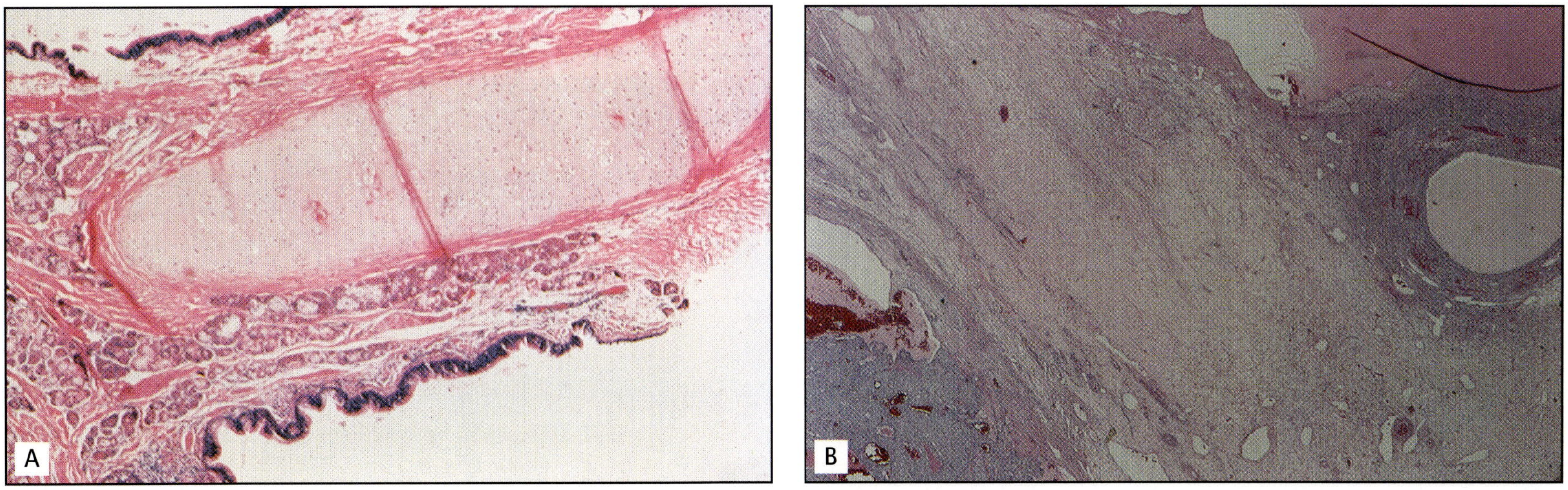

FIGURE 9-15.

Mature cystic teratoma—microscopic appearance. **A**, The inner wall of the cyst is usually lined with keratinized squamous epithelium, often containing numerous pilosebaceous units. Hair is usually present. Other types of epithelium, when present, are often arranged in organoid fashion, respiratory epithelium being found adjacent to cartilage for instance. Neural tissue is common, and must be examined closely for the presence of immature elements. Endocrine elements are relatively uncommon, with the exception of thyroid tissue. The term *struma ovarii* is used for those teratomas composed predominantly of thyroid tissue (**B**). Because these areas may be functional, patients may present with signs of hyperthyroidism.

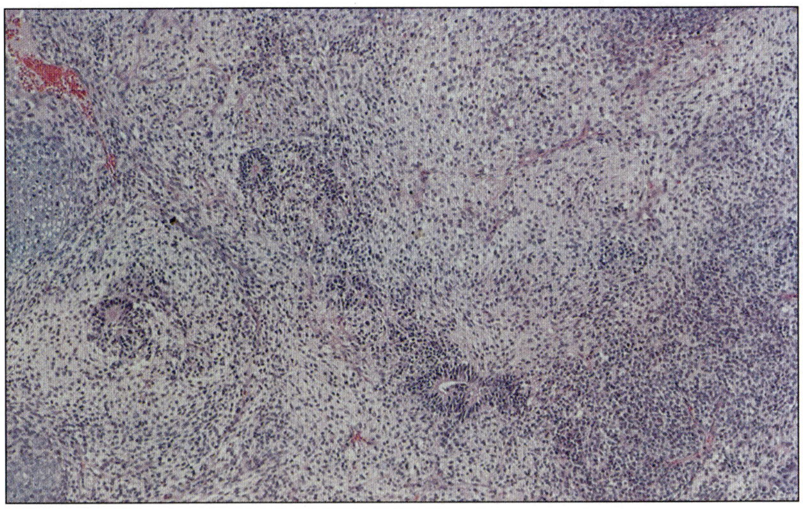

FIGURE 9-16.

Immature teratoma. The immature, or malignant, teratoma, similar to its benign counterpart, is composed of tissues derived from the three germ layers: ectoderm, mesoderm, and endoderm. However, the immature form contains embryonal tissues. Risk for recurrence and metastases increases with the amount of immature tissue; therefore, adequate histologic sampling is crucial. The immature teratoma, although malignant, is not to be confused with malignant transformation of tissues found in a mature teratoma. The main embryonal component in immature teratomas is usually neural in origin. Glial tissue may be abundant. However, prognosis is a function of the grade of the tumor, which is based on the volume of immature neuroepithelium. These elements are usually found in clusters or rosettes. In contrast to the relatively orderly organoid distribution of mature teratoma tissues, immature elements are more typically irregularly arranged. Areas of hemorrhage or necrosis may be present. Immature teratomas comprise approximately 1% of all teratomas. They occur in younger patients. Nearly four fifths of all patients present with stage IA disease.

GRADING OF IMMATURE TERATOMA

Grade 0	All mature elements
Grade 1	Immature neuroepithelium occupying 1 low-power microscopic field on any one slide
Grade 2	Immature neuroepithelium occupying between 1 and 4 low-power microscopic fields on any one slide
Grade3	Immature neuroepithelium occupying >4 low-power microscopic fields on any one slide

FIGURE 9-17.

Immature teratoma—classification. Grading of immature teratomas is based on volume of immature neuroepithelial elements. Although some immature teratomas may contain areas of other immature tissues, prognosis is a factor of the amount of neural tissue. Immature teratomas may also contain foci of other malignant germ cell tumors, thereby forming a mixed germ cell tumor.

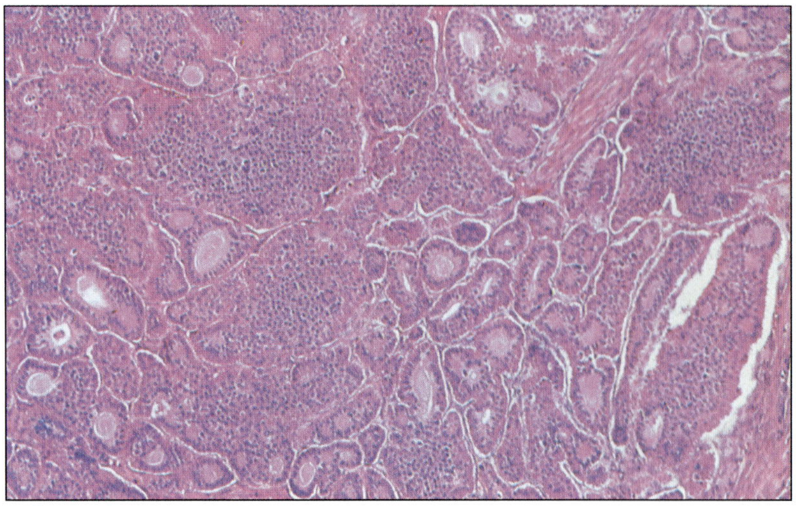

FIGURE 9-18.
Carcinoid tumors of the ovary. Carcinoid tumors may occur as a primary or metastatic lesion in the ovary. The most common pattern for primary and metastatic lesions is the midgut, or insular, pattern. Unlike carcinoid tumors of the intestinal tract, ovarian primaries present earlier in their clinical course, as the venous drainage from the ovary bypasses the portal circulation. Therefore ovarian carcinoids are capable of causing the carcinoid syndrome without metastasis. Serum serotonin levels may be used to monitor response to therapy. Not all tumors are functional.

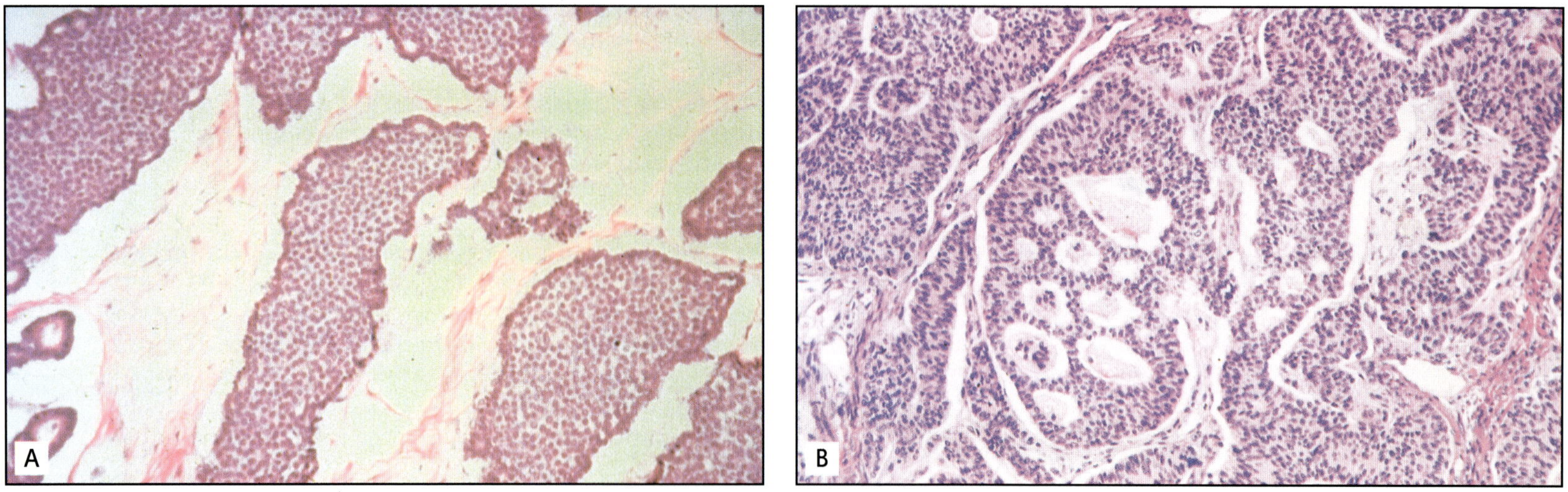

FIGURE 9-19.
Carcinoid—microscopic appearance. Histologically, carcinoids of the ovary resemble those of the intestinal tract. Islands of uniform small cells with little mitotic activity are surrounded by hyalinized connective tissue. The nuclei are small, round, and uniform, and cytoplasm is abundant (**A**). Neurosecretory granules are argentaffin positive. They may also be demonstrated using immunocytochemistry, staining for chromogranin, S-100, and neuron-specific enolase. Serotonin may be be demonstrated using immunoperoxidase. Acini with eosinophilic secretions may be noted, resembling Call-Exner bodies. However, the nuclei are rounded, regular, and basally oriented, whereas in granulosa cell tumor (**B**), the nuclei are typically grooved, and not basally oriented.

CHORIOCARCINOMA

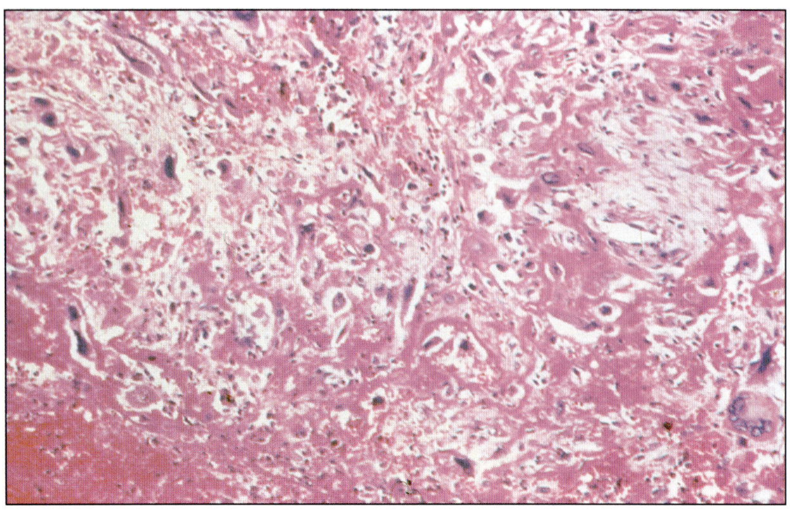

FIGURE 9-20.
Choriocarcinoma. Nongestational primary choriocarcinoma of the ovary is rare. It carries a worse prognosis than do gestational choriocarcinomas with spread to the ovary. As a primary lesion in the ovary, it is usually composed of a mixed germ cell tumor. It occurs in younger patients; many present with signs of precocious puberty. Histologically, these tumors are composed of both syncytiotrophoblasts and cytotrophoblasts.

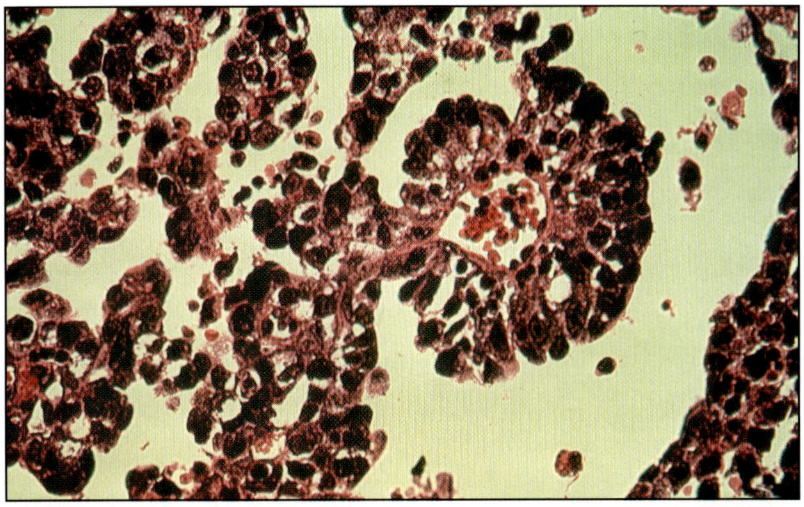

FIGURE 9-21.

Embryonal carcinoma. A considerable controversy has surrounded the embryonal carcinoma, a rare germ cell tumor often confused with yolk sac tumor. This entity represents less than 3% of malignant ovarian germ cell tumors and resembles the ebryonal carcinoma seen in the adult testicle. It is characterized by elevations of both β-human chorionic gonadotropin (β-hCG) and α-fetoprotein (AFP). The extreme rarity of this lesion renders significant statistical evaluation impossible. The close relationship of embryonal carcinoma to choriocarcinoma is demonstrated by the presence of β-hCG and syncytiotrophoblastic cells and the occasional coexistence of both tumors in combination. Embryonal carcinoma also has a tendency to differentiate toward a teratoma, as suggested by its primitive stroma and by the cartilage and squamous epithelium found in some pathologic specimens. It is considered a primitive germ cell tumor, intermediate between dysgerminoma and the others, and capable of both embryonic (teratoma) and extraembryonic (yolk sac tumor, choriocarcinoma) differentiation. The prognosis and treatment are similar to those of the endodermal sinus tumor. Histologically, solid sheets of large, primitive pleomorphic cells with amphophilic vacuolated cytoplasm and vesicular nuclei with one or more nucleoli. These cells may form glandlike spaces and clusters resembling glomeruli as seen here. (Hematoxylin-eosin stain: 100(magnification.) (*From* Breen JL, Sadural E, eds: *Pediatric and Adolescent Gynecology*. Edited by AF Goldfarb. Philadelphia: Current Medicine; 1998:9.13.)

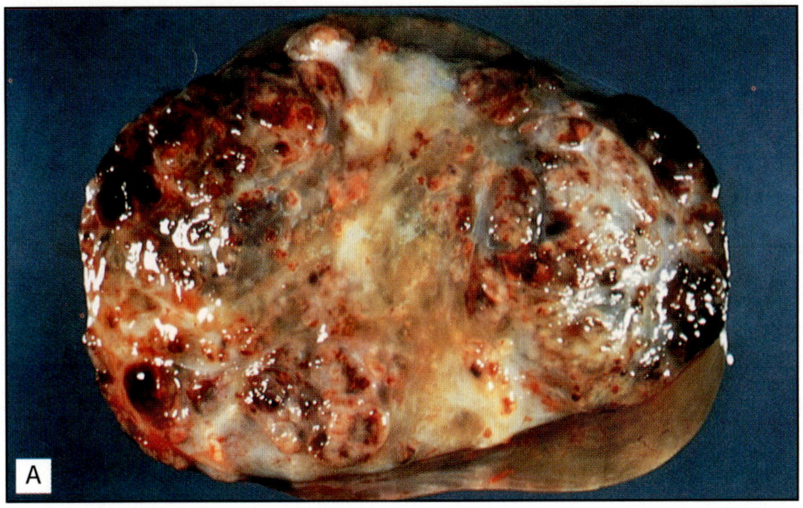

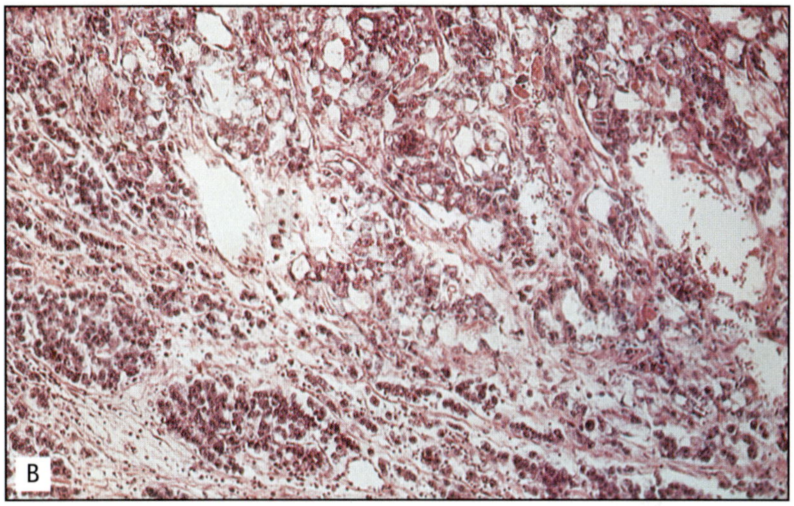

FIGURE 9-22.

Mixed germ cell tumors. These are neoplasms containing two or more germ cell tumors. The yolk sac tumor is seen in 88% of mixed germ cell tumors, and choriocarcinoma is the second most frequent germ cell element and is seen in 25%. These aggressive components are most often found in conjunction with a dysgerminoma. Adequate sampling of all ovarian germ cell tumors is necessary to make this diagnosis, with most pathologists recommending at least one section for every centimeter of tumor diameter. α-Fetoprotein and human chorionic gonadotropin (β-hCG) may be produced; however, the regression of tumor markers may not be predictive of the clinical course, since not all elements necessarily respond in a similar manner. The risk of bilaterality of mixed germ cell tumors is determined by the presence of dysgerminoma elements. The tumors are large and solid averaging 16 cm in diameter (**A**) and usually reveal a dysgerminoma with an asociated yolk sac carcinoma (**B**). (Hematoxylin-eosin stain: 100(magnification.) (*From* Breen JL, Sadural E, eds: Pediatric Ovarian Malignancies. In *Pediatric and Adolescent Gynecology*. Edited by AF Goldfarb. Philadelphia: Current Medicine; 1998:9.14–9.15.)

GONADOBLASTOMA

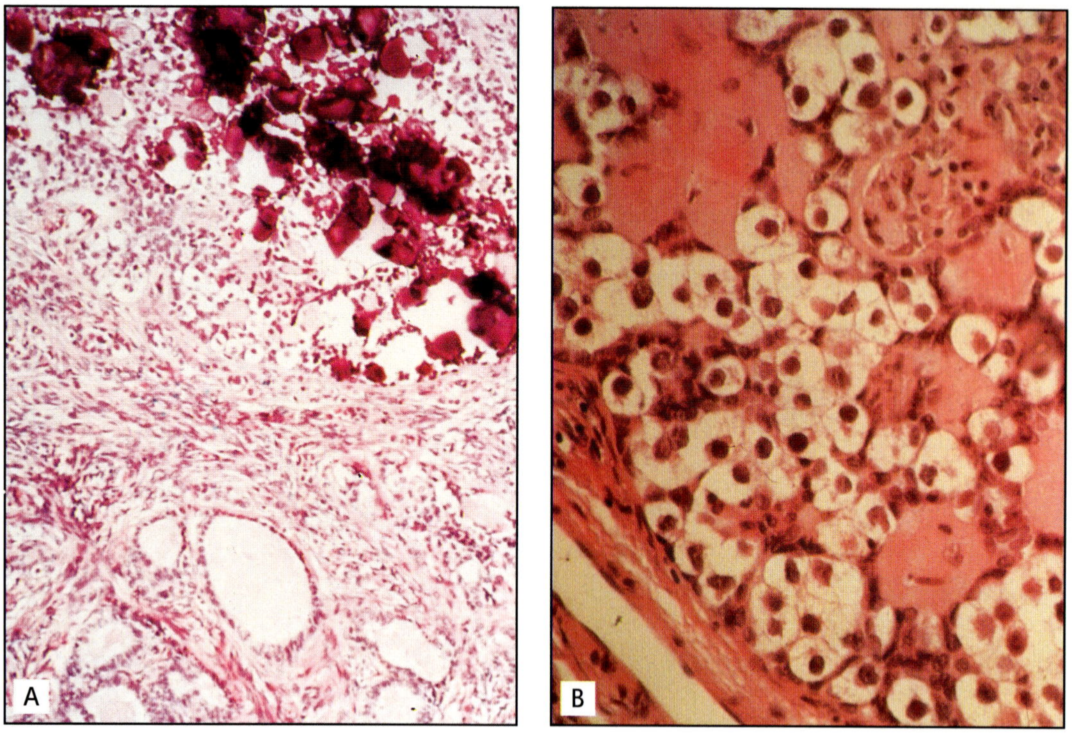

FIGURE 9-23.

Gonadoblastoma. Gonadoblastomas are rare tumors which are usually found in dysgenetic gonads, primarily in individuals with an XY karyotype. The tumors are solid and microscopically are composed of islands of large germ cells with smaller cells of sex cord origin. Areas of calcification are routinely found (**A**). Gonadoblastomas are benign ovarian tumors, but they can give rise to dysgerminomas. If gonadoblastomas are not removed, more than 50% will develop into ovarian malignancies. **A**, Low power and **B**, high power photomicrograph.

SEX CORD–STROMAL TUMORS

CLASSIFICATION OF SEX CORD–STROMAL TUMORS

A. Granulosa-stromal cell tumors
   1. Granulosa-cell tumor
      Adult type
      Juvenile type
   2. Thecoma-fibromas
      Thecoma
      Fibroma
B. Sclerosing stromal cell tumor
   1. Sertoli-Leydig cell tumor
   2. Sertoli-cell tumor
   3. Leydig-cell tumor
C. Sex cord tumor with annular tubules
D. Gynandroblastoma
E. Unclassified
F. Steroid cell tumors
   1. Stromal luteoma

FIGURE 9-24.

Sex cord–stromal tumor classification. Ovarian sex cord–stromal tumors account for approximately 5% of all malignant ovarian neoplasms. These tumors have the ability to produce a variety of hormones, and the clinical presentation of these tumors is related to the endocrine abnormalities that they produce. (*From* Hartman LC, Yound RH, Evans MP, Pooratz KC: Ovarian sex cord–stromal tumors. In *Principles and Practice of Gynecologic Oncology*, edn. 2. Edited by Hoskins WJ, Perez CA, Yound RC. New York: Lippincott-Raven, 1996.)

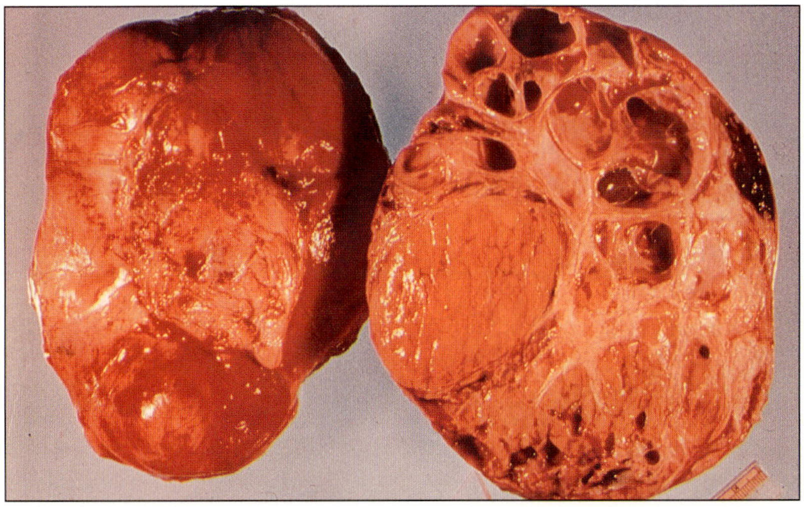

FIGURE 9-25.

Granulosa cell tumor—gross appearance. Granulosa cell tumors are usually solid with a smooth, lobulated surface. These tumors can also be multicystic, with numerous locules filled with fluid or clotted blood. They are rarely bilateral, and range in size from 1 to 2 cm up to 20 cm. Five percent of granulosa cell tumors are found in prepubertal females. The remainder are distributed throughout the reproductive and postmenopausal years. Granulosa cell tumors usually produce estrogen. In prepubertal girls, this can be associated with precocious puberty. In pre- and postmenopausal women, estrogens from granulosa cell tumors are associated with bleeding irregularities, endometrial hyperplasia, and endometrial cancer. Rarely, granulosa cells will secrete androgens.

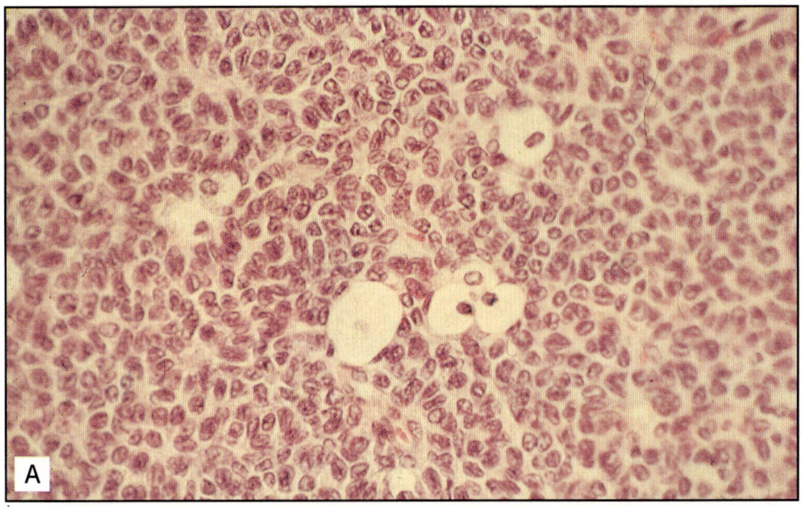

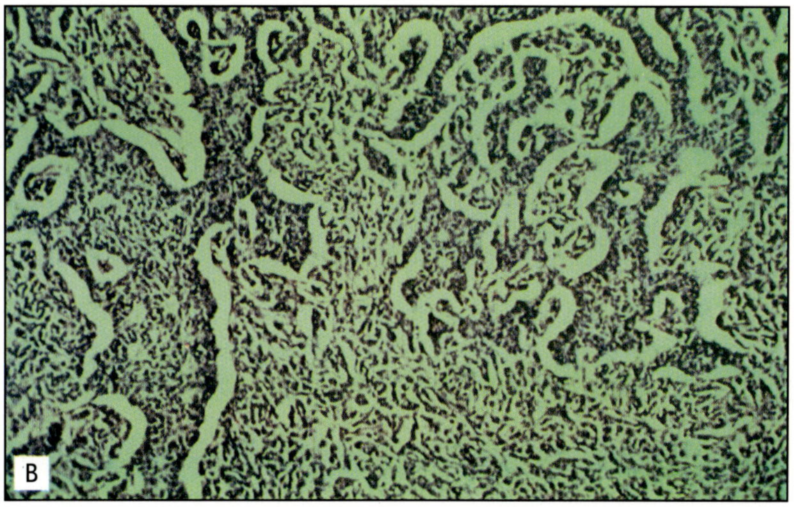

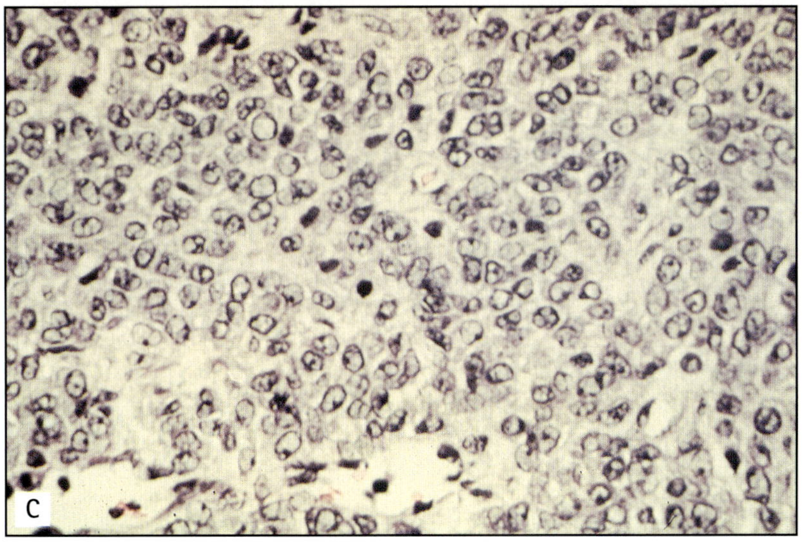

FIGURE 9-26.

Granulosa cell tumor—microscopic appearance. Microscopically, the granulosa cells are round with scant cytoplasm. The nucleus is angular or oval, and often grooved ("coffee-bean" nuclei); mitoses are also common. Several histologic patterns are seen . The most common variety is microfollicular. In this histologic pattern, the granulosa cells arrange themselves in small rosettes around a central empty space. These are Call-Exner bodies, and they resemble primordial follicles (*A*). Other histologic varieties of granulosa cell tumor include macrofollicular, which is characterized by cysts lined with well-differentiated granulosa cells; trabecular, (*B*) which is characterized by bands of granulosa cells separated by fibrous stroma; gyriform, which is characterized by rows of granulosa cells, usually in single file; and sarcomatoid, which is characterized by a patternless growth of granulosa cells (*C*). (*A courtesy of* Marit Ek, MD).

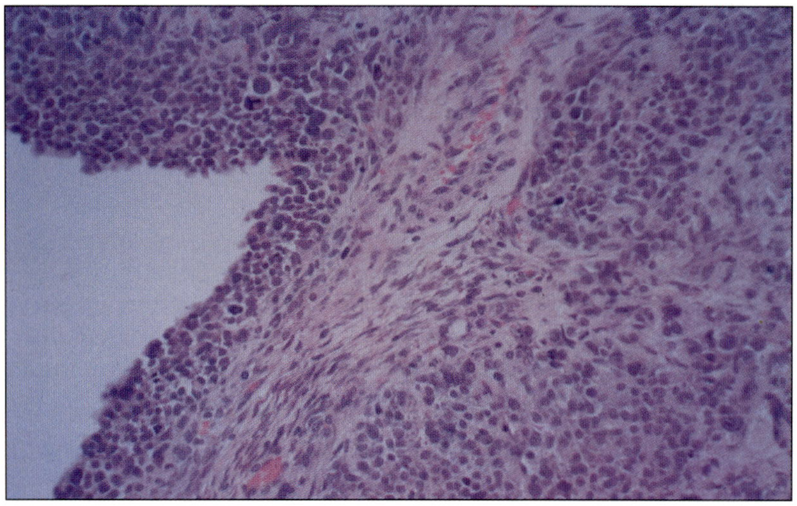

FIGURE 9-27.
Juvenile granulosa cell tumor—microscopic appearance. The juvenile variant of granulosa cell tumors accounts for 85% of granulosa cell tumors found in prepubertal girls. Grossly, the tumors can be solid or multicystic. Microscopically, the tumors contain nodules of granulosa cells with a central cavity containing mucin. These follicles vary in size, and Call-Exner bodies are rarely encountered. Features that distinguish juvenile granulosa cell tumors from the adult type are the rounded nuclei which lack grooves, and the moderate to abundant eosinophilic cytoplasm. (*Courtesy of* Marit Ek, MD).

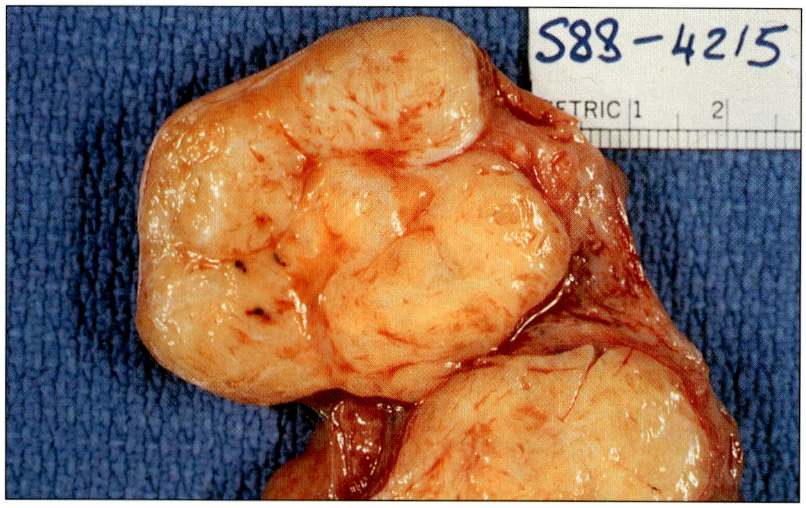

FIGURE 9-28.
Thecoma—gross appearance. Thecomas are solid tumors that grossly appear smooth with lobulated surfaces. Tumors can take on a yellowish appearance as a result of active hormone production. Thes tumors are usually unilateral and occur in the fifth and sixth decades of life. Thecomas rarely are malignant. (*Courtesy of* Marit Ek, MD).

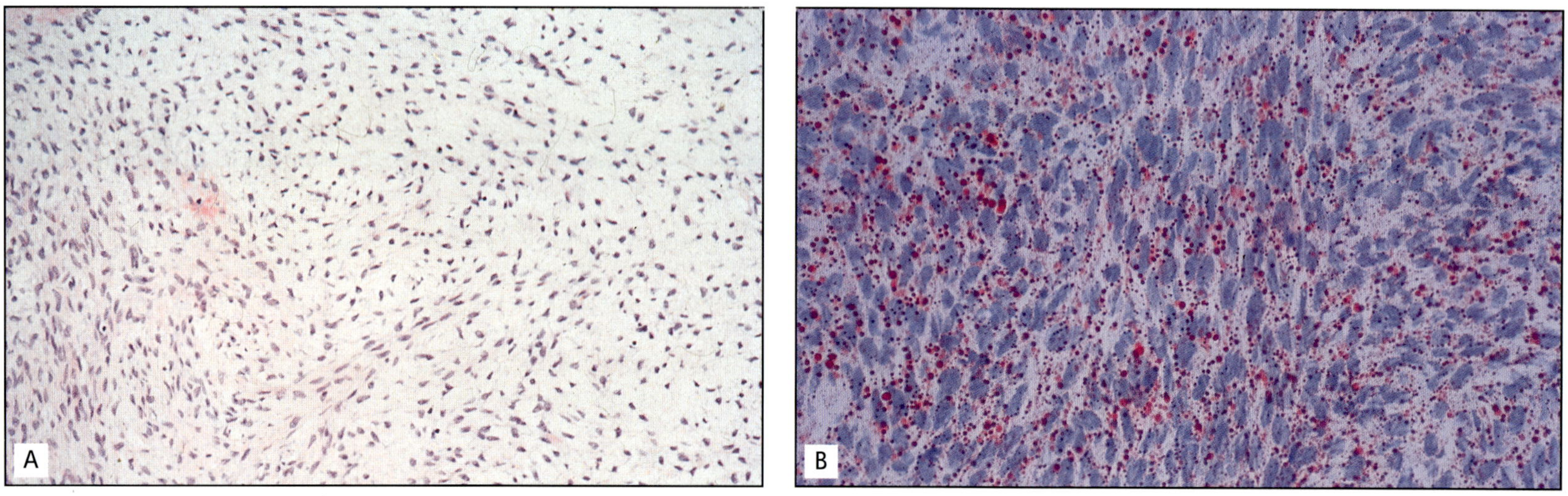

FIGURE 9-29.
Thecoma—microscopic appearance. Microscopically, thecomas have plump spindle cells with abundant cytoplasm. The cells are interlaced and separated by connective stromal tissue (**A**). Thecomas are very similar to fibromas except that thecomas contain lipid in the cytoplasm. This can be demonstrated with an oil red O stain (**B**). (*Courtesy of* Marit Ek, MD).

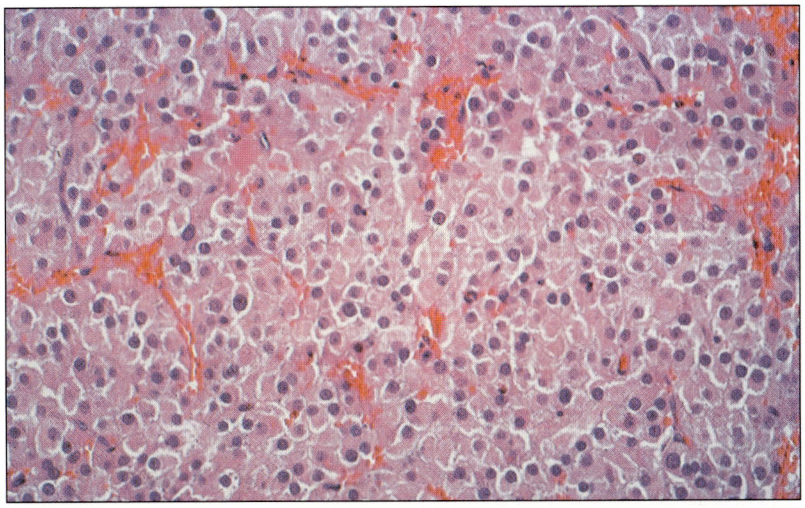

FIGURE 9-30.
Luteoma of pregnancy. This is a solid tumor consisting of nodular hyperplasia of ovarian lutein cells. It occurs during pregnancy and is associated with fetal and maternal virilization. Spontaneous regression occurs post partum. (*Courtesy of* Marit Ek, MD).

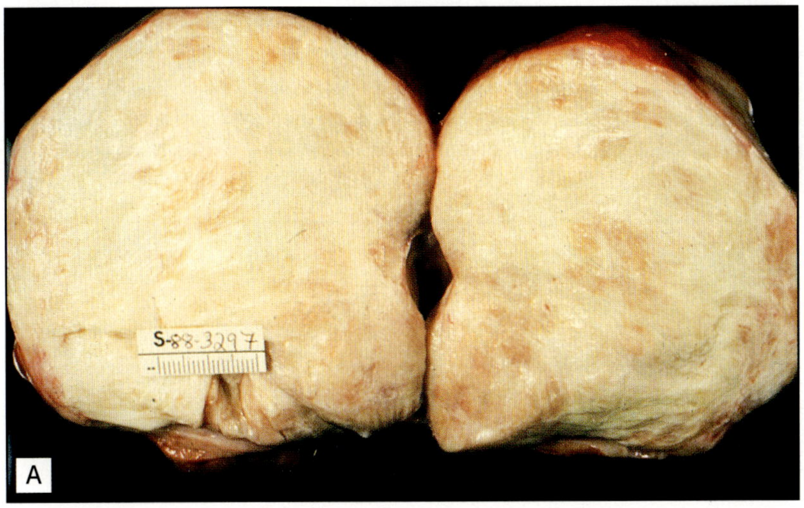

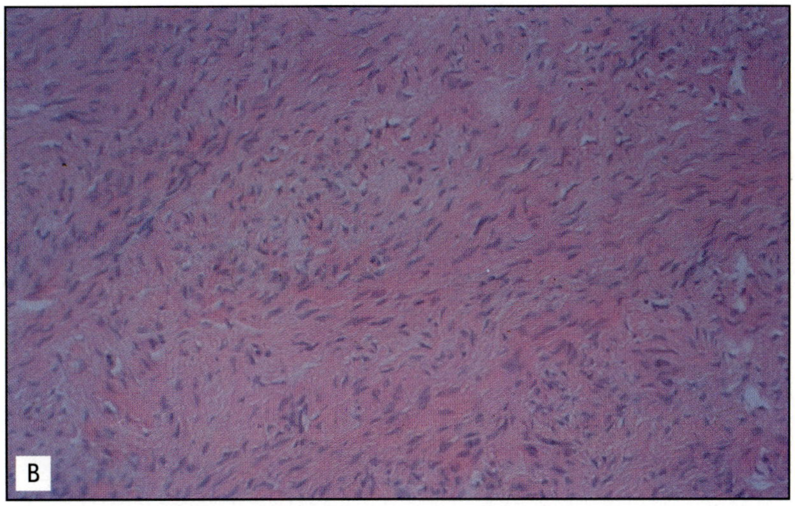

FIGURE 9-31.
Fibroma. Fibromas are benign connective tissue tumors. They are solid and 10% are bilateral. This tumor is associated with Meigs' syndrome (ascites, hydrothorax, and pelvic mass). The average size is 6 cm, but tumors can grow to be quite large. Grossly, the tumors are white and smooth (**A**). Cystic degeneration can be seen. Microscopically, tumors appear very similar to thecomas, with interlacing spindle cells containing small nuclei and abundant cytoplasm (**B**).

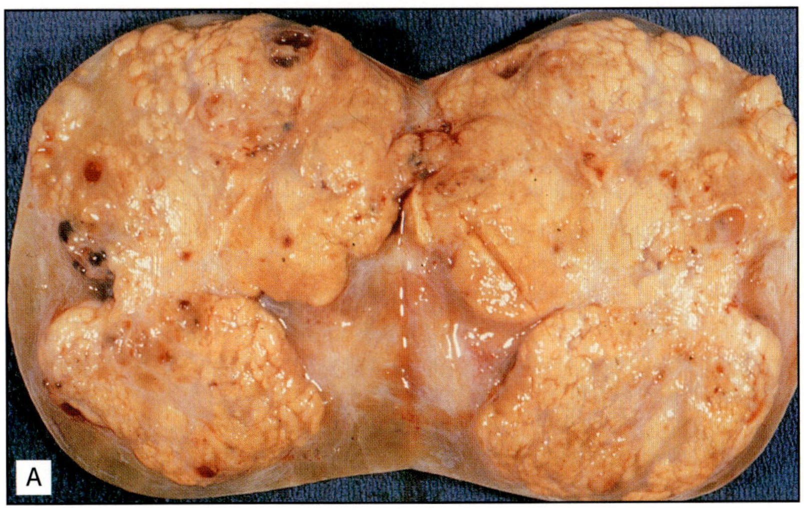

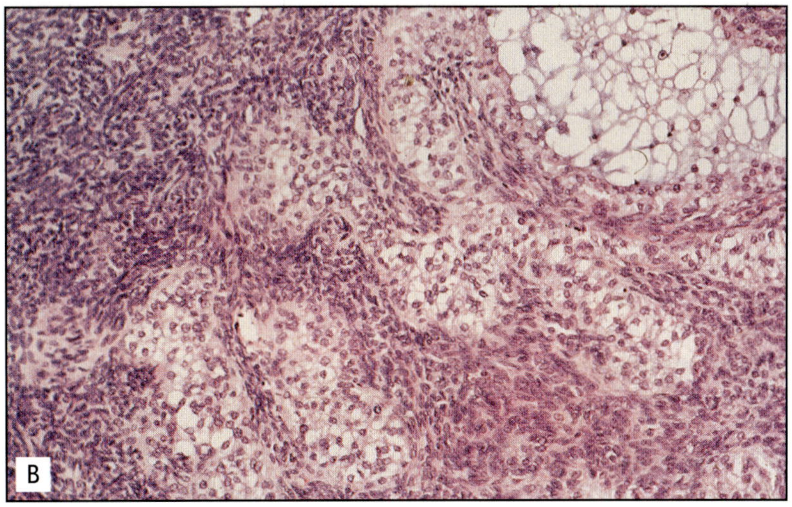

FIGURE 9-32.
Sertoli-Leydig cell tumor. Sertoli-Leydig cell tumors are solid tumors that are usually unilateral. They occur in the third or fouth decade of life. These tumors are usually associated with virilization; however, 5% secrete estrogen. Grossly, these tumors are smooth, with a grayish-yellow surface. Tumors vary in size, but most are between 5 to 10 cm in diameter (**A**). Microscopically, the tumor consists of Sertoli cell tubules with intervening Leydig cells (**B**). Reinke crystals may be seen. Sertoli-Leydig cell tumors may be graded as intermediate or poorly differentiated. Malignant behavior is exhibited only by the less well differentiated tumors. Heterologous elements are found in approximately 20% of Sertoli-Leydig cell tumors. Endodermal elements such as intestinal epithelium, or mesenchymal elements such as cartilage and skeletal muscle, are typically seen when heterologous elements are present. (*Courtesy of* Marit Ek, MD).

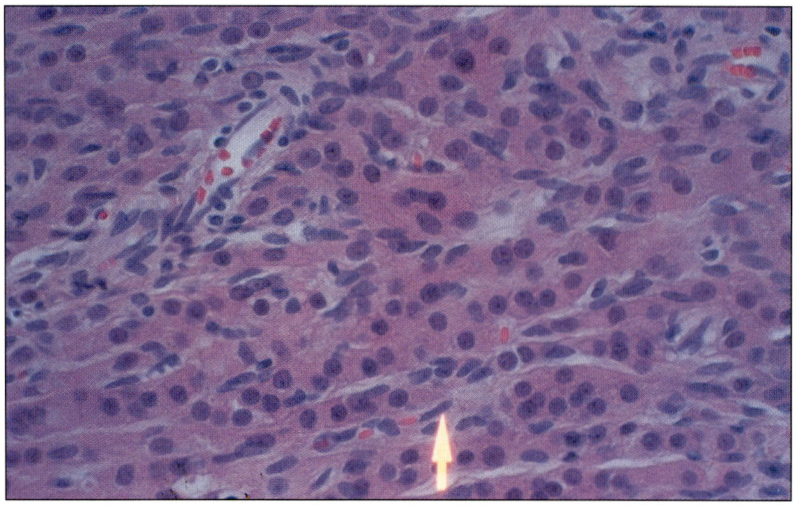

FIGURE 9-33.
Hilus cell tumors. Hilus cell tumors are located in the ovarian hilum and composed entirely of Leydig cells. The tumors usually produce testosterone. They are small, occur after age 50, and are almost always benign. Reinke crystals are present. (*Courtesy of* Marit Ek, MD).

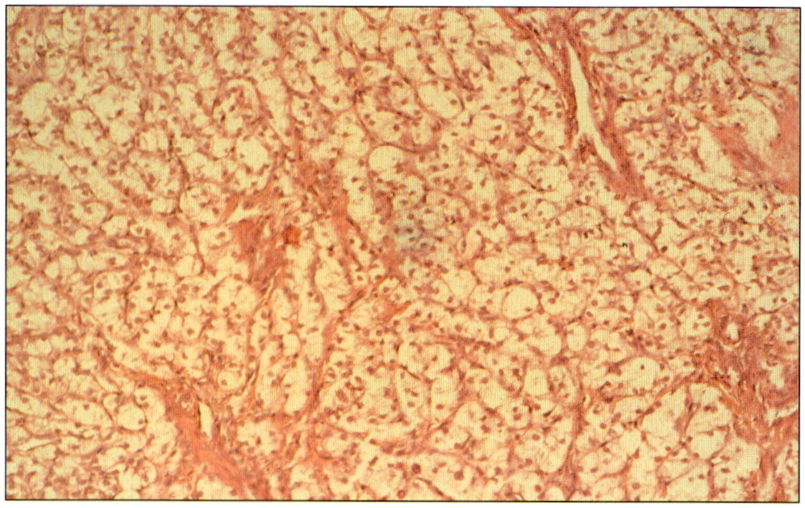

FIGURE 9-34.
Lipoid cell tumor. Lipoid cell tumors are solid tumors that usually occur in premenopausal women. Tumors are usually unilateral and greater than 8 cm in size. Microscopically, these tumors contain large rounded cells and luteinized ovarian stroma. Reinke cystals are not present. Approximately 20% of these tumors exhibit malignant behavior. (*Courtesy of* Marit Ek, MD).

METASTATIC TUMORS

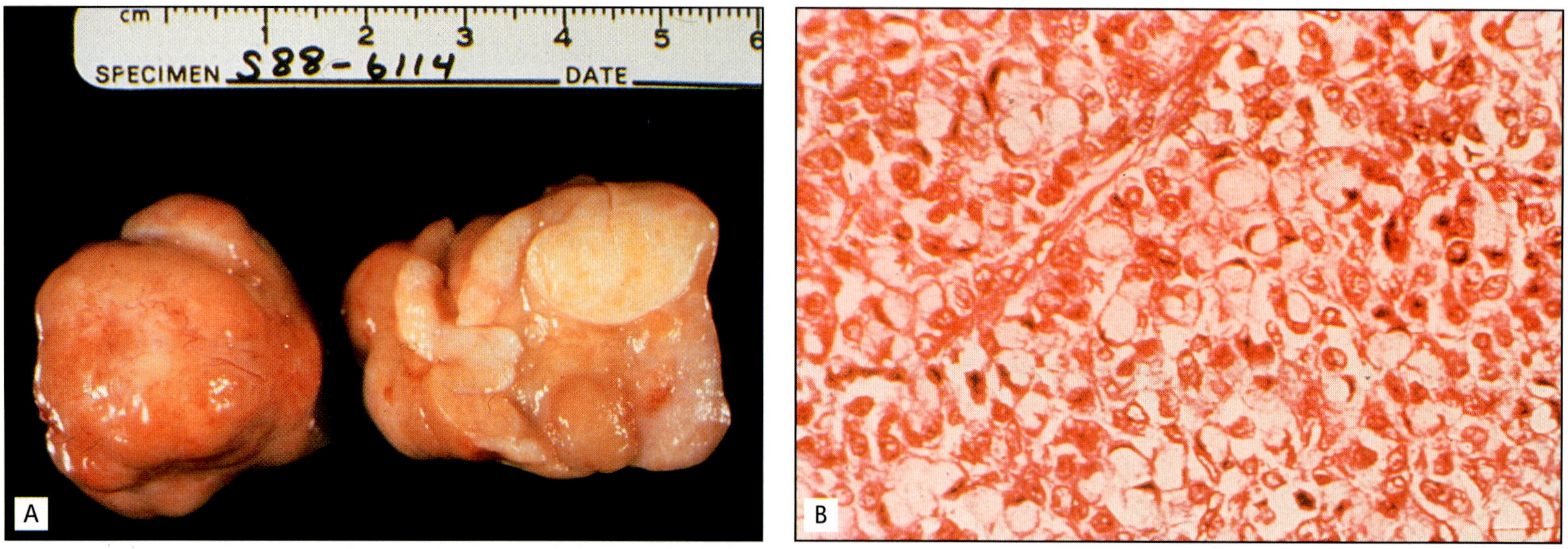

FIGURE 9-35.
Metastatic tumors. These tumors to the ovary occur most frequently from gynecologic malignancies that spread by direct extension, lymphatic spread, or hematogenous spread. Approximately 13% of tubal cancers and 5% of endometrial cancers involve the ovaries.

The most frequent nongynecologic tumor to spread to the ovaries is breast cancer. In advanced disease, ovarian involvement is found in 20% to 30% of cases, and is usually bilateral. Krukenberg tumors account for 30% to 40% of metastatic cancers to the ovaries.

Krukenberg tumors usually are metastatic from gastrointestinal primaries, the stomach, or the colon. However, rarely, metastasis from the breast, biliary tract, or bladder may result in a Krukenberg tumor. Grossly, the tumors are solid, smooth, and usually bilateral (**A**). Microscopically, signet ring cells are seen. In these cells, the nucleus is flattened against the cell by the accumulation of mucus (**B**).

(*Continued on next page*)

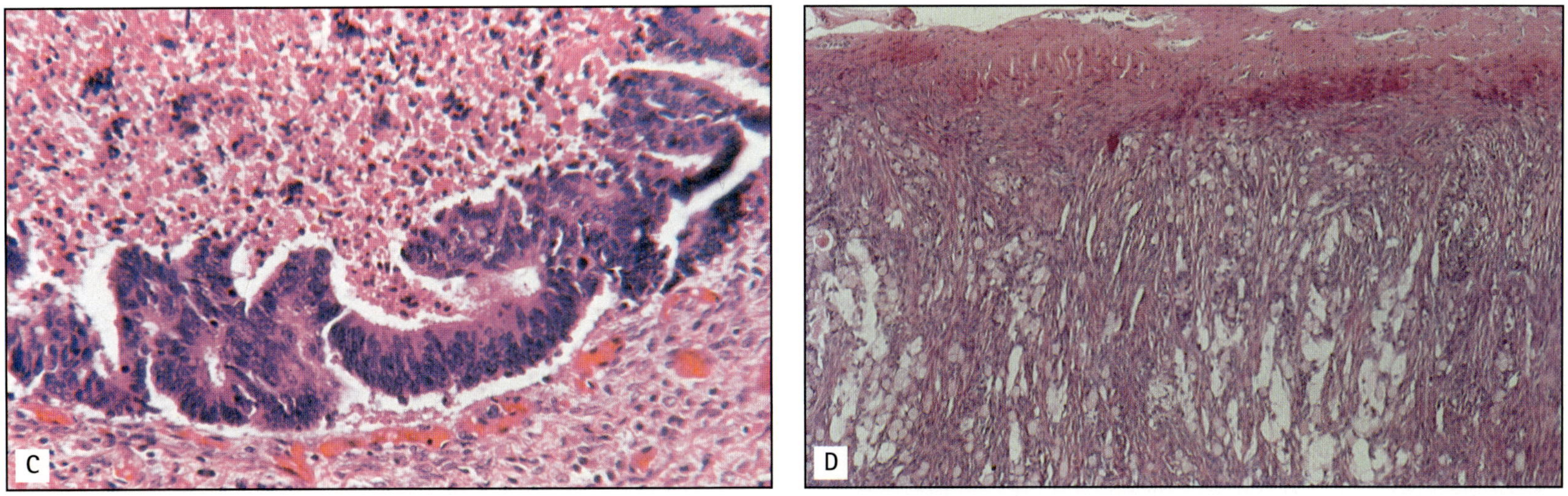

FIGURE 9-35. *(Continued)*

In other cases, metastasis from the gastrointestinal tract to the ovary will not have a Krukenberg histology, but will appear similar to a mucinous cystadenocarcinoma (**C**).

Other unusual tumors to involve the ovary include lymphomas and leukemias, with involvement usually being bilateral. With Burkett's lymphoma, ovarian involvement is common, and with Hodgkin's disease, approximately 5% of patients develop ovarian involvement. Melanoma (**D**) has also been reported to metastasize to the ovaries.

SUGGESTED BIBLIOGRAPHY

Aboud E: A review of granulosa cell tumours and thecomas of the ovary. *Arch Gynecol Obstet* 1997, 259:161–165.

Gershenson DM, Morris M, Burke TW, Levenback C, *et al.*: Treatment of poor-prognosis sex cord-stromal tumors of the ovary with the combination of bleomycin, etoposide, and cisplatin. *Obstet Gynecol* 1996, 87:527–531.

Gordon MD, Ireland K: New developments in sex cord-stromal and germ cell tumors of the ovary. *Clin Lab Med* 1995, 15:595–610.

Harman LC, Young RH, Evans MP, Pooratz KC: Ovarian sex cord–stromal tumors. In *Principles and Practice of Gynecologic Oncology,* edn 2. Edited by Hoskins WJ, Perez CA, Young RC. New York: Lippincott-Raven, 1996.

Rao BR, Slotman BJ: Ovarian tuors with endocrine manifestations. *Curr Ther Endocrinol Metab* 1997, 6:260–262.

CHAPTER 10

Placental Tumors

Hisham K. Tamimi

Gestational trophoblastic tumors are unique tumors derived from fetal tissue. They display a wide spectrum of malignant behavior, but, even in the presence of widespread metastasis, gestational trophoblastic tumors can be cured. The exquisite sensitivity of these tumors to chemotherapy allows a very high survival rate in all but the most advanced cases.

Gestational trophoblastic tumors are also unique because they are capable of elaborating steroid and protein hormones. These tumors have the capability of producing large amounts of human chorionic gonadotropin (hCG) which is an ideal tumor marker in that it is both extremely sensitive and specific for gestational trophoblastic disease. The development of sensitive tests to measure serum hCG levels has made dramatic advances possible in the diagnosis, treatment, and follow-up of patients with these diseases.

CLASSIFICATION, IDENTIFICATION, AND RISK FACTORS

HISTOPATHOLOGY CLASSIFICATION OF GESTATIONAL TROPHOBLASTIC DISEASE (GTD)

- Hydatidiform mole
  - Complete
  - Partial
- Invasive mole
- Choriocarcinoma
- Placental site trophoblastic tumor

FIGURE 10-1.
Histopathologic classification of gestational trophoblastic disease (GTD). GTD represents a spectrum of tumors which express various degrees of ability to invade, persist, and metasstasize. Hydatidiform moles should be defined as either partial or complete moles based on gross appearance, karyotype determination, flow cytometry analysis, and microscopic appearance. Invasive moles are characterized by invasion into the myometrium of edematous chorionic villi covered with layers of proliferative trophoblastic cells. Choriocarcinoma is characterized by the admixture of malignant cytotrophoblast and syncytiotrophoblast, and is often associated with hemorrhage or necrosis. Placental site trophoblastic tumors are an extremely rare entity, and are characterized by the absence of chorionic villi and the proliferation of intermediate cytotrophoblasts.

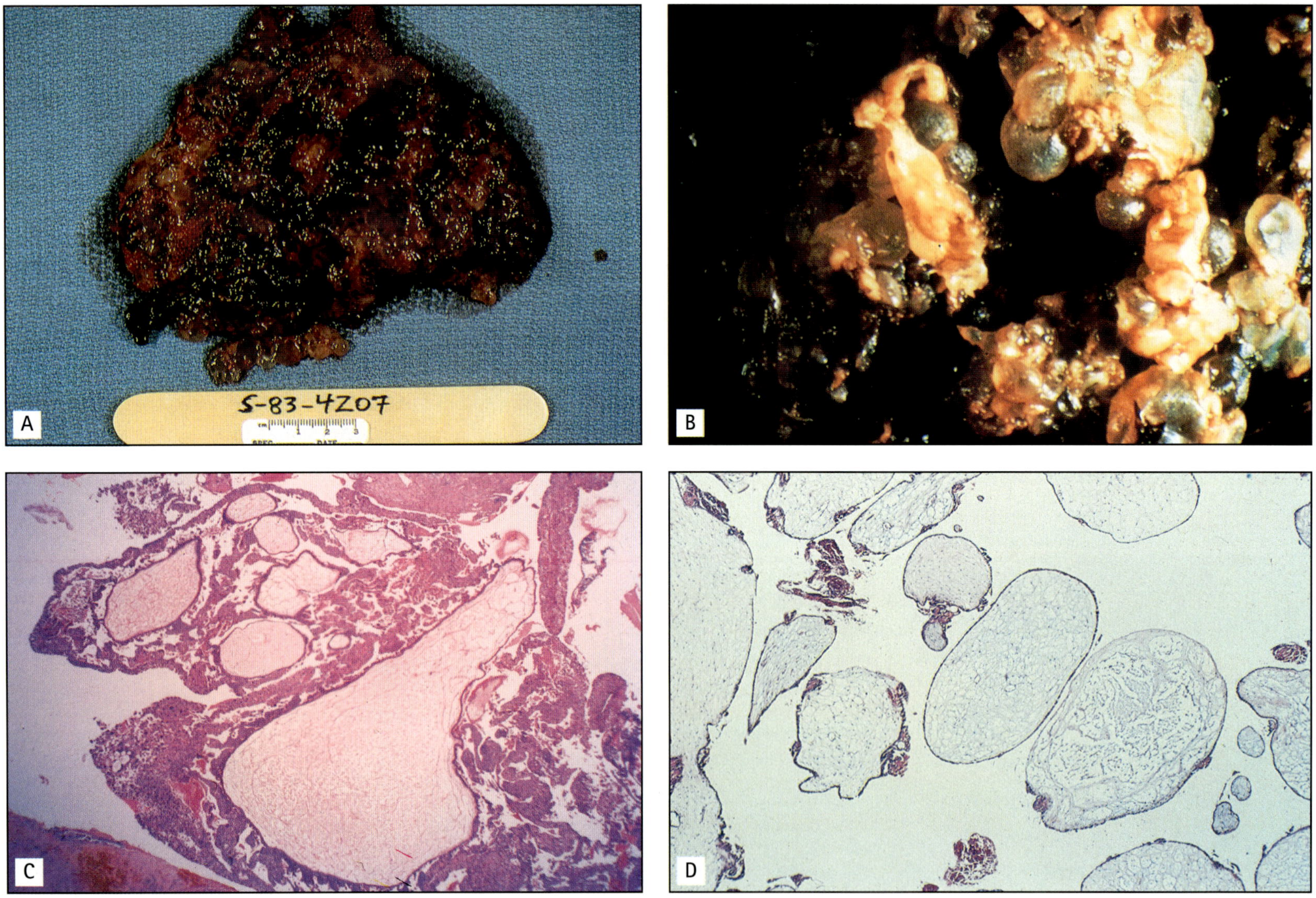

FIGURE 10-2.
Hydatidiform moles. Hydatidiform moles can be categorized as either complete or partial moles on the basis of gross morphology, histopathology, and karyotype. Grossly, complete moles are characterized by numerous thin-walled vesicles measuring 2 to 3 cm in diameter. The specimen resembles a cluster of grapes (**A** and **B**). Histologically, the characteristic features of a complete mole are diffuse trophoblastic hyperplasia, including syncytial and cytotrophoblasts, along with hydropic swelling of the villi. Frequently, many villi are necrotic and there is an absence of fetal tissue (**C**). Partial moles are characterized by the following pathologic features: chorionic villi of varying size with focal hydatidiform swelling, focal trophoblastic hyperplasia with or without atypia (**D**) and identifiable embryonic or fetal tissues.

RISK FACTORS FOR PERSISTENT GESTATIONAL TROPHOBLASTIC DISEASE (GTD)

Maternal age
hCG >100,000 mIU/mL
Uterine size > Gestational age
Theca lutein cysts >6 cm
Previous molar pregnancy

FIGURE 10-3.

Risk factors of persistent gestational trophoblastic disease (GTD). Following evacuation of a complete molar pregnancy, the risk of persistent GTD is approximately 20%. Factors that increase the risk of persistent trophoblastic disease include high levels of hCG, excessive uterine enlargement, and large theca-lutein cysts. In addition, older women have a higher incidence of persistent disease, and women with a previous molar pregnancy have a four-fold increased risk of developing persistent disease. Partial moles are rarely associated with persistent GTD. hCg—human chorionic gonadotropin; IU—inteinational units.

TYPES OF TUMORS

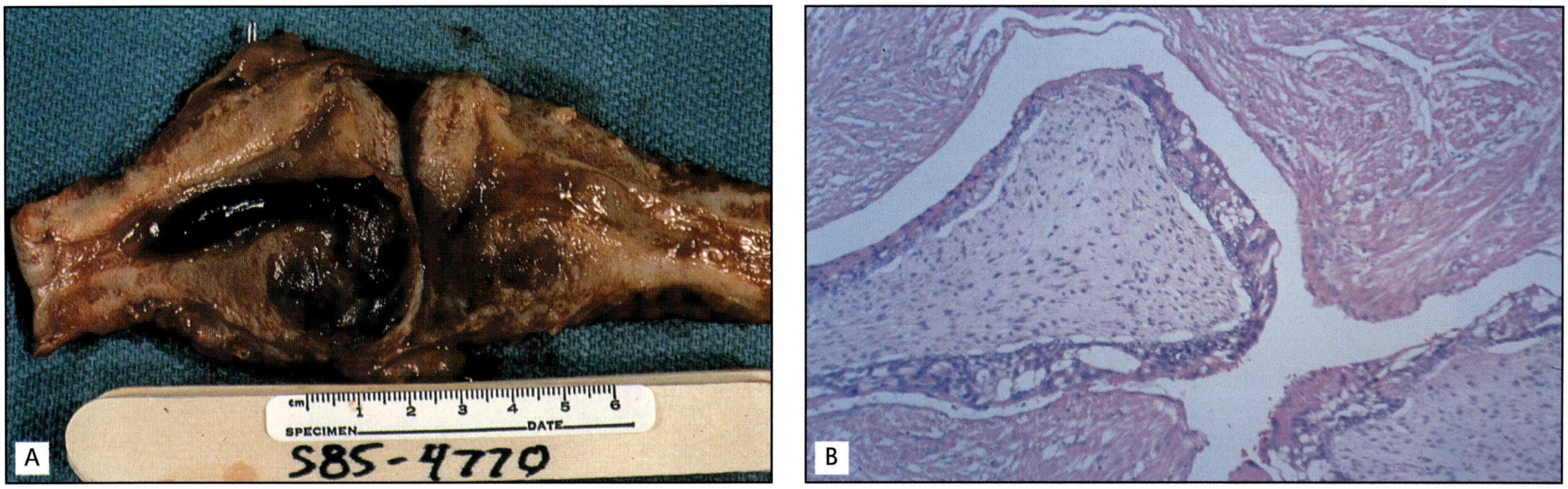

FIGURE 10-4.

Invasive moles. With the current successful use of chemotherapy, invasive moles rarely require a hysterectomy. In the case illustrated, molar vesicles are seen invading the myometrium, both grossly and microscopically (**A** and **B**). The extent of invasion can be significant, and even extend beyond the uterus into the parametrial tissues. Bleeding and infection represent major risks.

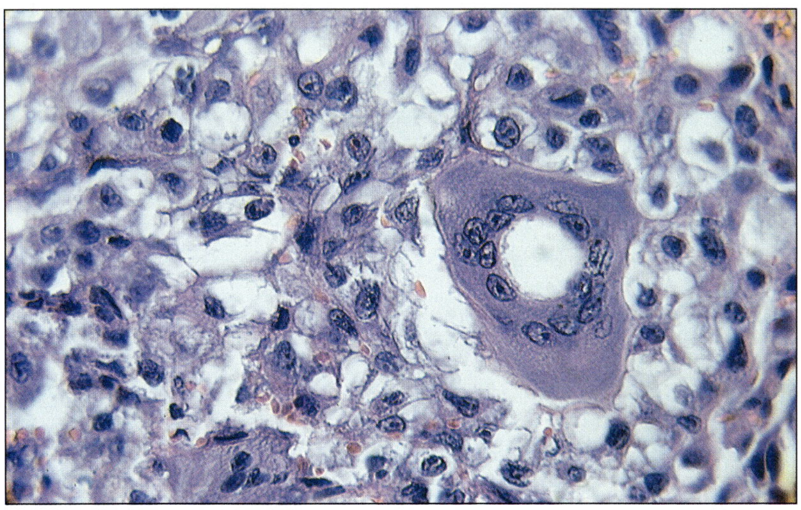

FIGURE 10-5.

Choriocarcinoma. Grossly, choriocarcinoma forms hemorrhagic nodules. Microscopically, columns of both syncytial and cytotrophoblastic tissues are evident, while chorionic villi are absent. Areas of hemorrhage and necrosis are common.

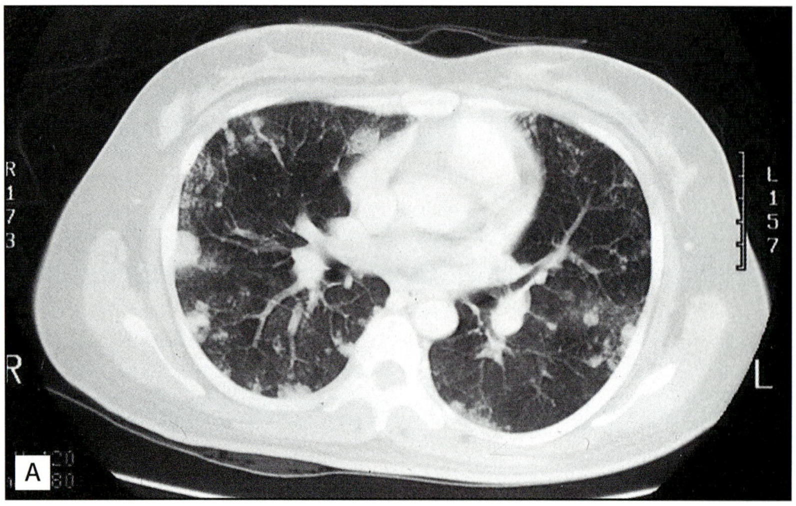

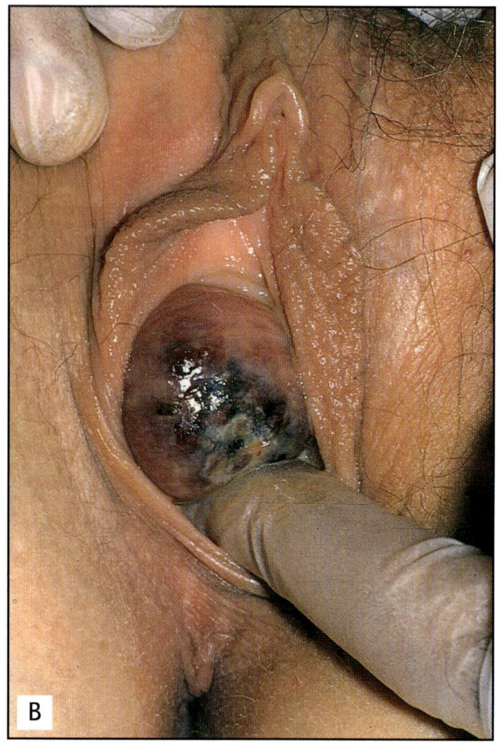

FIGURE 10-6.

Choriocarcinoma metastic to suburethral area. Metastic gestational trophoblastic disease, which can be widely disseminated, is usually associated with choriocarcinoma. Eighty percent of patients with metastatic gestational trophoblastic disease will have lung involvement. **A**, Representative chest computer tomography. Vaginal metastasis can also occur, including the suburethral area (**B**). Because trophoblastic tumors are perfused by an extensive network of blood vessels, they are frequently hemorrhagic. Significant bleeding can result if these lesions are biopsied.

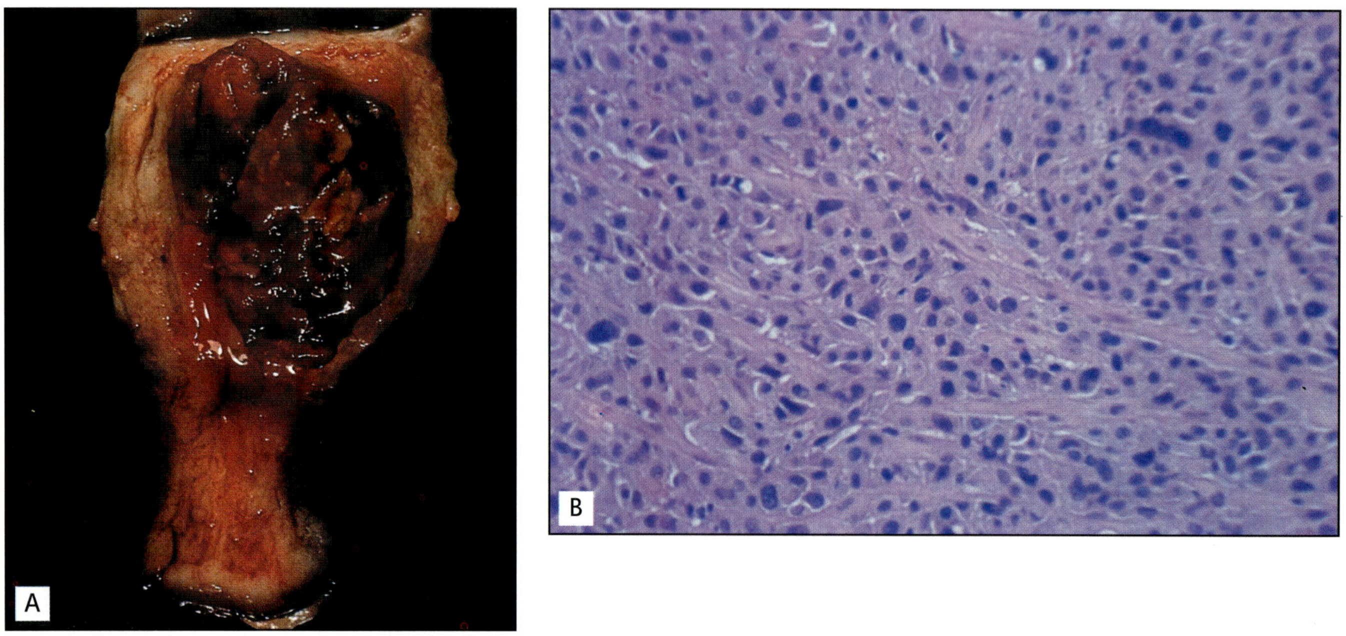

FIGURE 10-7.

Placental site trophoblastic tumor. These tumors are an uncommon variant of gestational trophoblastic disease. Grossly, these tumors appear as a fleshy mass without vesicles (**A**). Microscopically, the presence of the intermediate trophoblast is the hallmark of the diagnosis (**B**). Immunocytochemistry demonstrating the staining of human placental lactogen (HPL) is confirmatory evidence of the diagnosis. These tumors produce low levels of hCG and tend to remain confined to the uterus and metastasize late in their course. Placental site tumors are relatively insensitive to chemotherapy and hysterectomy is usually required for successful treatment.

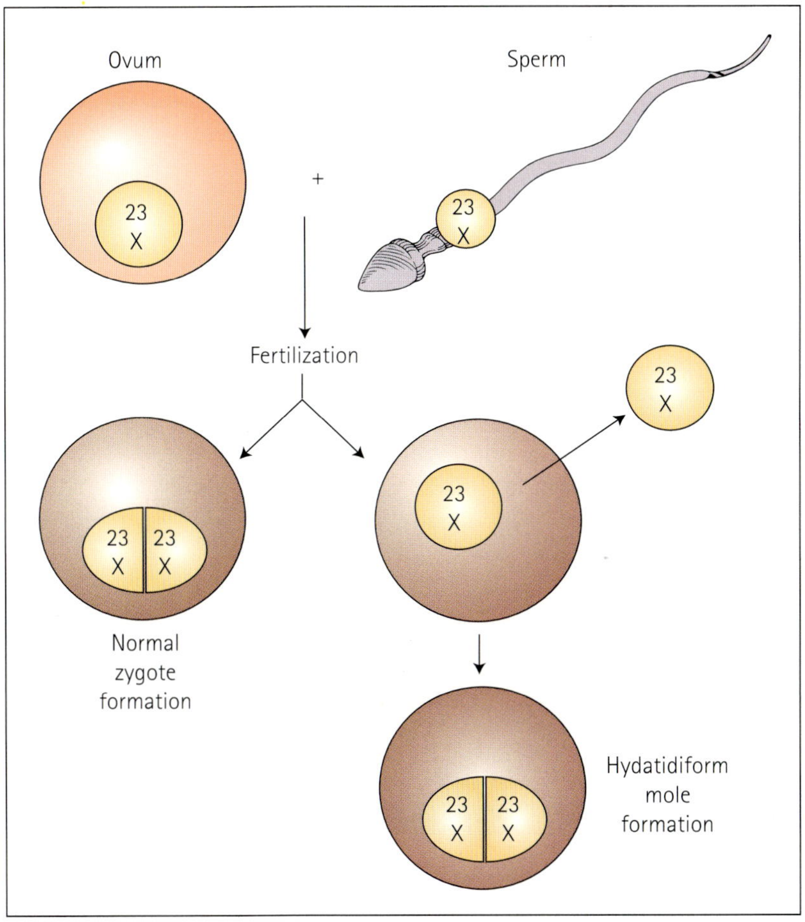

FIGURE 10-8.

Genetic constitution of molar preganacies—complete mole vs normal pregnancy. Schematic representation of the difference between complete molar pregnancy and nomal pregnancies. Complete molar pregnancies usually have a karyotype of 46XX owing to duplication of a haploid sperm and ejection of the oocyte genetic material; the molar pregnancy chromosomes are thus entirely paternal in origin. Dispermic molar pregancies are rare.

COMPLETE MOLE VS PARTIAL MOLE

	Partial Mole	Complete Mole
Karyotype	Triploidy (>90%) Tetraploidy	46XX (>90%) 46XY
Presence of fetal tissue	Present	Absent
Hydropic villi	Limited and focal	Extensive
Trophoblastic hyperplasia	Focal without mild atypia	Extensive with significant atypia

FIGURE 10-9.

Complete mole versus partial mole. The genetic constitution of complete molar pregnancy is usually of 46XX. Partial moles, on the other hand, are usually triploidy (triploidy: 69XXX or 69XXY or 69XYY), or rarely tetraploid. Complete moles are entirely of paternal origin. Complete moles appear to arise from an ovum that has been fertilized by a haploid sperm which then duplicates. The nucleus of the ovum is absent or inactivated. In partial moles, there are contributions from both mother and father; however, the extra haploid set of chromosomes is usually derived from the father.

FIGO STAGING OF TROPHOBLASTIC TUMORS

Stage I	Disease confined to the uterus
Stage Ia	Disease confined to the uterus with no risk factors
Stage Ib	Disease confined to the uterus with one risk factor
Stage Ic	Disease confined to the uterus with two risk factors
Stage II	GTT extends outside of the uterus but is limited to the genital structures (adnexa, vagina, broad ligament)
Stage IIa	GTT involving genital structures without risk factors
Stage IIb	GTT extends outside of the uterus but limited to genital structures with one risk factor
Stage IIc	GTT extends outside of the uterus but limited to the genital structures with two risk factors
Stage III	GTT extends to the lungs with or without known genital tract involvement
Stage IIIa	GTT extends to the lungs with or without genital tract involvement and with no risk factors
Stage IIIb	GTT extends to the lungs with or without gential tract involvement and with one risk factor
Stage IIIc	GTT extends outside to the lungs with or without genital tract involvement and has two risk factors
Stage IV	All other metastatic sites
Stage IVa	All other metastatic sites without risk factors
Stage IVb	All other metastatic sites with one risk factor
Stage IVc	All other metastatic sites with two risk factors

FIGURE 10-10.

FIGO staging. The FIGO staging system is a combination of anatomical staging and consideration of previously known risk factors. These risk factors are the level of pretreatment hCG and the duration of disease dated from termination of the antecedent pregnancy.

SELECTED BIBLIOGRAPHY

Azab M, Droz JP, Theodore C, *et al.*: Cisplatin, vinblastine, and bleomycin combination in the treatment of resistant high-risk gestational trophoblastic tumors. *Cancer* 1989, 64:1829–1832.

Berkowitz RS, Goldstein DP: Chorionic tumors. *N Engl J Med* 1996, 335(23):1740–1748.

Gestational trophoblastic diseases: report of a WHO scientific group. *WHO Tech Rep Ser* 1983, 692:51.

Homesley HD: Development of single-agent chemotherapy regimens for gestational trophoblastic disease. *J Reprod Med* 1994, 39:185–192.

Kaji T, Ohama K: Androgenetic origin of hydatidiform mole. *Nature* 1977, 268:633–634.

Long LC, Choo YC, Ma HK: Primary oral etoposide therapy in gestational trophoblastic disease: an update. *Cancer* 1986, 58:14–17.

Lurain JR, Brewer JI, Torok EE, Halpern B: Natural history of hydatidiform mole after primary evacuation. *Am J Obstet Gynecol* 1983, 145:591–595.

Newlands ES, Bagshawe KD, Begent RHJ, *et al.*: Results with the EMA/CO (etoposide, methotrexate, actinomycin D, cyclophosphamide, vincristine) regimen in high risk gestational trophoplastic tumors, 1979–1989. *Br J Obstet Gynaecol* 1991, 98:550–557.

Schink JC, Singh DK, Rademaker AW, *et al.*: Etoposide, methotrexate, actinomycin D, cyclophosphamide, and vincristine for the treatment of metastatic, high-risk gestational trophoblastic disease. *Obstet Gynecol* 1992, 80:817–820.

Szulman AE, Surti U: The clinicopathologic profile of the partial hydatidiform mole. *Obstet Gynecol* 1982, 59:597–602.

CHAPTER 11

Cytology

Rochelle L. Garcia and Nancy B. Kiviat

Fifty years after its inception, the cervical Pap smear remains the most effective and widely used cancer screening assay. In the United States, the establishment of widespread Pap screening in the 1960s has resulted in a 78% decrease in the incidence of and mortality from invasive cervical carcinoma [1–3]. Today, not having had a Pap smear within the last 10 years is the most important risk factor, other than exposure to human papillomavirus (HPV), for the development of invasive cervical carcinoma. Not surprisingly, in developing countries where Pap screening is largely unavailable, the incidence of cervical cancer has remained high [4,5].

This chapter focuses on cervical cytology and provides examples of normal and abnormal cytologic findings. The abnormal findings concentrate on neoplastic and inflammatory conditions arising in the cervix but also include examples of neoplastic disease arising elsewhere. Common, potentially confusing artifacts and specific infectious agents are also included.

Cervical cytology is a *screening* assay with a well established, moderately high, false-negative rate that ranges from 1.1% to 62.5% for the detection of carcinoma *in situ* [4,5]. This error rate is dependent on sampling errors (the lesion is present in the patient but not on the slide), screening errors (diagnostic cells are present on the slide but are not seen by the screener), and interpretation errors (abnormal cells are present on the slide and seen but are incorrectly interpreted). It is generally accepted that the true false-negative rate is about 50% due to sampling errors and about 50% due to other errors and that the irreducible false-negative rate for screening errors is about 5%. If a patient has a clinical abnormality, and a Pap smear is negative, further workup is required. Communication between the cytology laboratory and the clinician is essential and additional material—preferably a biopsy—should be obtained whenever a cytologic diagnosis does not fit the clinical picture.

CLASSIFICATION SYSTEMS

COMPARISON OF PAST AND PRESENT SYSTEMS FOR CLASSIFYING CERVICAL CYTOLOGY FINDINGS

Papanicolau system (approximately 1954–1980s)	Dysplasia/carcinoma in situ	CIN system (1987 to present for histology)	Bethesda system (1988–to present)
Class I: Normal cells *Class II*: Some abnormal cells present but probably reactive	*Negative*: Normal cells or cells with benign cellular changes including reactive, infectious, and repair	*Negative*: Normal cells or cells with benign cellular changes including reactive, infectious, and repair	*Negative*: Normal cells or cells with benign cellular changes including reactive, infectious, and repair
Class II: Some abnormal cells present but probably reactive	*Atypical*: Descriptive diagnosis	*Atypical*: Descriptive diagnosis	*Atypical squamous cells of undetermined significance (ASCUS)*: Does not include clearly reactive or neoplastic changes
Class III: Dyskaryotic cells present, malignancy cannot be ruled out	*Low-grade dysplasia*: Condyloma, HPV-associated changes	*Cervical intraepithelial neoplasia (CIN) grade I*: HPV changes, koilocytotic atypia, condyloma	*Low-grade squamous intraepithelial lesion (LGSIL)*: including HPV effect and "low-grade dysplasia"
Class III: Dyskaryotic cells present, malignancy cannot be ruled out *Class IV*: Dyskaryotic cells present, high probability of malignancy	*Moderate dysplasia, severe dysplasia, carcinoma in situ*	*CIN grades II and III*	*High-grade squamous intraepithelial lesion (HGSIL)*
Class V: Malignant cells present	*Specific diagnosis*: (*eg*, squamous cell carcinoma, adenocarcinoma)	*Specific diagnosis*: (*eg*, squamous cell carcinoma, adenocarcinoma)	*Positive* with specific diagnosis as to type of malignancy (*eg*, squamous, adenocarcinoma)

FIGURE 11-1.

Comparison of past and present systems for classifying cervical cytology findings. The table shows the corresponding diagnoses for each of the classification schemes noted. Until the Bethesda conference in 1988, Pap smear diagnoses were based on the Papanicolau class system. This system was initially designed to include a descriptive diagnosis and to predict the probability of existing cancer. The descriptions were often omitted, and the use of this system gradually changed, because the original terminology did not fit with the evolving understanding of cervical neoplasia. The dysplasia/carcinoma *in situ* system next gained general acceptance. It was originally based on histologic rather than cytologic material. It focused on the degree of cellular differentiation, nuclear detail, and numbers of "atypical" cells on the slide. In the 1960s the cervical intraepithelial neoplasia (CIN) system was proposed by Richart [6], initially for evaluating tissue biopsies and then adapted later for cytology. Subsequent studies, however, showed that the distinction between CIN I and human papillomavirus (HPV) effect (without "dysplasia"), and the distinction between CIN II and CIN III were not reproducible on Pap smears. As a result the term "lesion" was substituted for "neoplasia," since it appeared that many low-grade lesions not only do not progress but in fact spontaneously resolve. The Bethesda system was developed in 1988 and modified in 1991 [7] to attempt to standardize the diagnosis and reporting of cytologic findings.

THE 1991 BETHESDA SYSTEM

Adequacy of specimen

Satisfactory for evaluation

Satisfactory for evaluation but limited by... (specify reason)

Unsatisfactory for evaluation... (specify reason)

General categorization (optional)

Within normal limits

Benign cellular changes: see Descriptive diagnosis

Epithelial cell abnormality: see Descriptive diagnosis

Descriptive diagnosis

BENIGN CELLULAR CHANGES

Infection

- *Trichomonas vaginalis*
- Fungal organisms morphologically consistent with *Candida* species
- Predominance of coccobacilli consistent with shift in vaginal flora
- Bacteria morphologically consistent with *Actinomyces* species
- Cellular changes associated with herpes simplex virus
- Other*

Reactive changes

- Reactive cellular changes associated with:
  - Inflammation (includes typical repair)
  - Atrophy with inflammation ("atrophic vaginitis")
  - Radiation
  - Intrauterine contraceptive device
  - Other*

EPITHELIAL CELL ABNORMALITIES

Squamous cell

- Atypical squamous cells of undetermined significance: qualify†
- Low-grade squamous intraepithelial lesion (LGSIL) encompassing HPV*, mild dysplasia/CIN 1
- High-grade intraepithelial lesion (HGSIL) encompassing moderate and severe dysplasia, CIS/CIN 2 and CIN 3
- Squamous cell carcinoma

Glandular cell

- Endometrial cells, cytologically benign in a postmenopausal woman
- Atypical glandular cells of undetermined significance: qualify†
- Endocervical adenocarcinoma
- Endometrial adenocarcinoma
- Extrauterine adenocarcinoma
- Adenocarcinoma, NOS

OTHER MALIGNANT NEOPLASMS: specify

HORMONAL EVALUATION (applies to vaginal smear only)

- Hormonal pattern compatible with age and history
- Hormonal pattern incompatible with age and history: specify
- Hormonal evaluation not possible due to: specify

**Cellular changes of human papillomavirus (HPV), previously termed* koilocytosis, koilocytotic atypia, *and* condylomatous atypia, *are included in the category of LGSIL.*
†Atypical squamous or glandular cells of undetermined significance should be qualified further, if possible, as to whether a reactive or premalignant/malignant process is favored.
CIN—cervical intraepithelial neoplasia; CIS—carcinoma in situ; *NOS—including adenocarcinoma of uncertain origin (not otherwise specified).*

FIGURE 11-2.
The Bethesda System is designed to give a general categorization and a descriptive diagnosis with well-defined criteria for each categorization.

THE NORMAL (NEGATIVE) PAP SMEAR

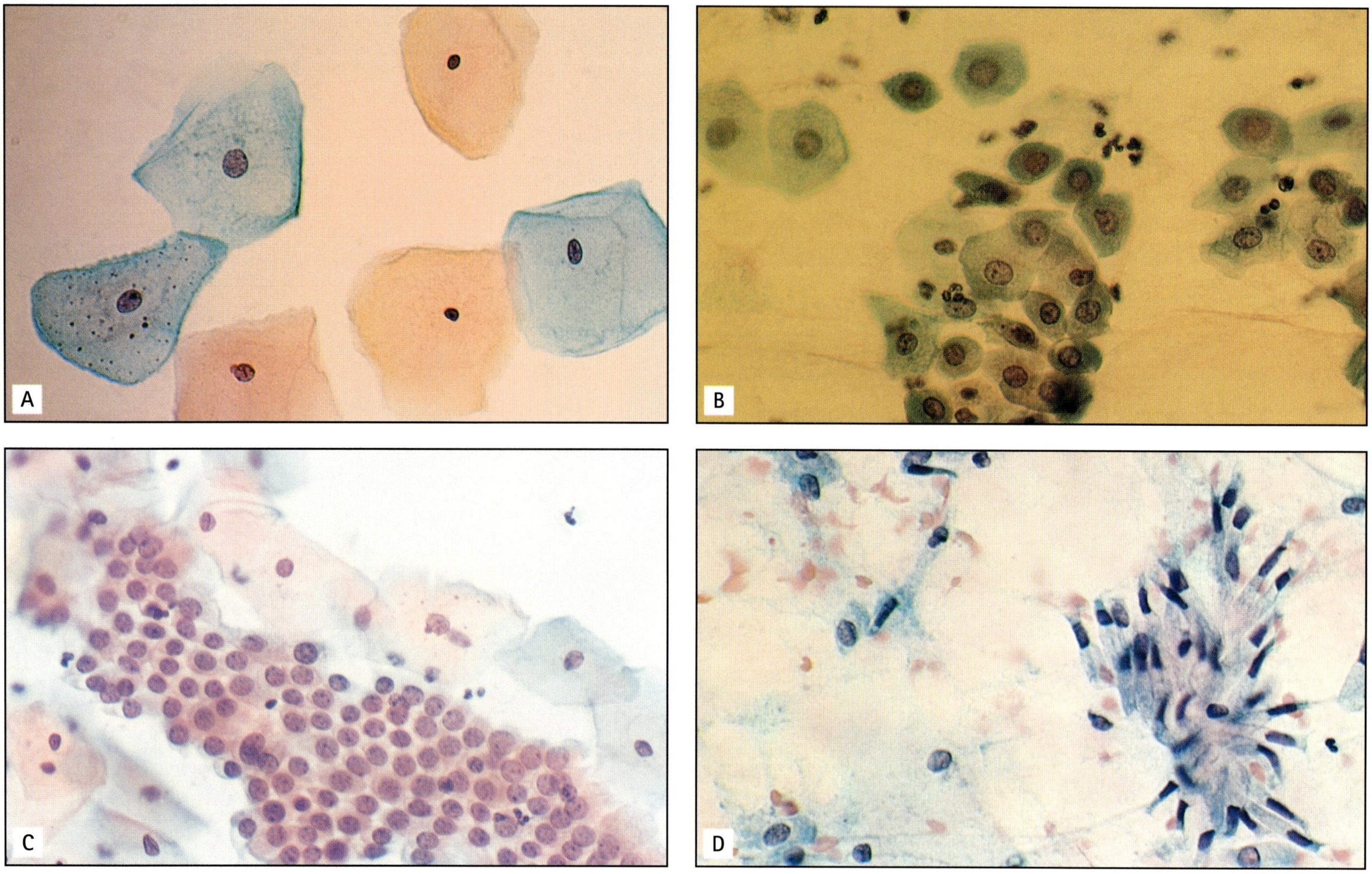

FIGURE 11–3.

Cell types from normal ectocervix and endocervix. The ectocervix is normally surfaced by nonkeratinizing stratified squamous epithelium. This multilayered epithelium forms a protective barrier between the external world and the cervix. The lowest, or basal cell layer, provides the dividing cell population whose progeny generally mature or differentiate to form additional epithelial cell layers. Cells "mature" as they proceed from the basal to the surface layers; their nuclei become smaller and more compact and cytoplasm becomes more abundant and more keratinized. The surface cells then exfoliate. Depending on a patient's age, hormonal status, and presence of inflammation-inducing conditions, the surface cells can express various stages of maturity. For example, in prepubertal, postmenopausal, and postpartum women, the exfoliated surface cells have immature and metaplastic forms. **A**, Superficial and intermediate squamous cells. The superficial squamous cell appears polygonal, is 40 to 50 µm in diameter, has abundant pink to green cytoplasm, and has a small (6 µm) and condensed (pyknotic) nucleus. Intermediate cells are approximately the same size and shape as superficial cells but have a slightly larger (10 µm), less condensed, and somewhat vesicular nucleus (in *center left* of figure). In general, greater numbers of superficial squamous cells are associated with higher estrogen levels (seen in early phase of menstrual cycle or in a postmenopausal woman on exogenous hormones).

B, Metaplastic/parabasal cells. Parabasal cells are located just above the basal cell layer. They are smaller (12 to 30 µm), have higher nuclear to cytoplasmic ratios and slightly larger nuclei than intermediate cells. They are generally not present in Pap smears. When similar cells form the surface layer, as in atrophic or immature metaplastic epithelia, they are referred to as metaplastic cells. These metaplastic cells cannot be cytologically distinguished from true parabasal cells, and are commonly seen in smears taken from women with low estrogen states (*eg*, prior to puberty, during pregnancy, after menopause), from areas of squamous metaplasia, from the transitional zone, and from areas of proliferative epithelial repair.

C, Endocervical cells. Glandular cells can originate either from the endocervix or, in a subset of women, from the vaginal wall. Normal endocervical cells are present either singly or in cohesive sheets. They have round, basally oriented nuclei and abundant vacuolated cytoplasm. Seen *en face*, they appear as honeycomb sheets with distinct cell borders, whereas viewed from the side they appear as strips of cells with basally oriented nuclei. **D**, "Ballerina" cells. Ballerina cells are endocervical cells that have been separated from one another and are stretched into columnar cells with slightly hyperchromatic and eccentrically placed nuclei, features reminiscent of ballerinas on point. More importantly, these altered cells may mimic adenocarcinoma *in situ* and care must be taken not to interpret them as dysplastic, although they prompt cytology technicians to search for high-grade squamous dysplasia. They are thought to be caused by the application of Lugol's solution before obtaining the Pap smear.

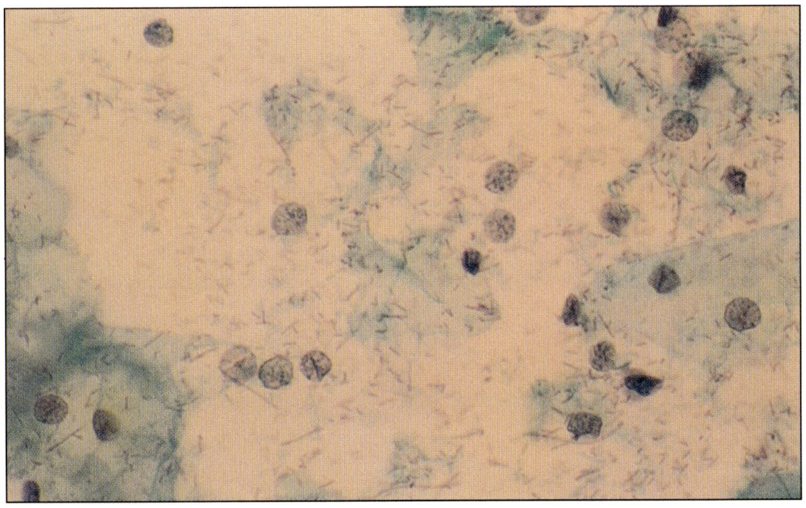

FIGURE 11-4.

Cytolysis. Cytoplasmic cytolysis of intermediate cells is a normal finding associated with the presence of lactobacillus which is characteristic of postovulation smears. Such smears may largely consist of naked, intermediate-sized nuclei such as those seen here. Extensive cytolysis may prompt a diagnostic interpretation of inadequate smear due to the inability to interpret the significance of naked nuclei.

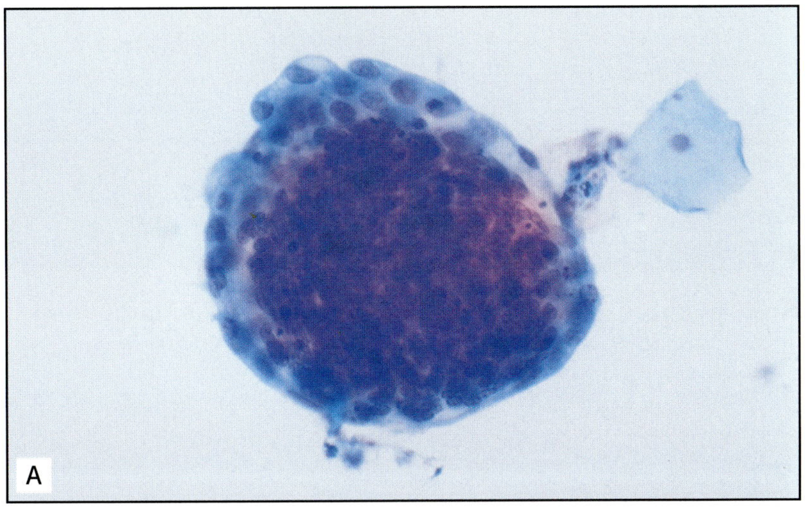

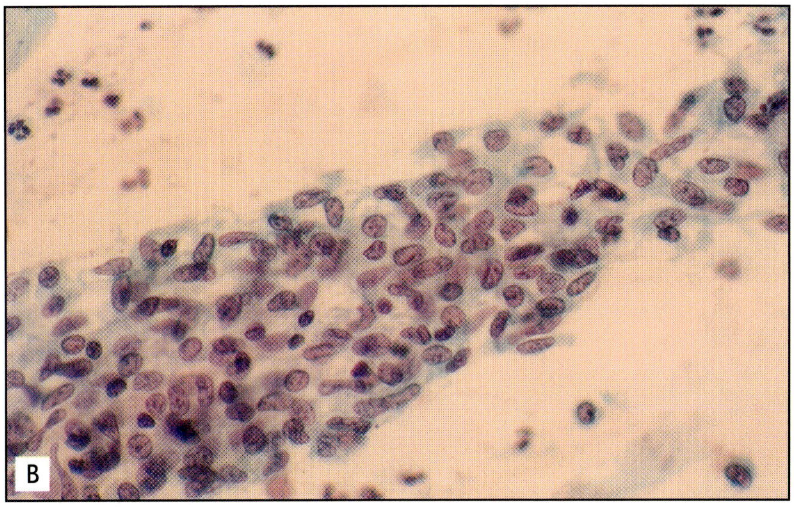

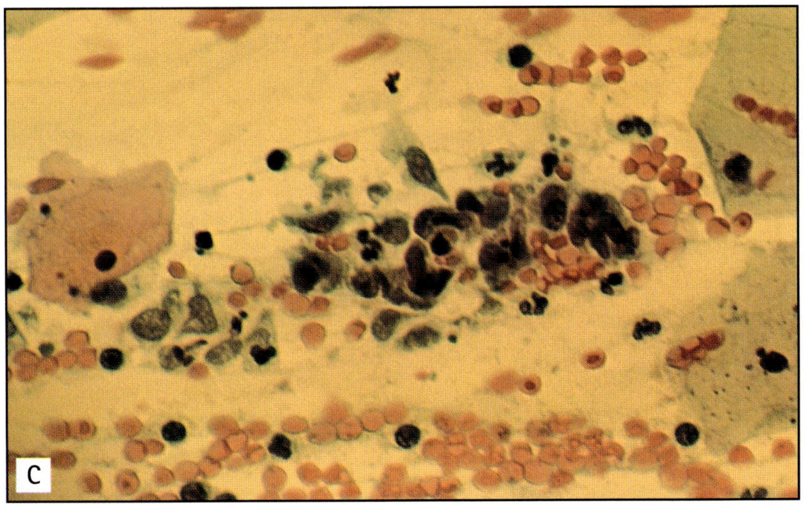

FIGURE 11-5.

Endometrial cells. Endometrial cells are normally present in smears taken during days 6 to 10 of the menstrual cycle (exodus). They commonly appear as compact balls comprised of condensed and degenerating stromal cells surrounded by rims of glandular cells (**A**). Superficial endometrial stromal cells are indistinguishable from histiocytes and therefore are often referred to as endometrial histiocytes; they tend to form loose aggregates and do not show as much variety as true histiocytes, but if seen in the absence of endometrial cell balls or other inflammatory cells, their exact etiology cannot be determined (**B**). Deep endometrial stromal cells commonly appear as somewhat loosely cohesive, hyperchromatic, and elongated spindle-shaped cells that must be differentiated from dysplastic cells (**C**).

ARTIFACTS, UNSATISFACTORY AND LESS THAN OPTIMAL PAP SMEARS

A. BETHESDA DEFINITIONS AND CRITERIA FOR SPECIMEN ADEQUACY

Specimens may be designated *Satisfactory, Satisfactory but limited by...* (specify), or *Unsatisfactory...* (specify)

Satisfactory for evaluation

The specimen has all of the following:

Appropriate labeling and identifying information

Relevant clinical information

Adequate numbers of well-preserved and well-visualized squamous epithelial cells

An adequate endocervical/transformation zone component (from a patient with a cervix)

Satisfactory for evaluation but limited by... (specifiy)

This designation applies if any of the following pertain to the specimen:

Lack of pertinent clinical patient information (age, date of last menstrual period as a minimum; additional information as appropriate)

Partially obscuring blood, inflammation, thick areas, poor fixation, air-drying artifact, contaminant, and the like that precludes interpretation of approximately 50% to 75% of the epithelial cells

Lack of an endocervical/transformation zone component

Unsatisfactory for evaluation... specify

The specimen receives this designation if any of the following applies:

Lack of patient identification on the specimen and/or requisition form

A technically unacceptable slide is defined as one that is broken and cannot be repaired, or cellular material that is inadequately preserved

Scant squamous epithelial component (well-preserved and well-visualized squamous cells covering less than 10% of the slide surface)*

Obscuring blood, inflammation, thick areas, poor fixation, air-drying artifact, contaminant, and so on that precludes interpretation of approximately 75% or more of the epithelial cells

The report must specify the basis for designating a specimen either *Satisfactory for evaluation but limited by...* or *Unsatisfactory for evaluation.* Any epithelial abnormality is of paramount importance and must be reported regardless of compromised specimen adequacy. If abnormal cells are detected, the specimen is never categorized as unsatisfactory.

**Criteria for thin preps may differ because of the smaller initial volume of cells. The current recommendation is to designate a case* Unsatisfactory *if less than 40% of the 20-mm cell deposit area contains well-preserved and well-visualized squamous epithelial cells.*

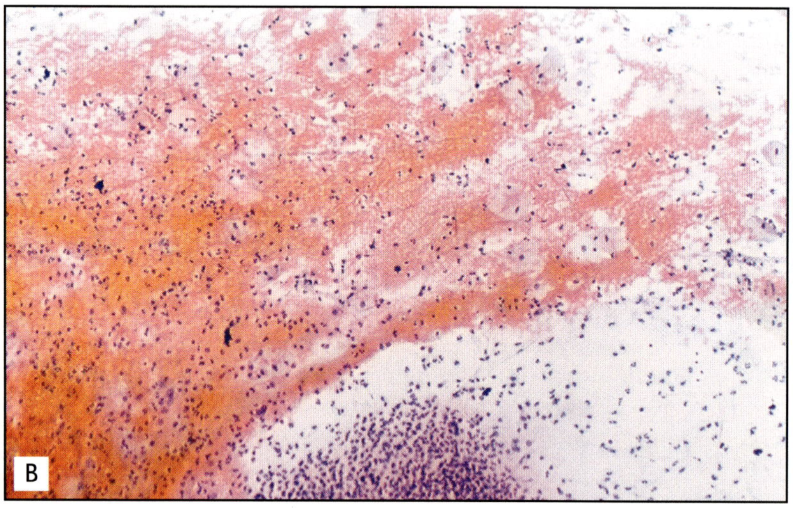

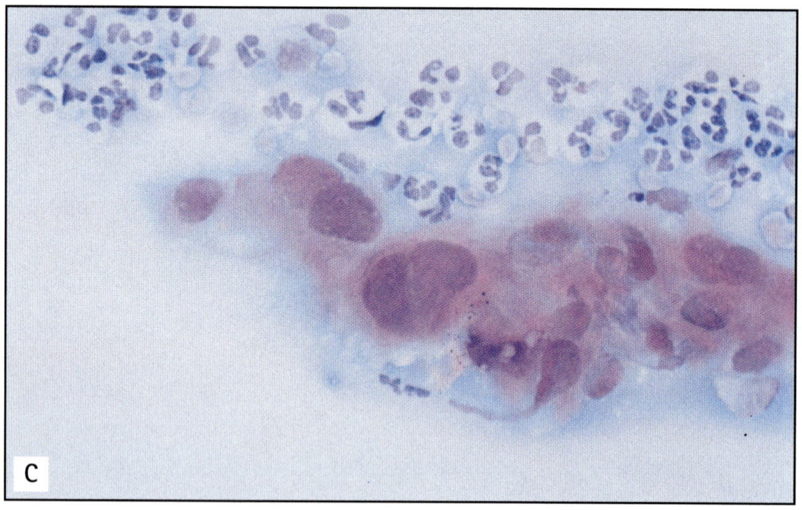

FIGURE 11-6.

Unsatisfactory and less than optimal smears. Conventional smears are considered to be unsatisfactory if (1) more than 75% of the squamous cells are obscured by blood or inflammatory elements; (2) most of the smear is thick, poorly fixed, or air-dried; or (3) less than 10% of the slide surface is covered by squamous epithelial cells. If such smears contain abnormal cells they should be categorized as abnormal but designated "less than optimal" with a comment explaining why. If blood, inflammation, poor preparation, or poor fixation are present but less extensive than that on smears designated unsatisfactory, the smear is classified as less than optimal. There are conflicting data on whether the presence of endocervical cells increases the likelihood of detecting dysplasia. The Bethesda system considers the presence of metaplastic cells and endocervical mucus equal in importance to the presence of endocervical cells for determination of the adequacy of a smear. The table (**A**) lists the Bethesda definitions and criteria for specimen adequacy. **B**, Unsatisfactory smear due to obscuring blood. The majority of the squamous cells in this unsatisfactory smear are obscured by blood. **C**, Air-dried artifact. Air-drying occurs when a slide is allowed to dry before fixing. This causes cellular enlargement with retained nuclear to cytoplasmic ratios but smudged chromatin patterns that interfere with diagnostic interpretation. These changes may mimic dysplasia causing the smear to be interpreted as atypical with a comment explaining that the atypia may be due to a mechanical artifact. Smears taken from atrophic epithelium or taken with an endocervical brush are especially prone to artifacts that mimic significant lesions.

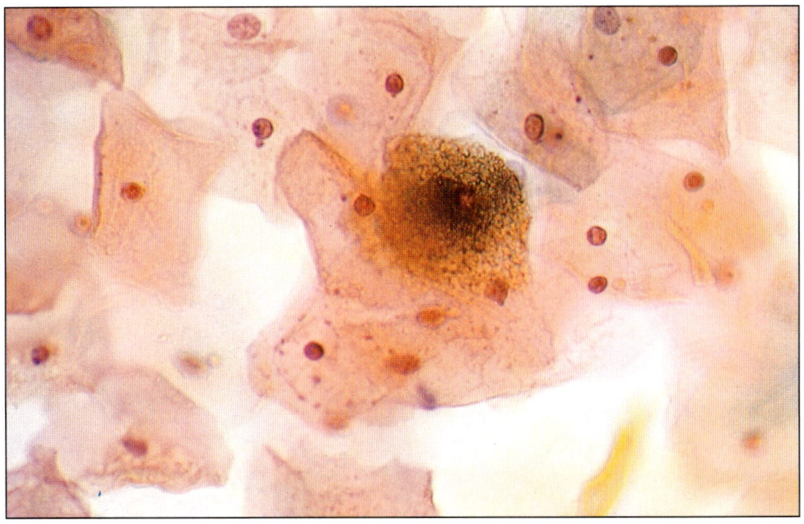

FIGURE 11-7.
Cornflaking. Cornflaking occurs when air is trapped on the cell surface during the coverslipping process. Affected squamous cells are covered by refractile, golden-brown, and relatively uniform dots reminiscent of a cornflake. These artifactual dots may be mistaken for keratohyaline granules, which are larger and stain blue-red. Cornflaked squamous cells are easily recognized by experienced technicians but may be mistaken for human papillomavirus–affected cells by less experienced observers.

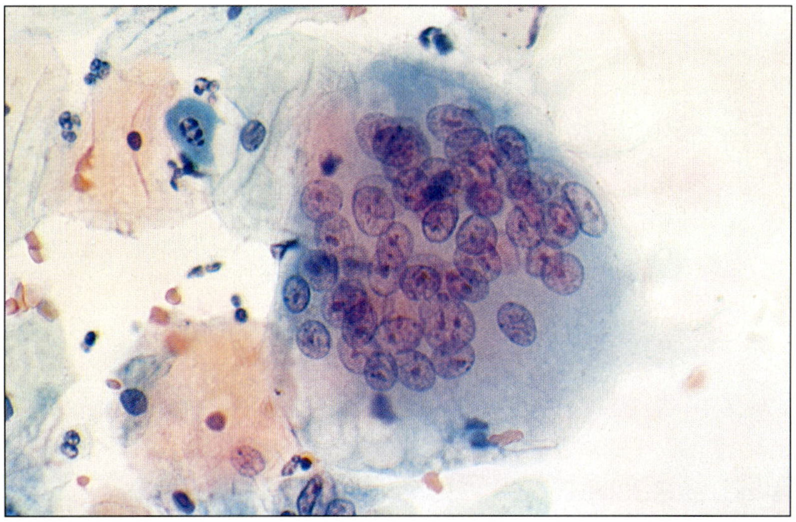

FIGURE 11-8.
Multinucleated histiocytes. Multinucleated histiocytes may be seen in a variety of inflammatory conditions, in smears obtained from postmenopausal women, and especially in smears obtained from women who have undergone previous radiation treatment. These large cells have abundant cytoplasm and numerous round to oval nuclei with vesicular chromatin.

REACTIVE CONDITIONS

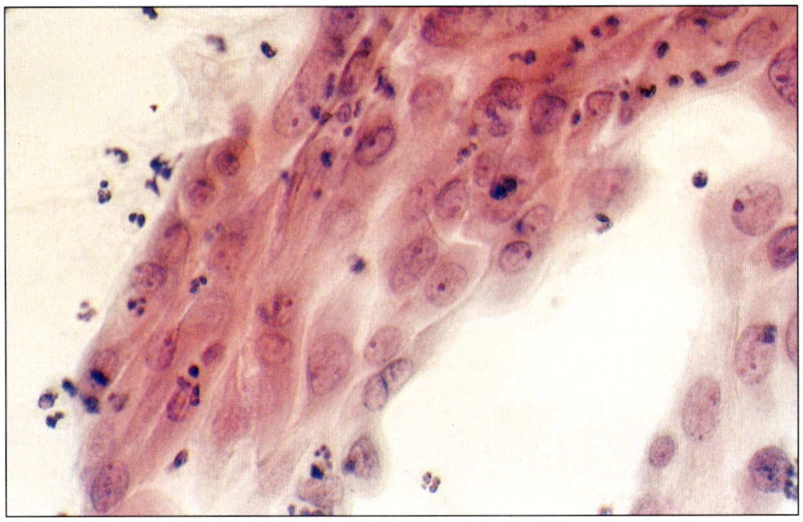

FIGURE 11-9.
Tissue repair. Smears from areas of tissue repair often include mixtures of reactive glandular, squamous, and metaplastic cells. These cells have enlarged nuclei with smooth nuclear membranes, fine to granular chromatin, and large, prominent nucleoli. Some may have two or more nuclei and more than one nucleolus. Cells from areas of repair characteristically form tightly cohesive sheets of amphophilic cells in orderly arrangements, although single cells can predominate. Reparative cells can usually be distinguished from malignant cells by their relatively low nuclear to cytoplasmic ratios and their orderly arrangements, although some anisocytosis can be present, and the distinction can be difficult to impossible in specific cases. In the latter, the smears should be diagnosed "atypical" with comments outlining possible etiologies.

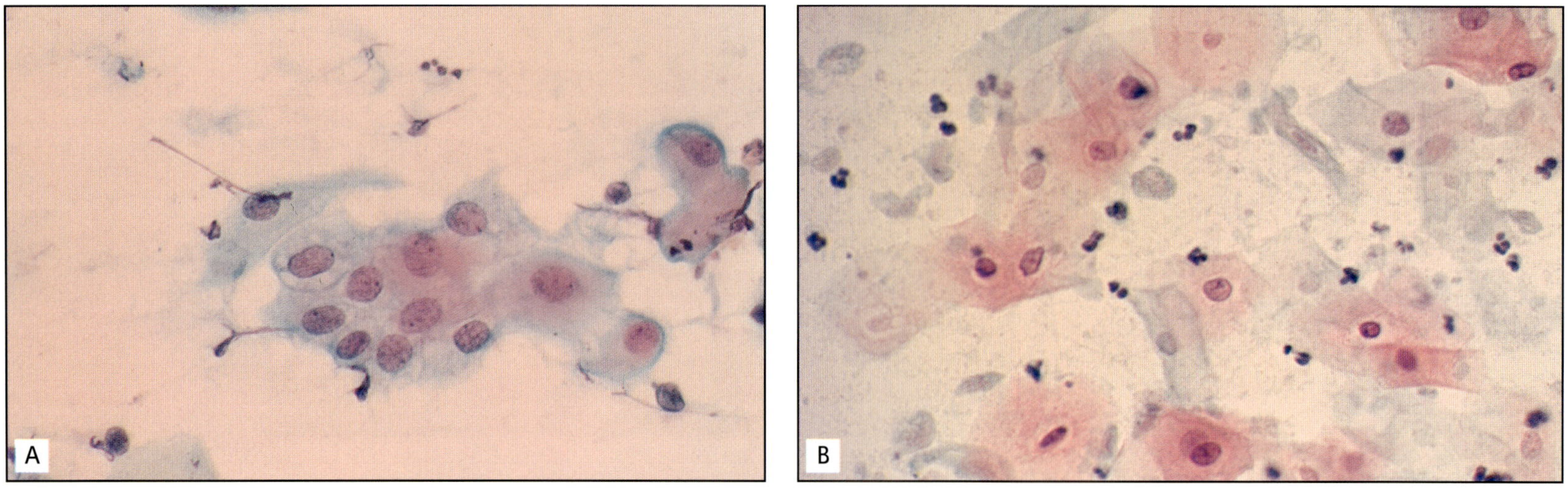

FIGURE 11-10.
Inflammatory conditions induce local epithelial cell changes and usually initiate defense cell infiltrates. The cell types present in such infiltrates determine the various patterns of inflammation, and these patterns often provide clues to the nature of the threatening agents. For example, *Chlamydia trachomatis* infection induces a predominantly immunologic reaction comprised of lymphocytes, immunoblasts, histiocytes, occasional plasma cells, and some polymorphonuclear leukocytes (PMNs), while *Neisseria gonorrhoeae* induces largely nonimmunologic inflammation characterized by PMN-rich infiltrates. Inflammatory epithelial cell changes include cytoplasmic vacuolization, nuclear enlargement, multinucleation, and staining variations (**A**). Affected squamous cells may demonstrate small perinuclear halos, especially with trichomonas (**B**) and candida organisms, but without the peripheral condensation typical of human papillomavirus effect. Metaplastic cells affected by *C. trachomatis* infection reportedly have mild changes, and squamous epithelium involved in reparative hyperplasia may exhibit hyper or parakeratosis (*see* Fig. 11-11 and 11-12).

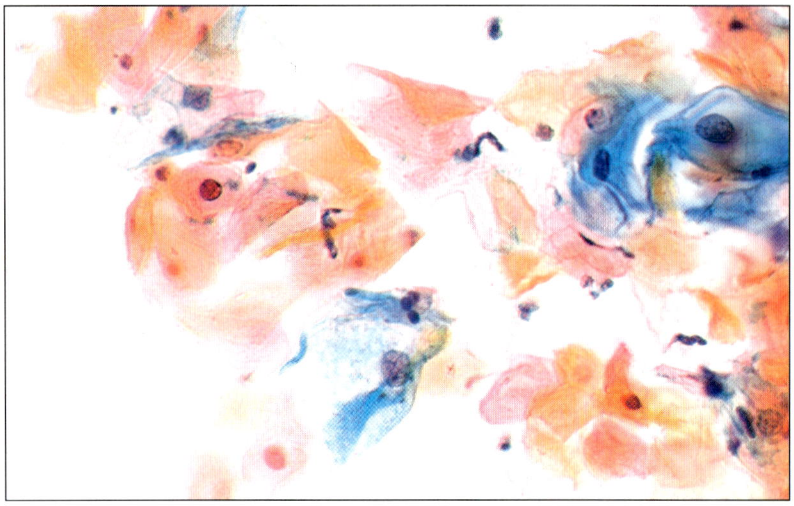

FIGURE 11-11.
Hyperkeratosis. Hyperkeratosis refers to the production of a densely keratinized anucleate surface cell layer by the normally nonkeratinized cervical squamous epithelium. It is a normal defensive response to many irritants, including physical, chemical, and microbiologic ones. Hyperkeratotic cells resemble the normal, superficial squamous cells but lack a nucleus and are frequently found in groups or plaques. The original nucleus location in such cells is sometimes identifiable as a clear spot. Hyperkeratosis can be found in association with human papillomavirus infection, dysplasia, or carcinoma, and the detection of hyperkeratosis should prompt a careful search for dysplastic cells in the smear.

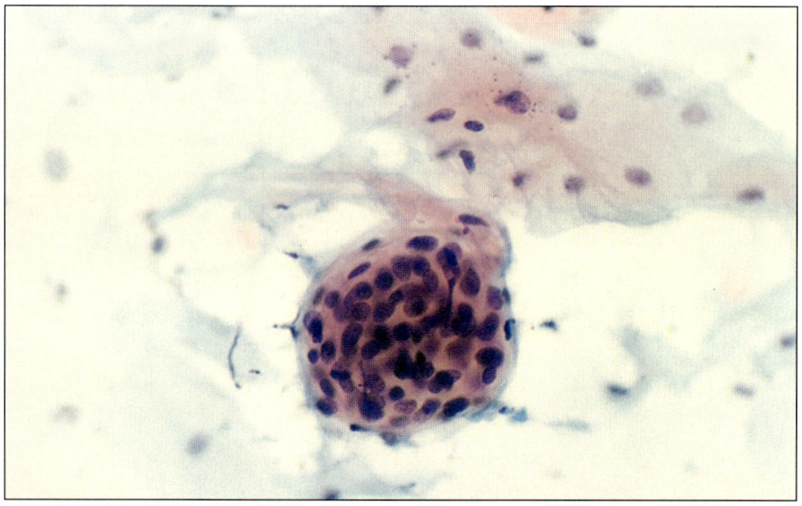

FIGURE 11-12.
Parakeratosis. Parakeratosis refers to the production of a surface layer made up of relatively small, polygonal or rounded cells with condensed ("pyknotic") nuclei. It is a normal defensive response to many irritants. Parakeratotic cells are similar to superficial cells, but are smaller, have higher nuclear to cytoplasmic ratios, and are characteristically extremely orangophilic. They often appear in sheets or rounded groups, and the parakeratotic cells in groups sometimes surround hyperkeratic cells ("keratin pearl"). They are not classified as atypical unless their nuclei are irregular and pleomorphic; atypical parakeratosis or dyskeratosis is commonly associated with human papillomavirus infection.

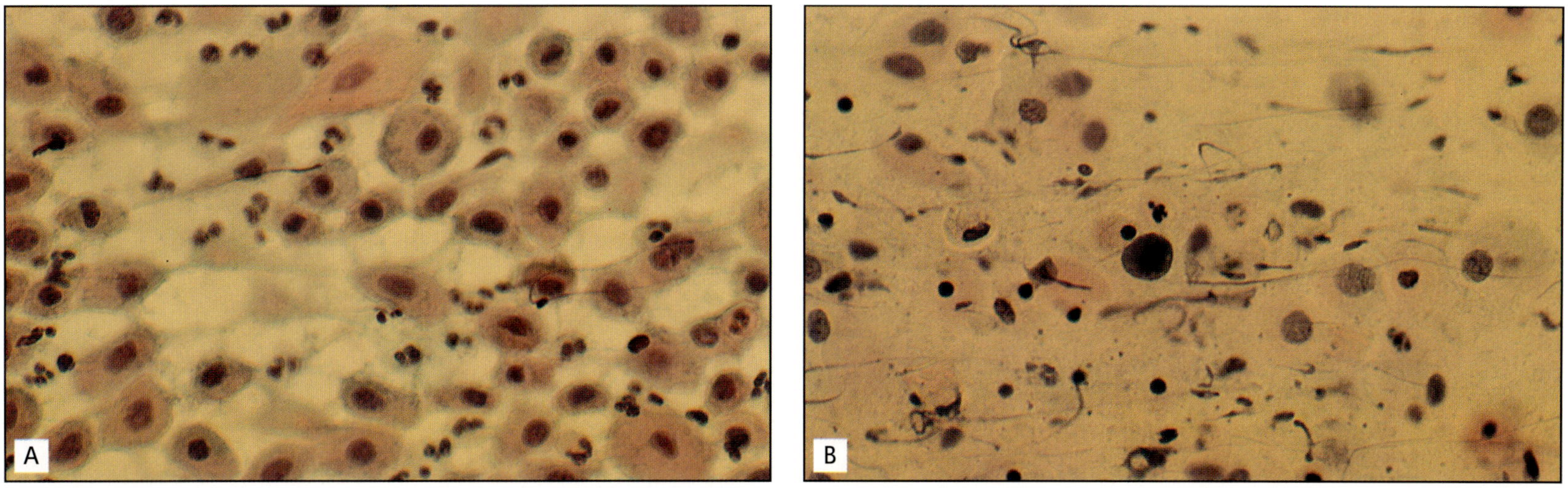

FIGURE 11-13.
Atrophic vaginitis/atrophic changes. Epithelial atrophy associated with diminished estrogen levels is characterized by a decreased number of cell layers and a lack of squamous cell maturation. An atrophic smear contains predominantly basal or parabasal cells. If these cells are uniform and unaltered by inflammation, this pattern does not present a diagnostic dilemma (**A**); however, inflammatory, reactive, and degenerative changes in these cells can blur the distinction between atrophy and dysplasia. These more worrisome changes can include generalized nuclear enlargement and increased nuclear to cytoplasmic ratios, although the chromatin pattern generally remains uniform and benign-appearing. In some smears, a background of amorphous granular material suggests a tumor diathesis, and in combination with many naked or stripped nuclei, and "blue blobs" (basophilic amorphous material from degenerated parabasal-like cells), the presence of malignancy (**B**) is suggested. A trial of topical estrogen (*eg*, 2 weeks) can help resolve the nature of the atypical changes in atrophic smears, as estrogen induces squamous cell maturation and regression of atrophy-associated atypia but will not affect changes associated with true cellular dysplasia (discussed later). After such treatment the dysplastic cells are more clearly evident against the background of mature squamous cells.

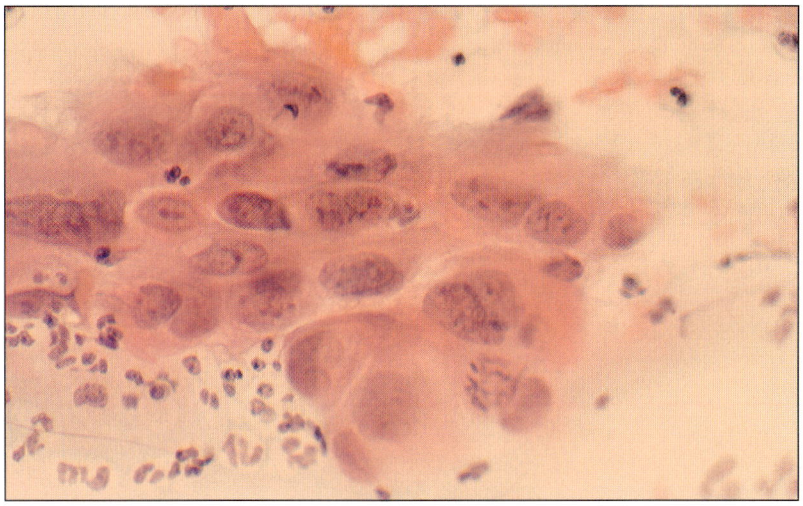

FIGURE 11-14.
Radiation effect. Radiation and some chemotherapeutic agents can cause changes worrisome for dysplasia or carcinoma. Nuclei can be markedly enlarged and have pleomorphic contours; however, there is almost always a corresponding increase in the amount of cytoplasm, little change in the nuclear to cytoplasmic ratios, and usually no overt nuclear hyperchromasia. In contrast, high-grade dysplasia and carcinoma cells typically have increased nuclear to cytoplasmic ratios and nuclear hyperchromasia. Radiation frequently induces characteristic cytoplasmic and nuclear vacuolization.

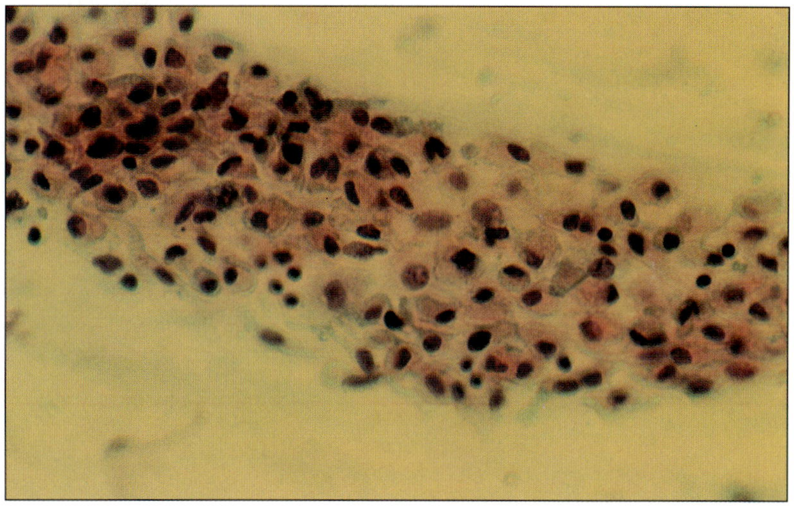

FIGURE 11-15
Pill effect. Exogenous hormones frequently induce microglandular hyperplasia associated with degenerative endocervical cell changes, which are commonly referred to as "pseudoparakeratosis." These degenerate cells resemble parakeratotic squamous cells because they have pyknotic nuclei and orangophilic cytoplasm; however, they typically also have vacuolated cytoplasm and disrupted nuclear membranes indicative of their degenerate state.

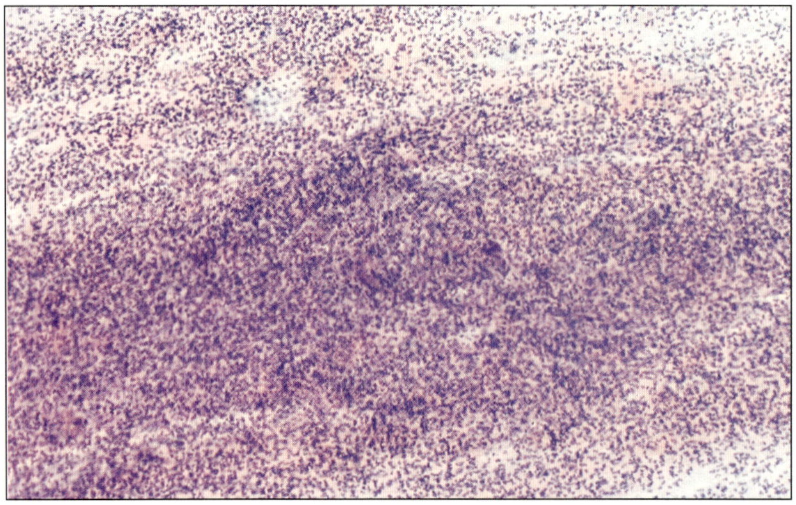

FIGURE 11-16.
Neutrophilic inflammation. A small number of neutrophils is common in Pap smears, but a large number suggests a clinically significant reaction and may hinder adequate evaluation of such smears. Dense neutrophil-rich infiltrates have been associated with *Chlamdyia trachomatis, Neisseria gonorrhoeae, Herpes simplex,* and *Trichomonas vaginalis* infections and can be seen in noninfectious and radiation-induced cervicitis.

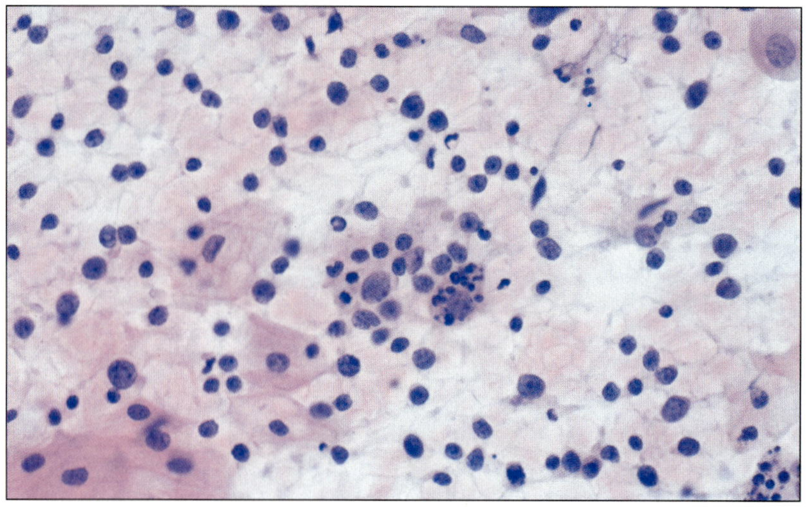

FIGURE 11-17.
Follicular cervicitis. Follicular cervicitis, which is strongly associated with *Chlamydia* infections, is an inflammatory reaction pattern that features subepithelial, B-lymphocytic follicles with mitotically active germinal centers. Smears from patients with this reaction pattern contain many small and large transformed lymphocytes, plasma cells, and histiocytes including "tingle body macrophages" that have ingested the abundant necrotic cell debris that accumulates in germinal centers.

INFECTIOUS AGENTS

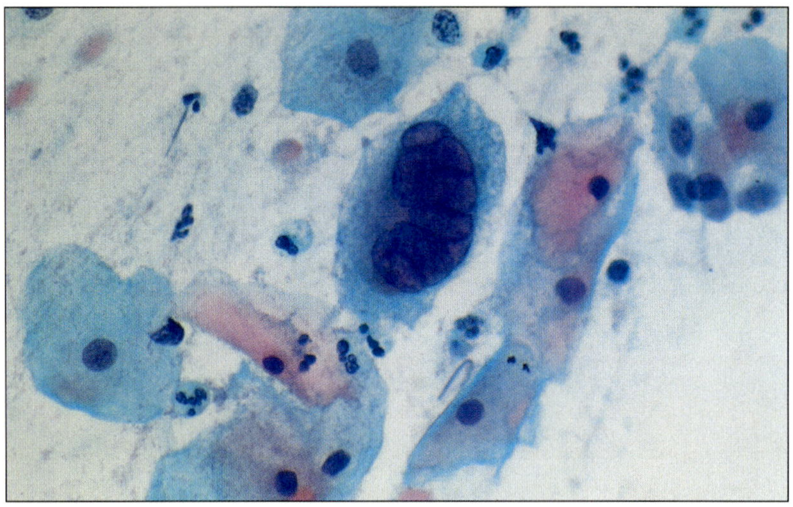

FIGURE 11-18.
Herpes simplex virus (HSV) infection. HSV replicates in the squamous or glandular epithelial cell nuclei, and the associated changes in nuclear appearance are responsible for the highly specific HSV-cytopathic effects. Early in the process of intracellular infection, the cells have a "ground glass," "opaque," or "glassy" nuclear appearance. Affected cells may become multinucleate, and when they do, the compacted individual nuclei are molded against one another. Later in the process of infection, when the cell has used up all or most of the DNA constructing new virions and has an excess of intranuclear viral protein, the excess condenses and appears as a cherry red aggregate ("nuclear inclusion") surrounded by a zone of clearing ("Cowdry type A inclusion"). Epithelial infections often lead to ulcerations, and although cytology is relatively insensitive, the likelihood of seeing the specific cytopathic effects is greatest when smears are made from scrapings taken along the edges of such ulcers.

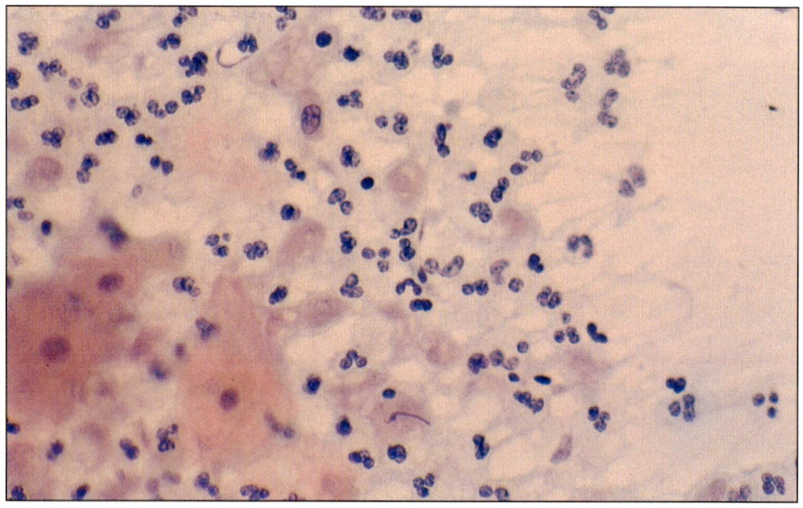

FIGURE 11-19.
Trichomonas vaginitis. On Pap smears, *Trichomonas vaginalis* organisms have somewhat triangulate or round to oval forms that may be mistaken for debris. They have relatively small vesicular nuclei, may have reddish cytoplasmic granules, and generally stain green to lavender.

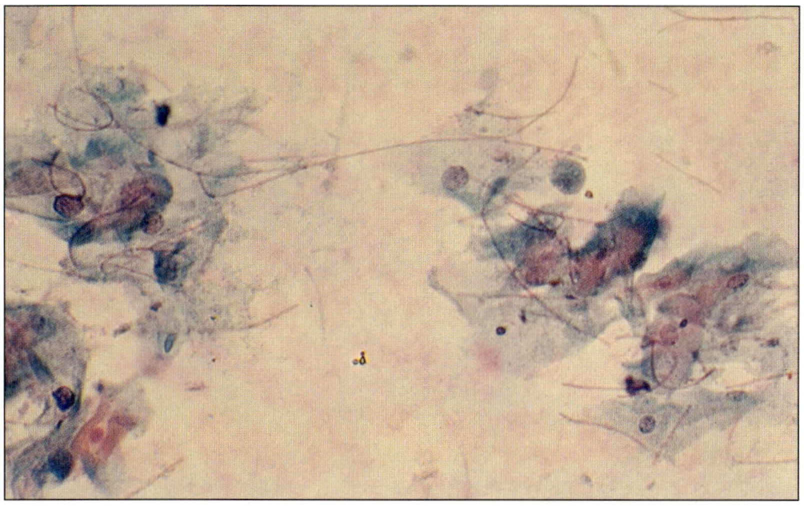

FIGURE 11-20.
Leptothrix "infestation." *Leptothrix*, a long filamentous bacterium, is commonly present in association with trichomonas infections; therefore, its detection on smears should prompt a search for the other organism.

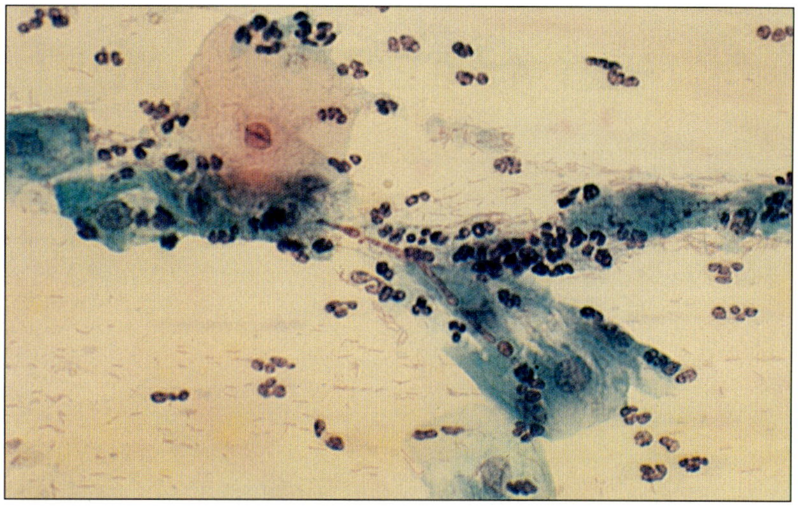

FIGURE 11-21.
Candidiasis. *Candida albicans* and *Candida glabrata*, fungal components of the normal vulvar and vaginal microbial flora in many women, can initiate clinically symptomatic infections whenever the normal microbial balance is disturbed. As components of the normal flora, these fungal organisms tend to grow as budding yeast forms, and as components of clinically symptomatic infections, they tend to grow also as filamentous ("pseudohyphal") forms. These various forms can be detected either on routine Pap smears or on specific potassium hydroxide preparations; however, they are more clearly identified when their cell walls are stained with special silver or periodic acid–Schiff preparations. Smears from patients with symptomatic infections commonly include evidence of inflammatory changes, including reactive squamous cell atypia that can be confused with dysplasia and numerous fragmented neutrophils that are clues to look for the various fungal forms.

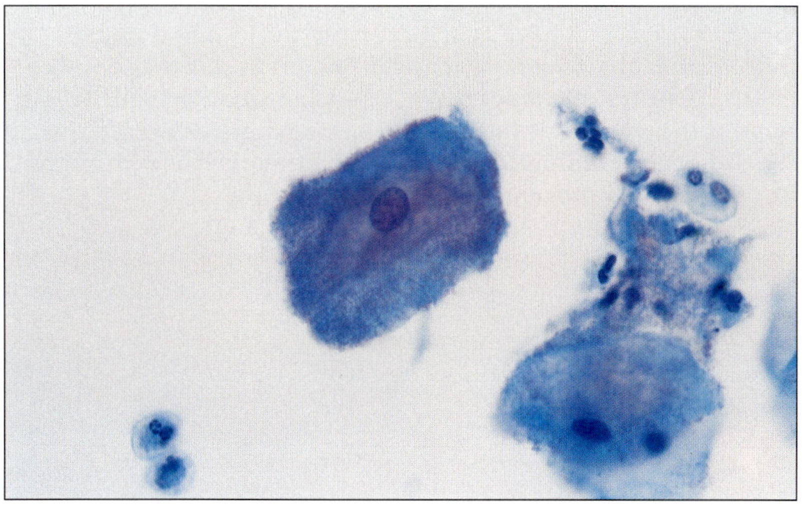

FIGURE 11-22.
Bacterial vaginosis. Multiple bacterial organisms (*eg, Gardnerella vaginalis, Mobiluncus*, and *Bacteroides*), alone or in combinations, have been implicated as causes of this infection, one of the most common causes of vaginal discharge and discomfort. On Pap smears, coccobacillary organisms are numerous; they tend to appear either as a "blue haze" against the general background and as numerous bacteria on or in superficial squamous cells ("clue cells"—the accepted "diagnostic" cell), whose basic features tend to be obscured by the organisms.

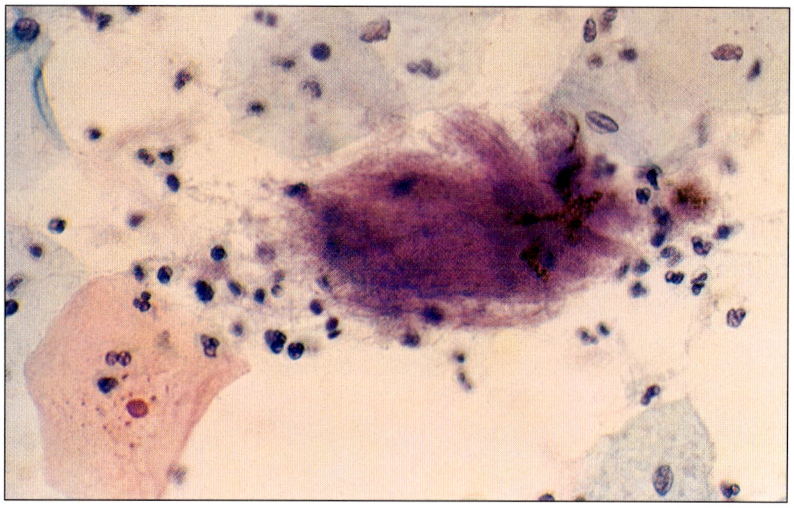

FIGURE 11-23.
Actinomycosis. *Actinomyces* spp, filamentous bacteria, have been associated with infections in combination with intrauterine contraceptive devices (IUDs). As the usage of IUDs has diminished, such infections have become less common. On Pap smears, the organisms appear as compact aggregates or "hazy purplish balls" of bacillary forms, some of which have long filamentous forms.

ATYPICAL CELLS OF UNDETERMINED SIGNIFICANCE

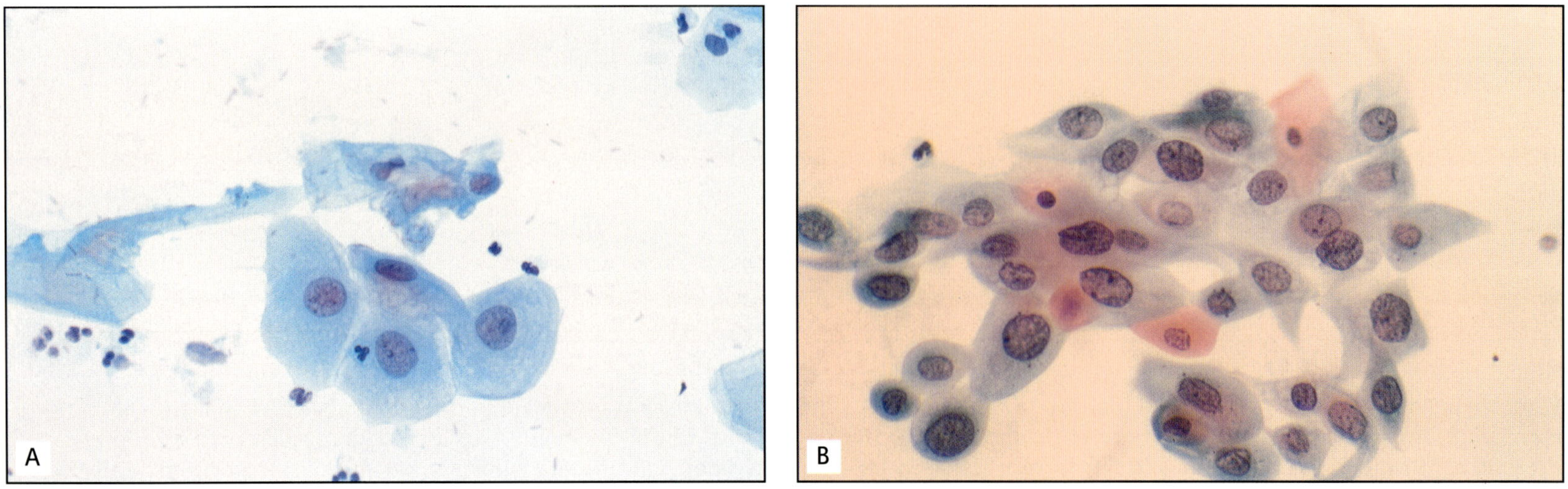

FIGURE 11-24.

Atypical squamous cells of undetermined significance (ASCUS). ASCUS, according to the Bethesda system, are cellular abnormalities that are more marked than those attributable to reactive changes but quantitatively or qualitatively less definitive than those required for the diagnosis of squamous intraepithelial lesion (SIL). The atypical findings need to be explained as completely as possible, and the term *ASCUS* should only be used when dysplasia is suspected but the specific changes noted and/or the number of abnormal cells present do not allow one to make a definitive distinction between reactive or neoplastic processes. **A**, ASCUS, possibly low-grade SIL. **B**, ASCUS worrisome for high-grade SIL.

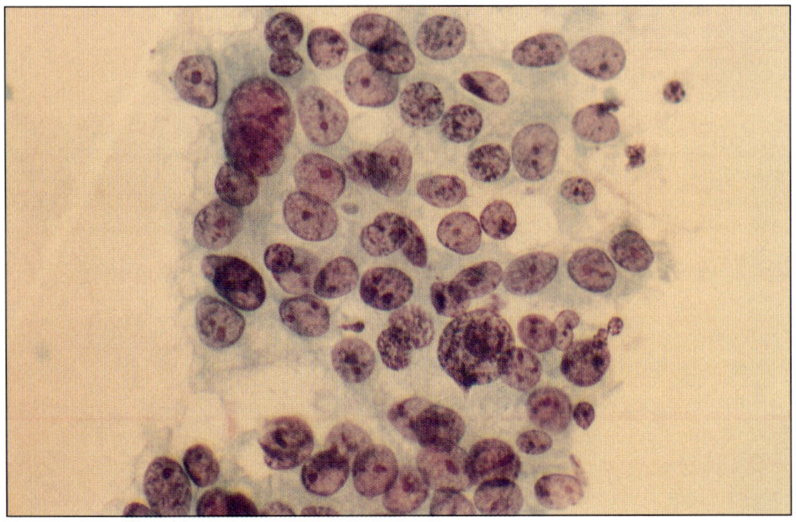

FIGURE 11-25.

Atypical glandular cells of undetermined significance (AGUS). AGUS, according to the Bethesda system and used in a manner similar to ASCUS, are atypical glandular cells with changes worrisome for, but not diagnostic of, neoplasia. These might include but are not limited to cells that have enlarged round nuclei and prominent nucleoli and are moderately crowded when in sheetlike arrangements. Features that favor neoplasia include markedly increased nuclear to cytoplasmic ratios, nuclear membrane irregularities, the presence of multiple large nucleoli, or marked crowding and loss of orderly arrangements in cellular groups.

DYSPLASIA

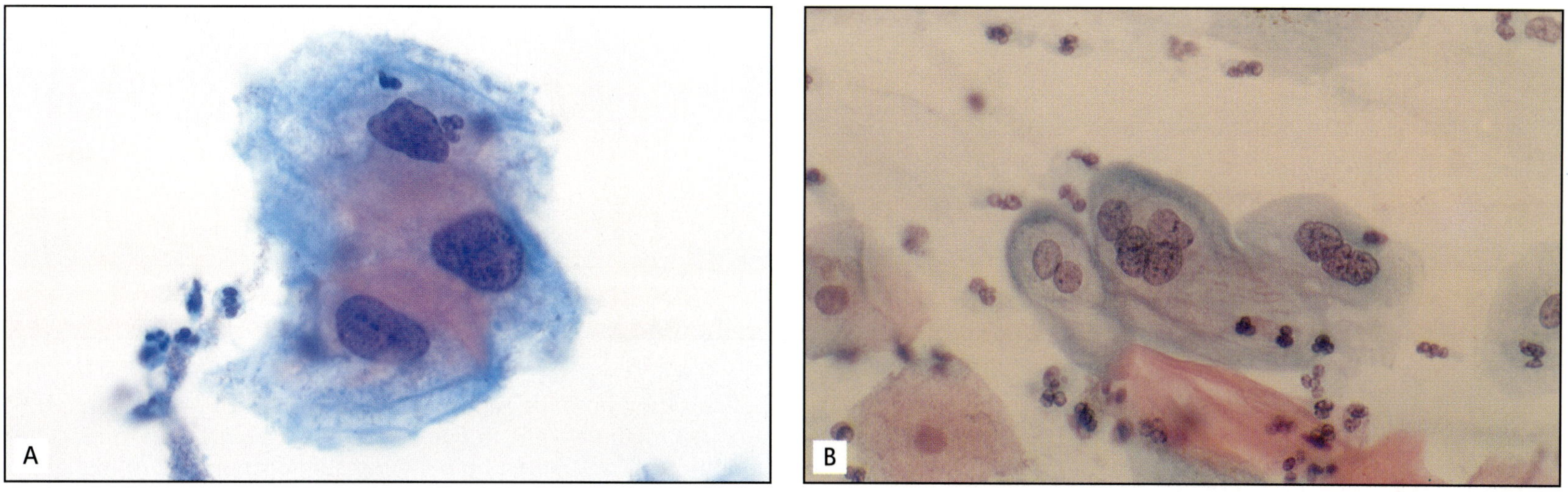

FIGURE 11-26.

Low-grade squamous intrepithelial lesion (SIL) and human papillomavirus (HPV) infection. Low-grade SIL, according to the Bethesda system, encompasses changes previously termed low-grade dysplasia and changes suggestive of HPV infection ("koilocytotic atypia"). These two conceptual entities were encompassed by the one term, because they could not be reliably differentiated in most studies, both are associated with HPV infection, and both appear to have the same relatively low risk of progressing to more worrisome entities. Low-grade SIL is characterized by cells with nuclei at least three or more times the size of a normal intermediate squamous cell nucleus, hyperchromatic and abnormally condensed chromatin, irregular nuclear outlines, and two or more nuclei (**A**). The "koilocyte"—a cell with dysplastic nuclear changes, an optically clear perinuclear halo, and a perihalo rim of dense cytoplasm—is considered to be an HPV effect (**B**).

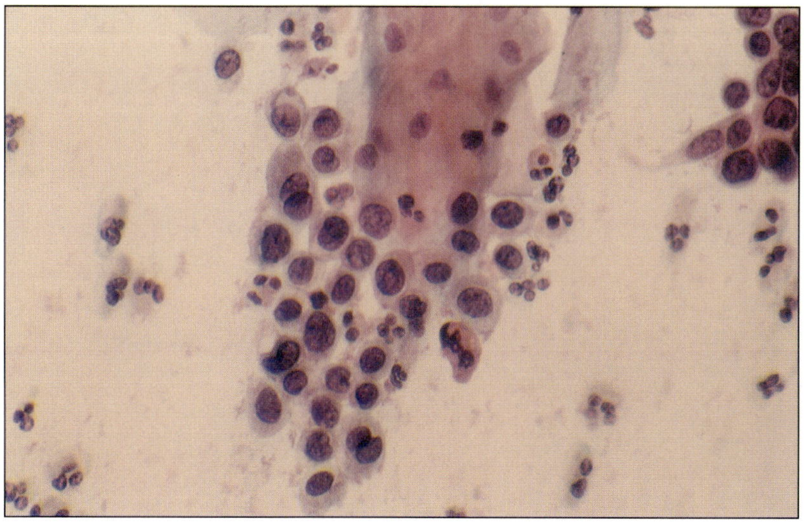

FIGURE 11-27.

High-grade squamous intrapithelial lesion (SIL). High-grade SIL, according to the Bethesda system, encompasses cervical intraepithelial neoplasia (CIN) II and CIN III/carcinoma *in situ*. These conceptual entities were encompassed by the one term, because studies have shown that they could not be reproducibly differentiated. According to both the World Health Organization system and the Bethesda system, a smear should receive the diagnosis of the worst cell(s) on the slide and not the diagnosis of the numerically dominant cells. Although most cases of low-grade SIL appear to regress, it is thought that 10% to 60% of patients with high-grade SIL will eventually develop invasive carcinoma within an expected lifetime. High-grade SIL is characterized by cells with nuclei that have higher nuclear to cytoplasmic ratios than those of low-grade SIL. The actual nuclear size may be fairly small compared with the more marked nuclear enlargement observed in low-grade SIL. Nuclear membranes are irregular and chromatin patterns commonly hyperchromatic and irregularly coarse.

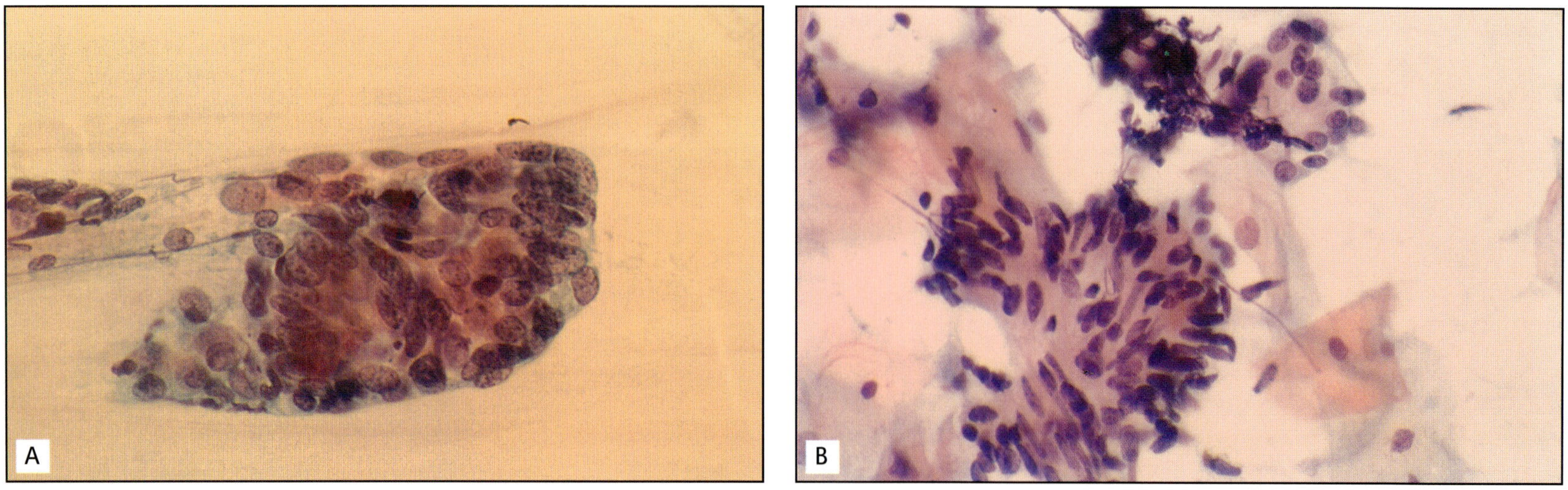

FIGURE 11-28.
Endocervical adenocarcinoma *in situ* is much less common than squamous cell carcinoma *in situ* and is strongly associated with squamous cell dysplasia. It is characterized by cells with enlarged, elongate, and hyperchromatic nuclei that tend to retain their basilar locations ("nuclear polarity"). Such cells are often arranged in crowded groups and appear to have overlapping nuclei (**A**); the groups often present as strips or rosette-like aggregates (**B**). Groups of cells with "feathered" nuclei—irregular protrusion of nuclei beyond the outer edges of their respective groups—are observed more characteristically in adenocarcinoma *in situ* than in reactive conditions. The distinction between adenocarcinoma *in situ*, glandular cells with marked reactive changes, and glandular cells with tubal cell metaplasia can be difficult [8,9], however, and if the diagnosis is uncertain the designation atypical glandular cells of undetermined significance (AGUS) with explanation as to possible etiologies is warranted.

CARCINOMA

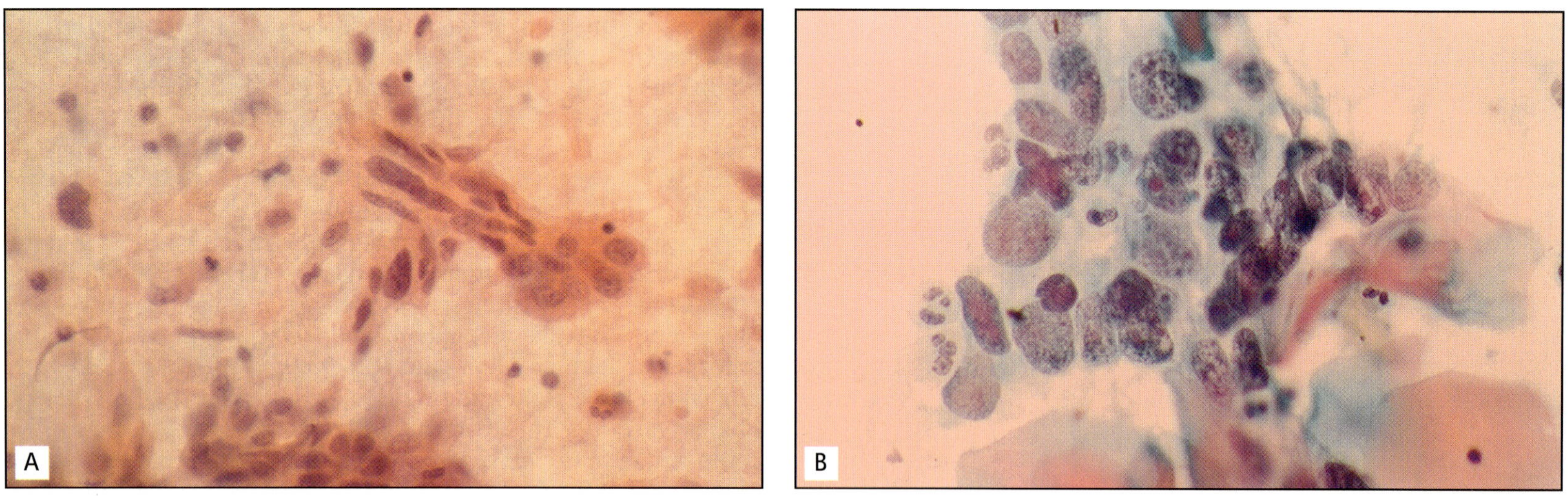

FIGURE 11-29.
Invasive squamous cell carcinoma. The hallmark of invasive squamous carcinoma is a "tumor diathesis" (**A**) along with malignant epithelial cells. This diathesis is characterized by the presence of old blood, necrotic cell debris, and neutrophil-rich inflammatory cells. Malignant squamous cells from an invasive carcinoma can take a variety of appearances. They may be similar in appearance to those from an *in situ* process, but typically are markedly pleomorphic and show greater "differentiation." In intraepithelial carcinoma the dysplastic cells migrate to and slough from the surface and tend to retain more immature or less differentiated appearances; in the invasive portions of the same lesions, the malignant cells cannot slough and therefore tend to age and mature irregularly (**B**). If the lesion is ulcerated as is frequently the case, the invasive component will appear on Pap smears. As they mature and grow, the invasive malignant cells often develop larger nuclei, more prominent nucleoli—a sign of stepped-up DNA transcription and increased protein production—and more abundant cytoplasm.

(*Continued on next page*)

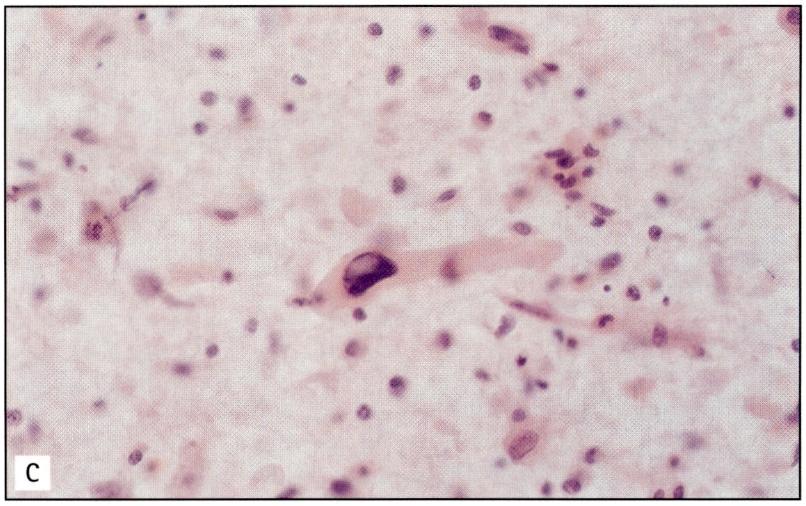

FIGURE 11-29. *(Continued)*
This cytoplasm may or may not be hyperkeratotic, but when it is, it is deeply orangophilic and commonly associated with markedly hyperchromatic and irregular nuclei, the usual cytologic features of "keratinizing" squamous cell carcinomas. Certain atypical cell forms such as "tadpole" and "fiber" are commonly observed in smears from an invasive carcinoma (**C**). The tadpole cell has the shape of a tadpole and a hyperchromatic nucleus with irregular chromatin pattern; the fiber cell has a prominently elongated shape; neither of these cell forms is specific, but the observation of either is a clue to look for more specific evidence of an invasive carcinoma. These various cytologic findings can only suggest the possibility of an invasive carcinoma; the actual proof of the invasive process requires histologic studies, *ie*, the evaluation of tissue biopsies. Histologic confirmation should always be obtained before specific treatment plans for "invasive carcinomas" are developed and implemented.

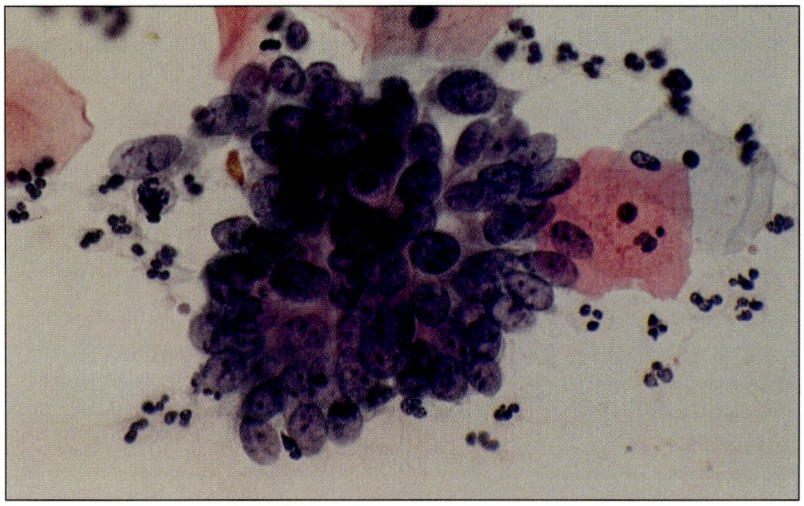

FIGURE 11-30.
Invasive endocervical adenocarcinoma. The cytologic features of well-differentiated endocervical adenocarcinoma (called microinvasive adenocarcinoma) and endocervical adenocarcinoma *in situ* overlap, and these entities are not reliably distinguished by cytology. The cytologic features of more poorly differentiated adenocarcinoma are reasonably distinctive and include enlarged and often pleomorphic cells in crowded aggregates, increased nuclear to cytoplasmic ratios, and irregular nuclear contours. These features do not identify an endocervical origin, and the possibilities of endometrial, ovarian, and more distant metastatic origins must be considered. Again, the proof of invasive carcinomas requires histologic evaluations.

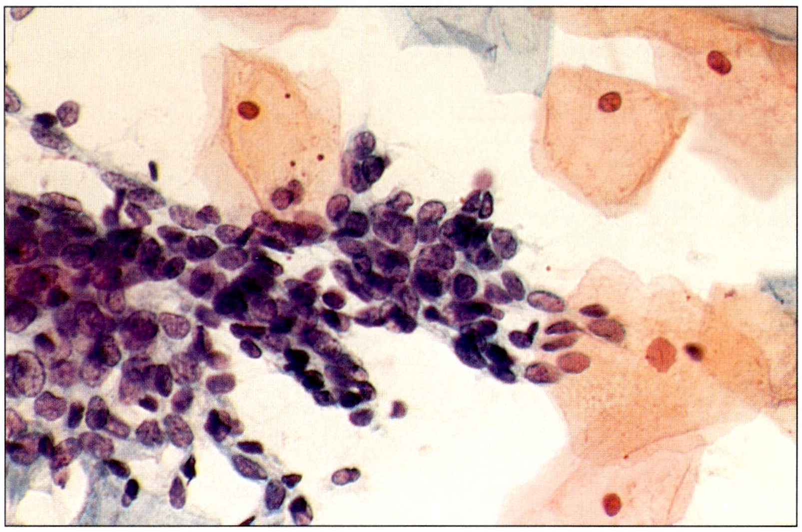

FIGURE 11-31.
Small cell carcinoma. Small cell carcinoma is a term for the most primitive or least differentiated appearing malignant neoplasm derived from any epithelial cell population. The malignant cells are generally smaller than the malignant cells of differentiated (*eg*, squamous, glandular) neoplasms and somewhat larger than normal small lymphocytes; they are similar in size to larger transforming and many malignant lymphocytes, from which they must be distinguished. They tend to be monotonously similar with little but variable tendency to be adherent to one another; their cytoplasm tends to be scanty to unappreciable, their nuclear patterns hyperchromatic and coarse, and their nucleoli small to unappreciable. They may be distinguished from lymphocytic cell types by immunocytochemistry, as they have epithelial markers (*eg*, cytoplasmic keratin) and often neuroendocrine markers (*eg*, cytoplasmic chromogranin) and lack lymphocytic markers. On rare occasions, small cell carcinoma cells must be distinguished from better differentiated and clinically less aggressive "basaloid squamous carcinoma" cells, which are similar in size and cytoplasmic quantity but tend to have far more orderly and adherent cell-cell arrangements.

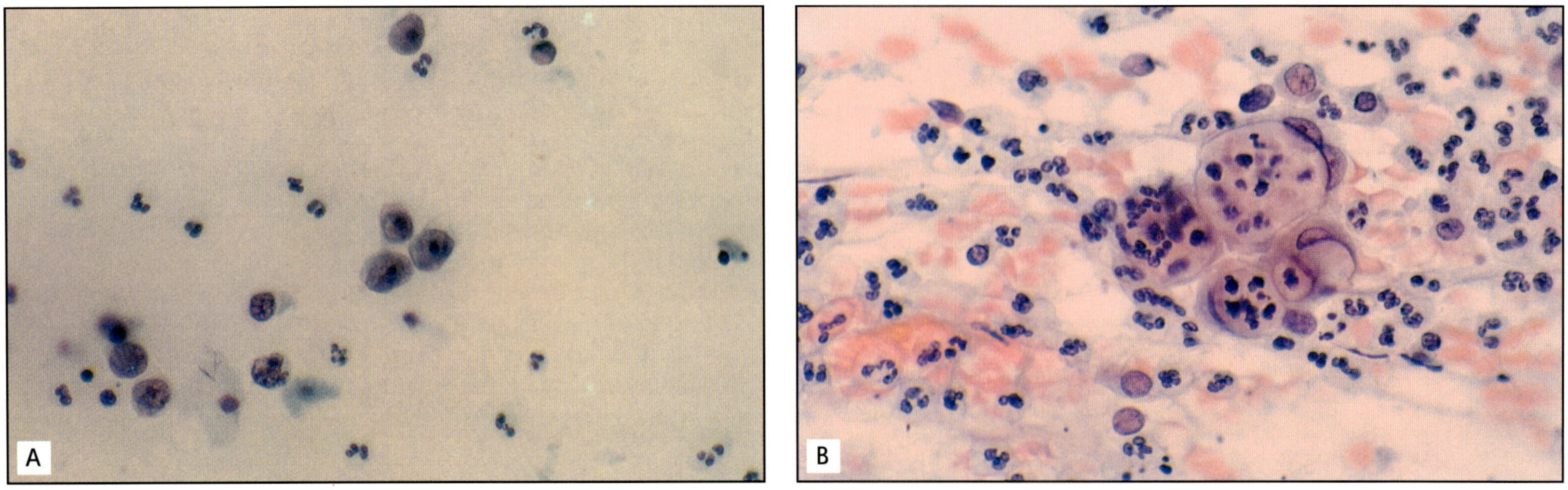

FIGURE 11-32.

Endometrial carcinoma. Cervical Pap smears are not sensitive methods for diagnosing endometrial carcinomas. On those occasions when endometrial carcinomas do shed cells that appear on Pap smears, the malignant cells usually are aggregated in three-dimensional balls; if the carcinoma is low grade (**A**), the cells have increased nuclear to cytoplasmic ratios, and their nuclei are typically small with small nucleoli; if the carcinoma is high grade (**B**), the cells are generally larger and often pleomorphic with pleomorphic and hyperchromatic nuclei and prominent nucleoli. The malignant cells may have vacuolated cytoplasm, and when such cells also have low-grade nuclear features, individual cells can be difficult to distinguish from histiocytic cells. The observation of neutrophils within the cytoplasm of malignant glandular cells is suggestive of an endometrial cell type. With endometrial and ovarian primaries, the Pap smears are typically "cleaner" than those derived from patients with primary cervical adenocarcinomas.

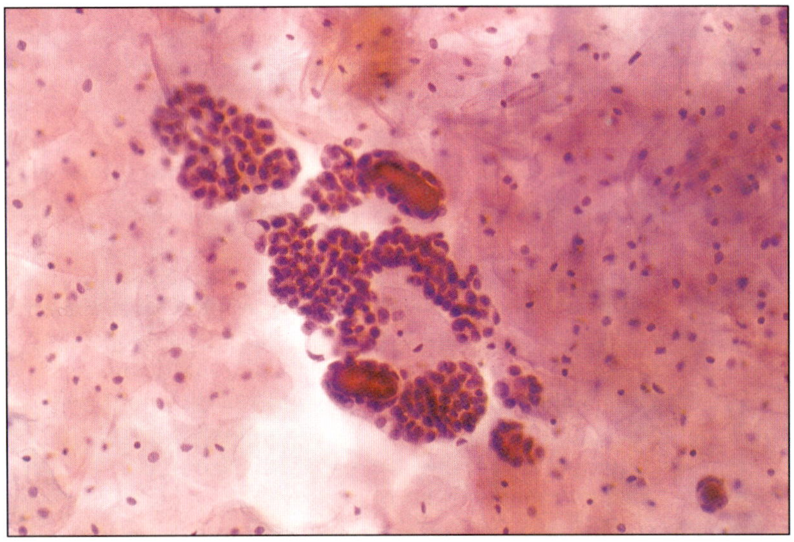

FIGURE 11-33.

Ovarian and tubal carcinoma. Ovarian and tubal carcinoma cells rarely appear on Pap smears, but when they do, they are generally associated with a clean background, as noted in Figure 11-32, unless cervical pathology is also present. Papillary serous carcinoma cells are usually aggregated in three-dimensional balls with features that depend on grade; low-grade carcinoma sheds cells that have bland nuclei but are abnormal in their configuration appearing as papillary balls, often with psamommatous calcifications (as seen in the figure). In ovarian or tubal carcinomas, it is usually the high-grade carcinomas that shed cells found on Pap smears, and these have the usual hallmarks of such malignancies, *ie*, cellular enlargement, cellular pleomorphism, high nuclear to cytoplasmic ratio, and nuclear pleomorphism, irregularities, and hyperchromatism. Again, cytologic studies cannot identify specific primary sites, and additional studies must be done to complete specific patient evaluations.

PERITONEAL CYTOLOGY

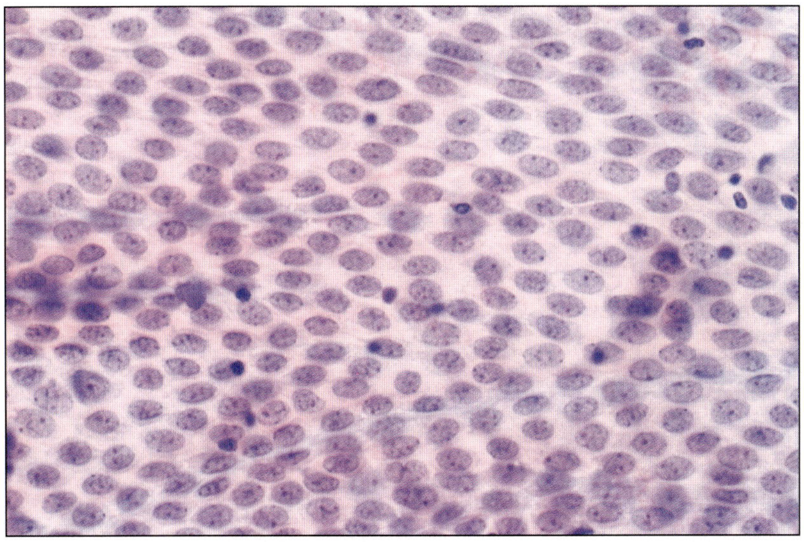

FIGURE 11-34.

Peritoneal cytology. This is most commonly used to assess extraovarian spread of papillary serous carcinoma, although it is also performed in the assessment of other gynecologic malignancies, including tubal, endometrial, and cervical malignancies. A negative peritoneal wash is shown in the figure. Benign peritoneal washes may contain a variety of cell types, but the principal cells are normal or reactive mesothelial types. These mesothelial cells can appear either as isolated cells, in which case they tend to be spherical, or as components of cohesive sheets, in which their shapes are determined by cell-cell relationships. Sheets of mesothelial cells are more common in washes than in ascitic fluid samples. Normal mesothelial cells tend to be uniform in appearance with single round nuclei and relatively small nucleoli, whereas reactive mesothelial cells may be moderately pleomorphic and multinucleate with prominent nucleoli. Mesothelial cells arranged in sheets have polygonal forms, orderly cell-cell relationships, and apparent intercellular "windows."

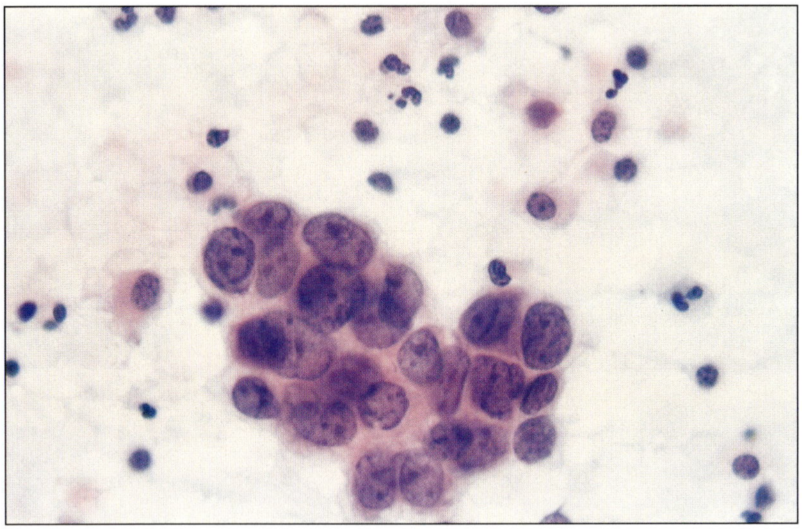

FIGURE 11-35.

Papillary serous carcinoma. The presence of malignant cells in smears of peritoneal washes may be obvious (*eg*, high-grade carcinomas) or remarkably subtle (*eg*, low-grade carcinomas) with epithelioid cells being difficult to distinguish from reactive mesothelial cells. The obviously malignant carcinoma cells are distinctly different in appearance from the normal and reactive mesothelial cells, and they have the usual cytologic features, including irregular hyperchromatic nuclei and high nuclear to cytoplasmic ratios. Lower grade carcinoma cells may have bland nuclear features similar to those of mesothelial cells; however, these cells tend to form abnormal cell-cell groups, wherein the aggregated malignant cells form papillary groups with smooth community borders as opposed to the flowerlike borders of mesothelial cells in otherwise similar groups.

REFERENCES

1. Harlan LC, Bernstein AB, Kessler LG, *et al.*: Cervical cancer screening: Who is not screened and why? *Am J Public Health* 1991, 81:885–890.
2. National Cancer Institute, Division of Cancer Prevention and Control: *1987 Annual Cancer Statistics Review*. NIHAU Publication No. 88-2789. US Department of Health and Human Services; 1988.
3. Kosary CL, Ries LAG, Miller BA, *et al.*: *SEER Cancer Statistics Review, 1973–1992: Tables and Graphs*. NIH Publication No. 96-2789. Bethesda, MD: National Cancer Institute; 1995.
4. Sherman ME, Kelly D: High-grade squamous intraepithelial lesions and invasive carcinoma following the report of three negative Papanicolaou smears: screening failures or rapid progression. *Mod Pathol* 1992, 5:337–342.
5. Bamford PN, Beilby JO, Steele SJ, Vlies R: The natural history of cervical intraepithelial neoplasia as determined by cytology and colposcopic biopsy. *Acta Cytol* 1983, 27:482–484.
6. Richart R: Causes and Management of Cervical Intraepithelial Neoplasia. *Cancer* 1987, 60:1951–1959.
7. National Cancer Institute Workshop: The revised Bethesda System for reporting cervical/vaginal cytologic diagnoses: Report of the 1991 Bethesda Workshop. *JAMA* 1991, 267:1892.
8. Jaworski R, Pacey F, Greenberg M, Osborn R: The histologic diagnosis of adenocarcinoma *in situ* and related lesions of the cervix uteri: *Cancer* 1987, 61:1171–1181.
9. Ayer B, Pacey F, Greenberg M, Bousfield L: The cytologic diagnosis of adenocarcinoma *in situ* of the cervix uteri and related lesions: I. *Acta Cytol* 1987, 31:397–411.

SUGGESTED BIBLIOGRAPHY

Bibbo, M: Comprehensive Cytopathology, edn. 2. Philadelphia: WB Saunders.

DeMay, R: The Pap Smear, In *The Art and Science of Cytopathology*. Chicago: ASCP Press; 1996.

CHAPTER 12

Immunocytochemistry

Allen M. Gown, Nan Ping Wang, and Douglas A. Hansen

Staining tissues with hematoxylin and eosin, or other empirical dyes, generally provides the pathologist with slide preparations that contain information sufficient to generate an accurate diagnosis in over 90% of cases. However, hematoxylin and eosin stains do not even begin to extract the incredible wealth of information that actually resides in a tissue section, and in the small percentage of cases in which hematoxylin and eosin stains do not provide enough information to enable the pathologist to reach a conclusive diagnosis, other techniques are required.

For the past 20 years or so, pathologists have had at their disposal the technique of immunocytochemistry, which is the application of antibodies to tissue sections combined with the use of sensitive detection systems to visualize bound antibodies. By the judicious selection of antibodies, detailed information regarding cell and tumor type can be obtained. Monoclonal antibody technology has permitted the development of panels of antibodies with predetermined specificities that can be applied to deparaffinized, formalin-fixed tissue sections. Given that tumor classification systems are still in large part determined by putative cell of origin, a large stable of cell type-specific antibodies can play a critical role in the immunocytochemical analysis of gynecologic tumors. Antibodies exist with both broad and narrow specificities: antibodies to low molecular weight cytokeratins exist which identify the entire range of carcinomas, and there are antibodies to proteins, such as inhibin alpha, which have the narrow specificity of granulosa and related cells. In practice, however, the pathologist is wise to employ panels of antibodies that can be used to fingerprint different types of tumors, rather than relying on a single marker, whatever its specificity and sensitivity.

The collection of images in this chapter highlights the clusters of markers that characterize a wide range of gynecologic malignancies and can assist in the positive identification of particular tumors in situations where hematoxylin and eosin–based histology alone is insufficient.

CERVICAL NEOPLASMS

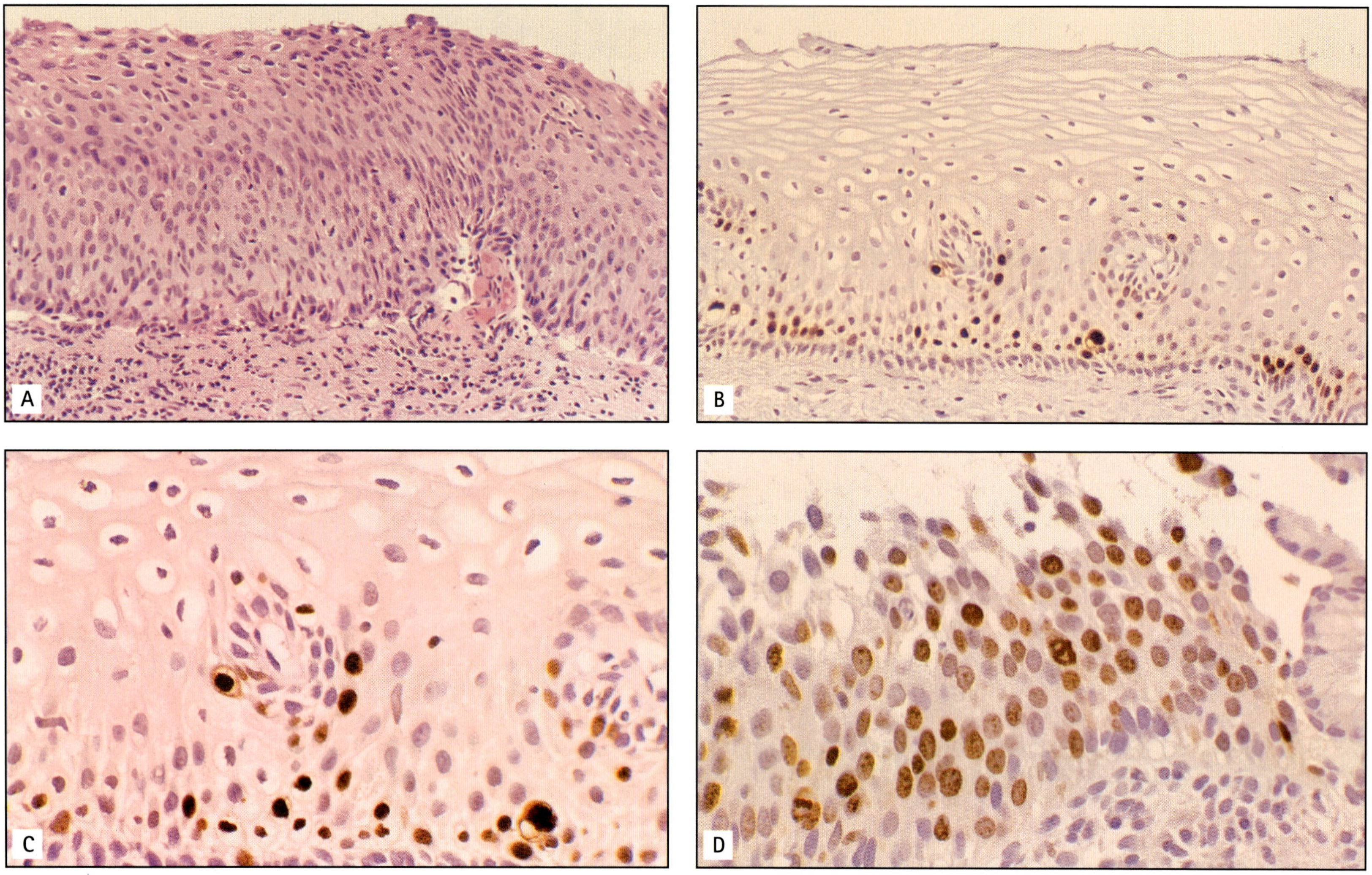

FIGURE 12–1.

Cervical intraepithelial neoplasia (CIN). CIN is a process of increasingly disordered and uncontrolled cell proliferation within the cervical epithelium, finally progressing, in a subset of cases, to invasive carcinoma. This process is driven, at least in part, by the human papillomavirus (HPV); in particular, HPV types 16 and 18 carry a high risk of progression to invasive carcinoma [1]. While localization of HPV subtypes using immunocytochemical techniques has inadequate sensitivity to be used diagnostically, it is possible to use immunocytochemical techniques to define, in a semiquantitative manner, the loss of cell proliferation control that characterizes this process [2,3]. This sequence of photomicrographs documents this finding using, as a marker of cell proliferation, the Ki-67 antigen, as identified by antibody MIB-1 (the latter having the property of identifying this marker in archival, formalin-fixed tissue). **A**, In normal cervical epithelium (hematoxylin and eosin, the proliferative compartment (brown positive nuclei) is restricted to the basal layer (**B**). As the degree of CIN increases, MIB-1–positive nuclei appear at a higher level above the basement membrane. In low-grade dysplasia, a subpopulation of cells with larger nuclei lying about the basal layer contain MIB-1–positive cells (**C**). In higher degrees of CIN, MIB-1–positive cells are found through almost the full thickness of epithelium. In moderately severe CIN, MIB-1–positive nuclei appear two thirds of the way to the superficial layers (**D**).

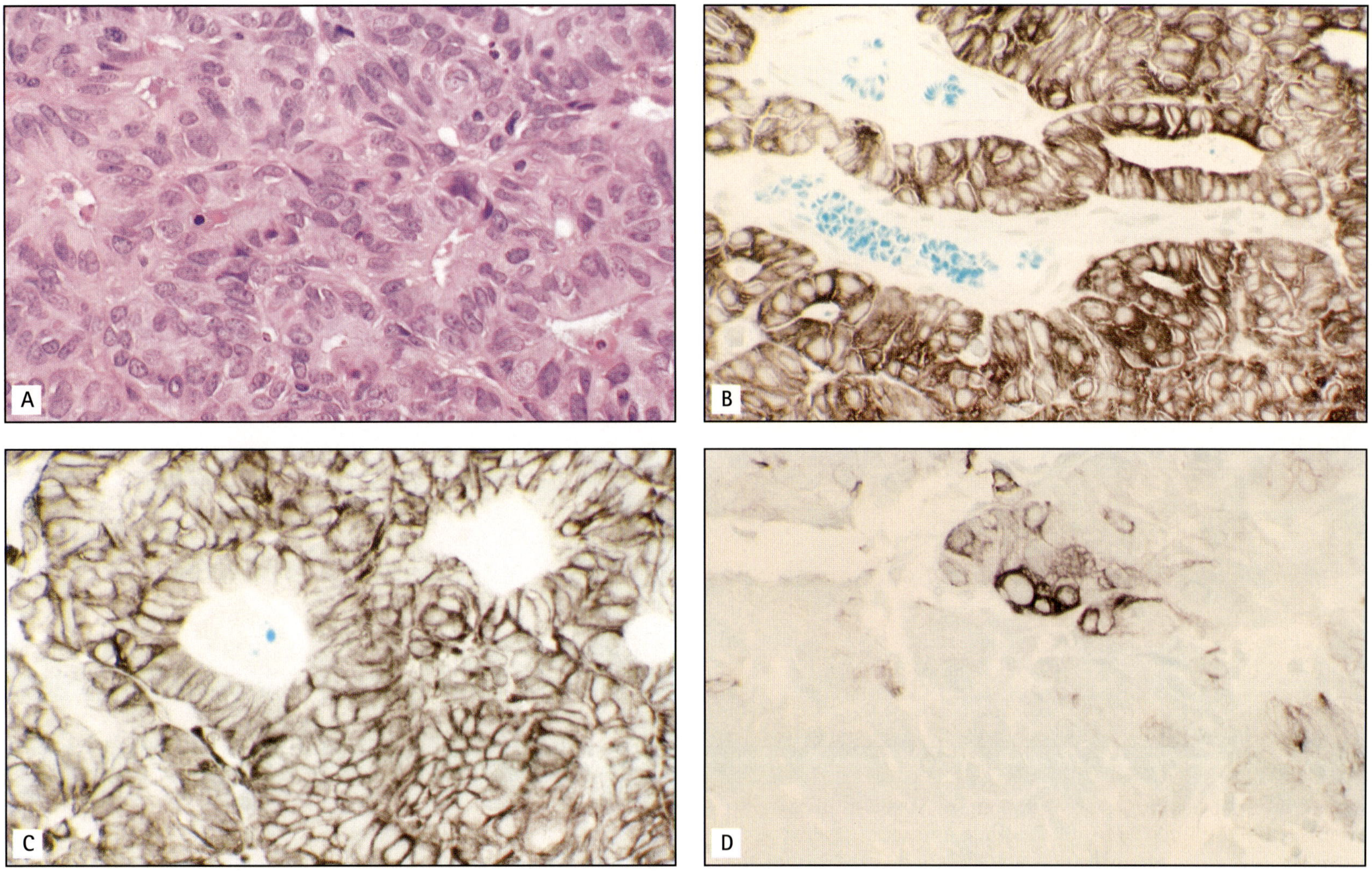

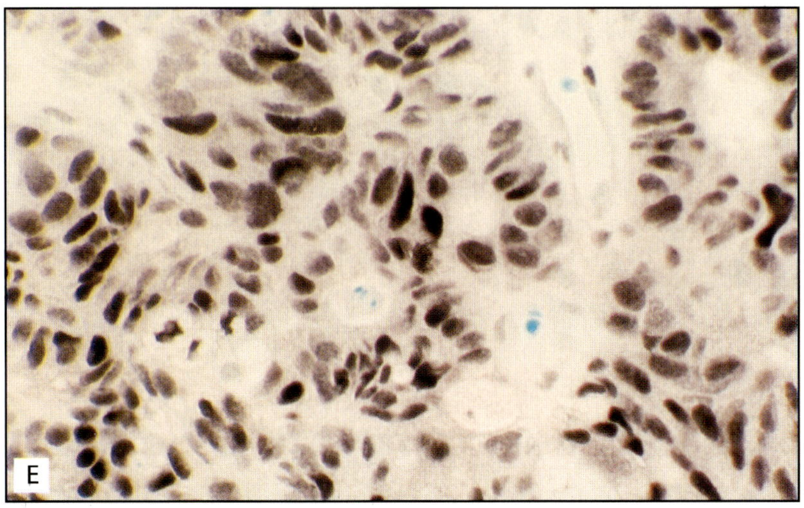

FIGURE 12-2.

Endometrioid endometrial carcinoma. This is the most common form of endometrial cancer. **A**, The neoplastic epithelium generally shows varying degrees of multilayering and squamous metaplasia is a very common finding (hematoxylin and eosin). In fact, virtually all endometrioid endometrial carcinomas display at least focal squamous metaplasia as revealed by immunocytochemical studies, shown in the following sequence of photomicrographs. The most characteristic feature, however, of endometrioid endometrial adenocarcinomas is an immunophenotype of coexpression of low molecular weight cytokeratin (**B**) (antibody 35βH11 to cytokeratin 8) and vimentin (**C**), the intermediate filament protein usually expressed exclusively by mesenchymal cells. This feature is useful in distinguishing endometrioid endometrial adenocarcinoma from other adenocarcinomas, particularly those from the endocervix and colon [4–6]. In addition, this case also shows very focal expression of high molecular weight cytokeratin (**D**); (antibody 34βE12), corresponding to foci of squamous differentiation. Approximately two thirds of well-differentiated endometrioid endometrial adenocarcinomas express the estrogen receptor (ER) protein, with the frequency of ER expression decreasing in less well differentiated tumors [7,8]. **E**, Expression of estrogen receptor can be elucidated using antibodies to ER, a nuclear protein (antibody 1D5 to estrogen receptor). Recent studies have also suggested that an absence of ER protein expression appears to define a subset of endometrial adenocarcinomas with a worse outcome, and that this prognostic information is independent of tumor stage and grade [9,10].

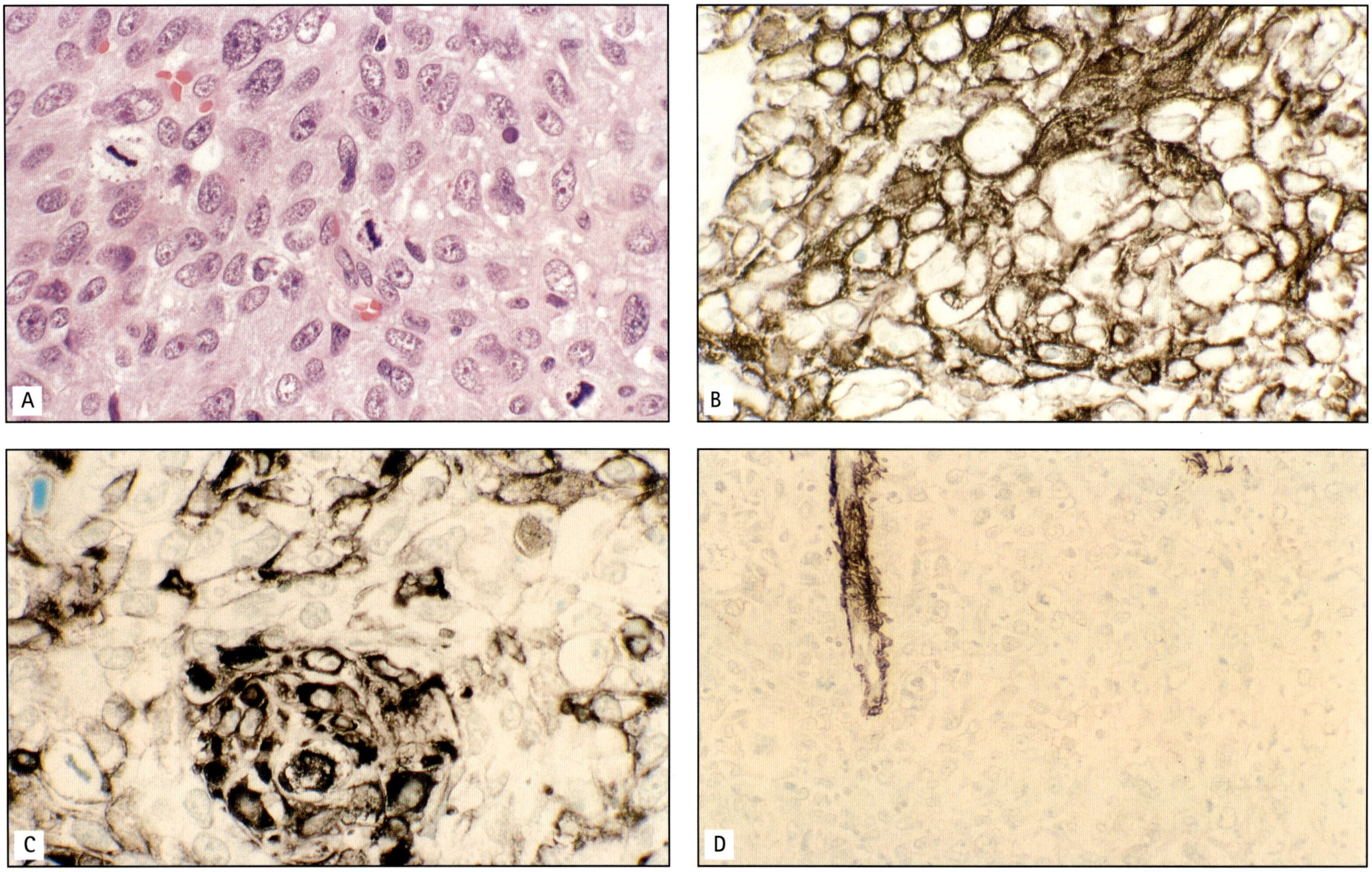

FIGURE 12-3.

A, Endometrial carcinosarcoma (malignant mixed müllerian tumor). Mixed müllerian tumors include a number of processes, including müllerian adenofibroma, atypical polypoid adenomyoma, müllerian adenosarcoma, and carcinosarcoma (the latter previously referred to as malignant mixed müllerian tumor [MMMT]). Carcinosarcoma of the endometrium usually arises in elderly females and presents as a bulky polypoid mass. By definition, this tumor contains two histologically (and immunophenotypically) disparate and distinct components: one carcinomatous and the other sarcomatous. Figures 12-3 *A* through *D* represent the carcinomatous component, and Figures 12-4 *A–D* represent the sarcomatous component of a single mixed müllerian tumor. The carcinomatous component (hematoxylin and eosin; *see* Fig. 12-3*A*) is composed of what appears to be sheets of undifferentiated cells. **B**, Endometrial carcinosarcoma (malignant mixed müllerian tumor)—carcinomatous component. Immunocytochemistry studies clearly show the carcinomatous portion of the tumor to represent carcinoma, *ie*, it is uniformly positive for expression of low molecular weight cytokeratin (identified by antibody 35βH11; seen in the figure) as well as high molecular weight cytokeratin (identified by antibody 34βE12; not shown). **C**, Endometrial carcinosarcoma (malignant mixed müllerian tumor)—carcinomatous component. The carcinomatous component also coexpresses vimentin (as shown in the figure), albeit not to the same degree as the endometrioid endometrial adenocarcinoma of (*see* Fig. 12-2C). **D**, Endometrial carcinosarcoma (malignant mixed müllerian tumor—carcinomatous component. The carcinomatous component, in contradistinction to the sarcomatous element, does not manifest any evidence of specific mesenchymal differentiation, *eg*, it is negative for desmin expression (as shown in the figure). Note positive internal control immunostaining of smooth muscle cells of small arteriole.

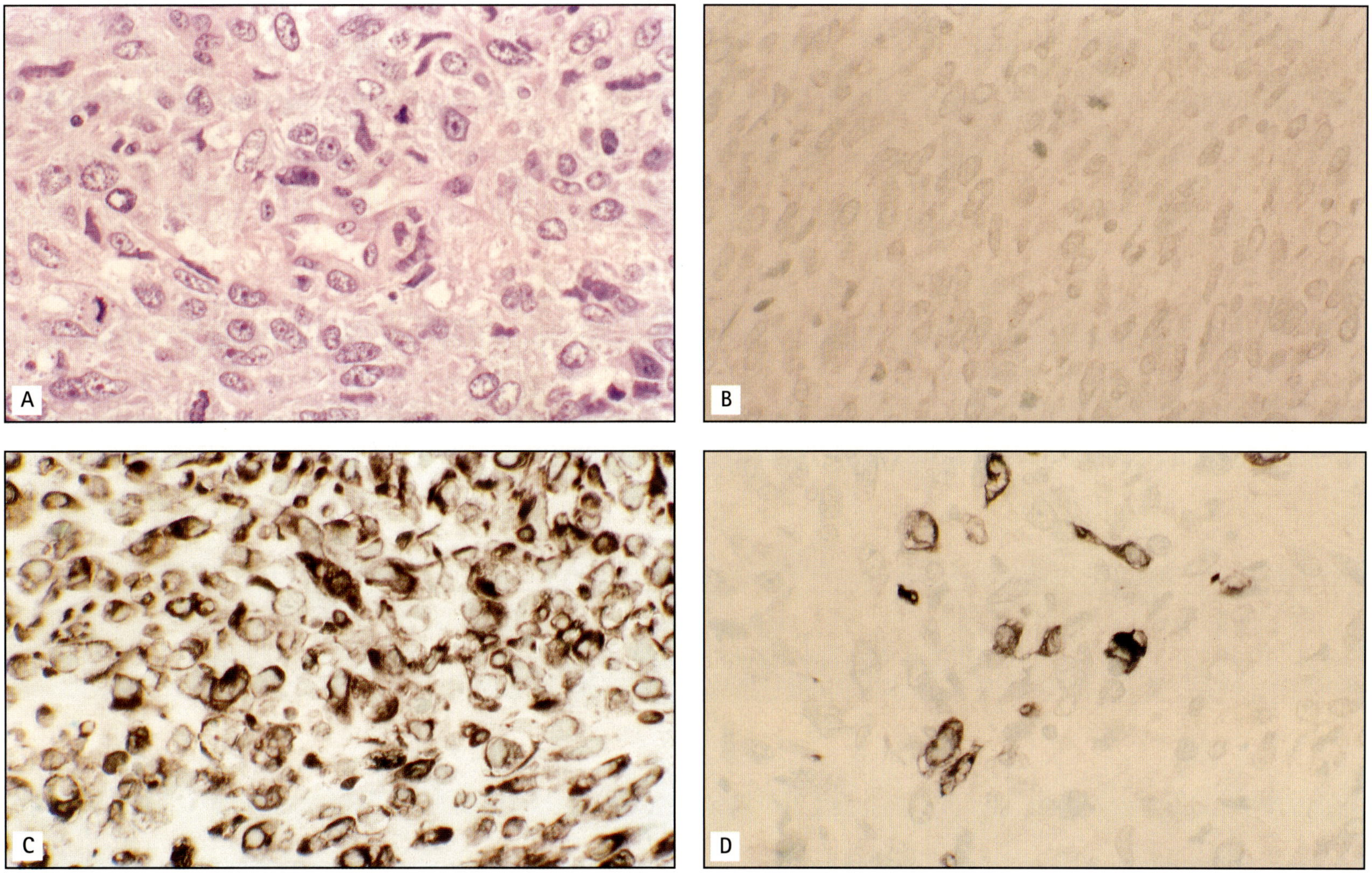

FIGURE 12–4.

Endometrial carcinosarcoma (malignant mixed müllerian tumor)—sarcomatous component. In contrast to the carcinomatous component, the sarcomatous element of the tumor **A**; hematoxylin and eosin), although also high grade and undifferentiated, does not express cytokeratin **B**; negative low molecular weight cytokeratin study), but strongly and uniformly expresses vimentin (**C**), revealing its sarcomatous nature. The sarcomatous component of these tumors may be undifferentiated, may resemble endometrial stromal sarcoma, or may manifest aspects of leiomyosarcoma, as in the case demonstrated here. **D**, This figure shows expression of desmin in a subset of the sarcomatous population, an indication of muscle differentiation. "Heterologous" elements may also present in approximately 50% of uterine carcinosarcomas, the most common being striated muscle, cartilage, bone, and fat. The presence of these heterologous elements does not convey any prognostic information, however [11]. It has been suggested by some that the immunohistochemical profile of carcinosarcomas ovelaps with that of endometrioid endometrial adenocarcinomas [12]; however, the finding of two immunohistochemically distinct components in a single malignant neoplasm is highly characteristic of carcinosarcoma.

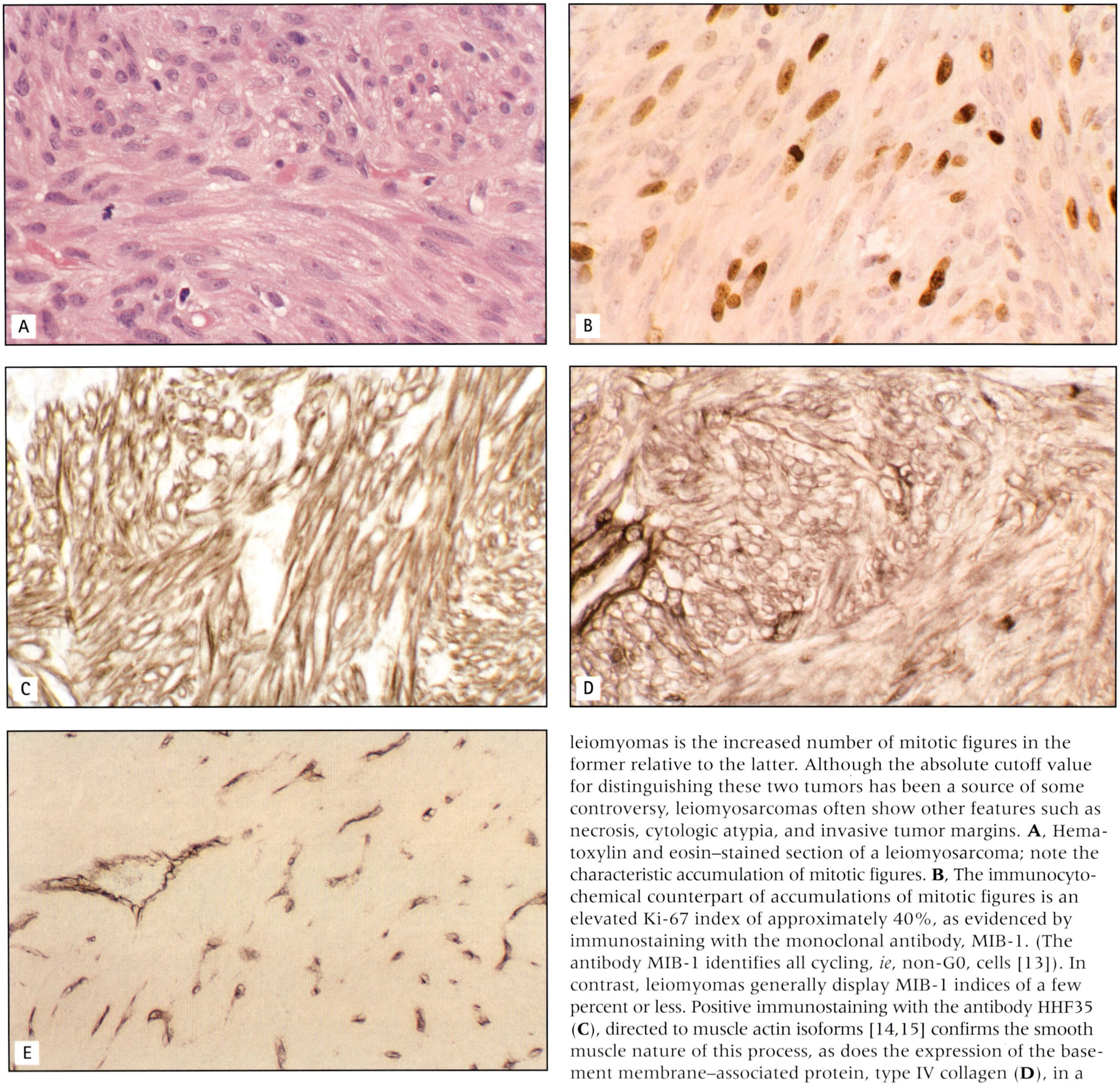

FIGURE 12-5.

Uterine leiomysarcoma. Although leiomyomas, composed of a benign proliferation of smooth muscle cells, are the most common neoplasm of the uterus (and of the entire female genital tract), their malignant counterpart (leiomyosarcoma) is relatively rare, generally occurring in women over the age of 40. One of the key microscopic features that distinguishes leiomyosarcomas from leiomyomas is the increased number of mitotic figures in the former relative to the latter. Although the absolute cutoff value for distinguishing these two tumors has been a source of some controversy, leiomyosarcomas often show other features such as necrosis, cytologic atypia, and invasive tumor margins. **A**, Hematoxylin and eosin–stained section of a leiomyosarcoma; note the characteristic accumulation of mitotic figures. **B**, The immunocytochemical counterpart of accumulations of mitotic figures is an elevated Ki-67 index of approximately 40%, as evidenced by immunostaining with the monoclonal antibody, MIB-1. (The antibody MIB-1 identifies all cycling, *ie*, non-G0, cells [13]). In contrast, leiomyomas generally display MIB-1 indices of a few percent or less. Positive immunostaining with the antibody HHF35 (**C**), directed to muscle actin isoforms [14,15] confirms the smooth muscle nature of this process, as does the expression of the basement membrane–associated protein, type IV collagen (**D**), in a characteristic pattern demonstrating layers of this latter protein around individual cells. Immunostaining with antibodies to CD34 (**E**), which labels the endothelial cells of the tumor [16,17], rather than the tumor population itself, demonstrates the intense vascularity characteristic of this malignant process (another feature that can help distinguish leiomyosarcomas from leiomyomas, as the latter usually have poor vascularity).

(*Continued on next page*)

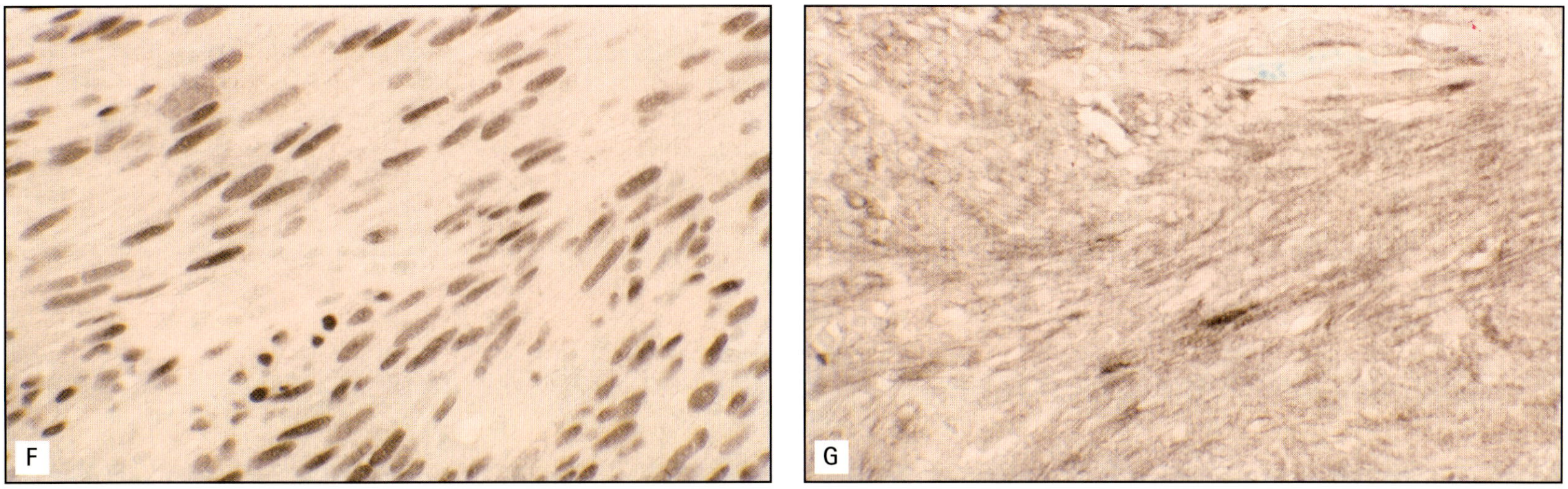

FIGURE 12-5. *(Continued)*

F, Uniform, nuclear expression of progesterone receptors by this tumor is seen, a feature present in a significant subset of leiomyosarcomas, in contrast to most other sarcomas. (Note also how, in contrast to the MIB-1 study shown in panel *B*, antibodies to progesterone receptor identify every tumor cell.) **G**, Another characteristic feature of approximately one third of leiomyosarcomas is anomalous cytokeratin expression [18–20], demonstrating expression, at low levels, and in a "wispy" fashion, of low molecular weight cytokeratin (antibody 35βH11).

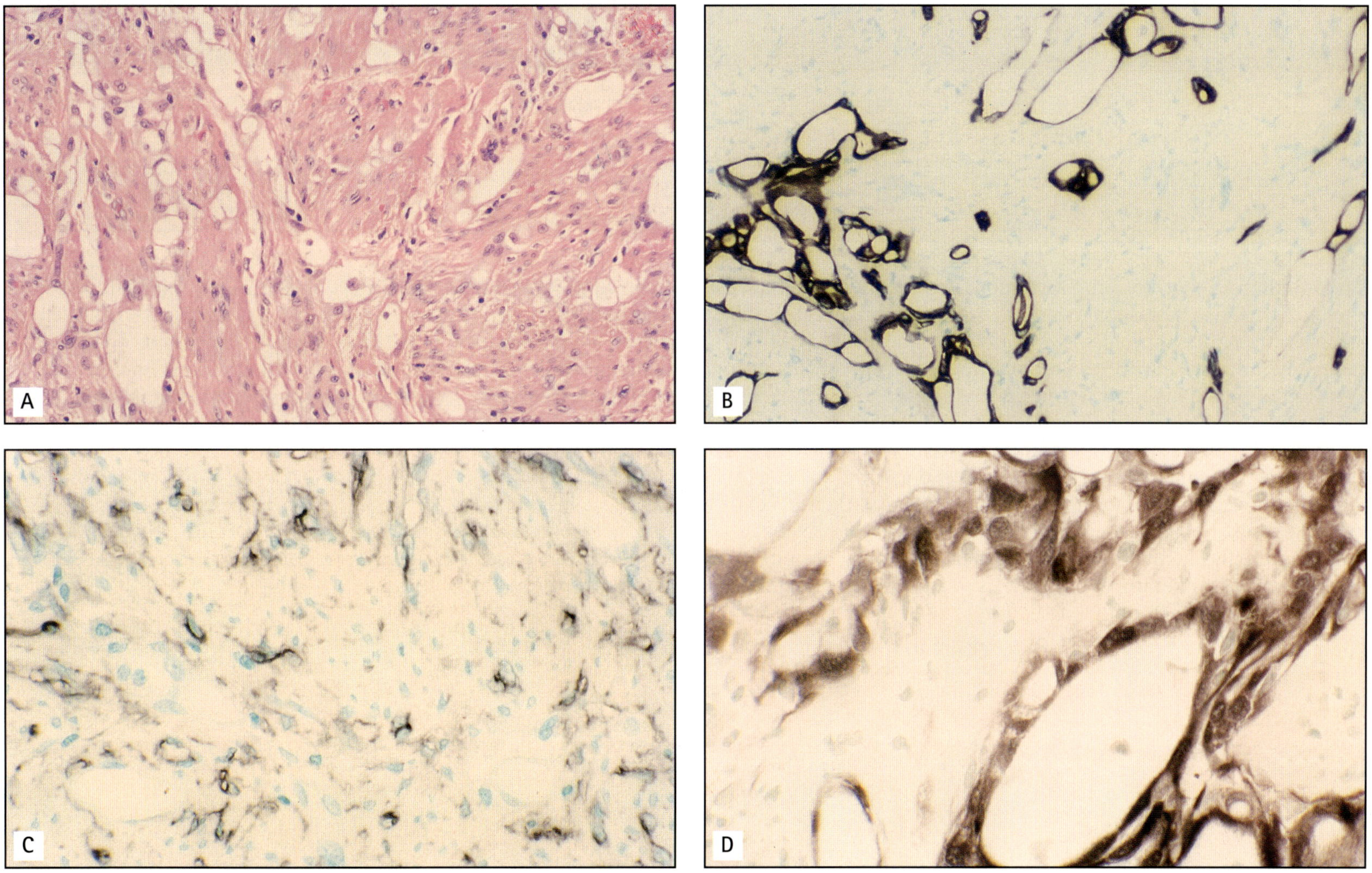

FIGURE 12-6.

Adenomatoid tumor. This is a benign tumor, generally occurring in women of reproductive age, which characteristically appears as a subserosal nodular process, sometimes mimicking the gross appearance of a leiomyosarcoma. **A**, A typical lesion contains "pseudovascular" spaces (hematoxylin and eosin), which are actually lined not by endothelium but mesothelium, which is a type of epithelium. **B**, The uniform positive immunoreactivity of these lining cells is shown with antibodies to low molecular weight cytokeratin (antibody CAM5.2). **C**, Demonstration of how antibodies to CD34 identify the intervening capillary endothelial cells, but not the cells lining the large "pseudovascular" spaces [16,17]. **D**, Proof of the mesothelial nature of the process is evidenced by immunolocalization of the mesothelial-associated protein, calretinin [21].

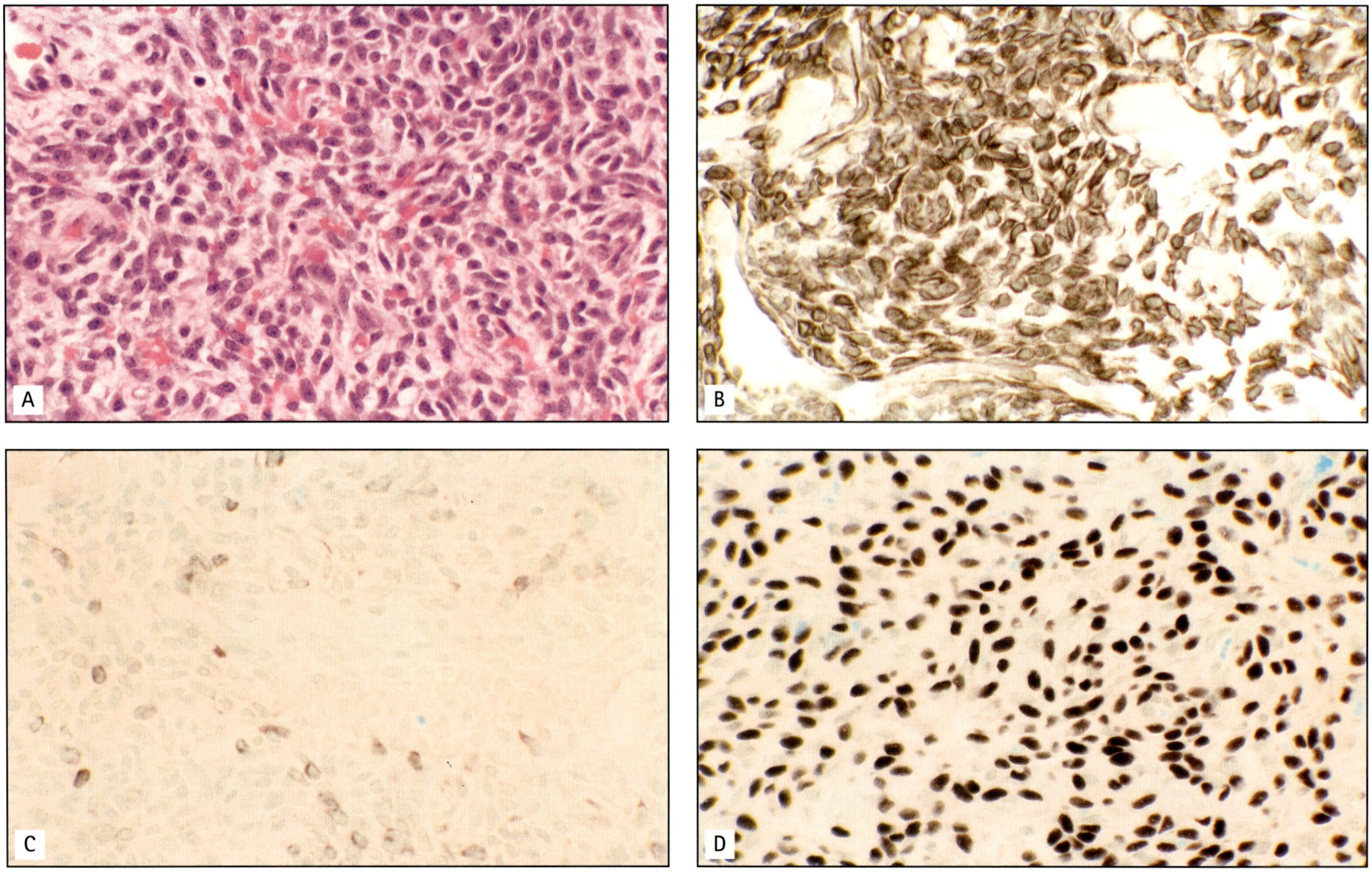

FIGURE 12-7.

Endometrial stromal sarcoma. **A**, Endometrial stromal sarcomas are mesenchymal neoplasms that have a histologic appearance resembling stroma of the normal proliferative endometrium, characterized by generally uniform cells with minimal nuclear pleomorphism and cytologic atypia, hyalinized connective tissue, and a rich vascularized background (hematoxylin and eosin). Unlike smooth muscle tumors of the uterus, the presence or absence of mitotic figures gives no prognostic significance [22]. Studies of endometrial stromal sarcomas have generally found these cells, similar to their normal endometrial stromal counterparts, to display to varying degrees a smooth muscle–like phenotype [23–25], *ie*, expressing desmin or muscle actin. Cytokeratin expression has also been described in these tumors, although it is not certain if this has implications for an origin in primitive totipotential stem cells, as has been suggested, or merely a manifestation of the known proclivity of smooth muscle malignancies to manifest anomalous cytokeratin expression [18]. **B**, Uniform expression of vimentin by endometrial stromal sarcoma is seen. **C**, As in most cases of endometrial stromal sarcoma, evidence of a partial smooth muscle phenotype, as evidenced by the expression of desmin, in this case, in a subset of the tumor cell population (antidesmin antibody). **D**, Finally, as evidence of this tumor's relationship to normal endometrial stroma, the tumor cells generally manifest uniform expression of estrogen and progesterone receptors (antiprogesterone receptor antibody PR88).

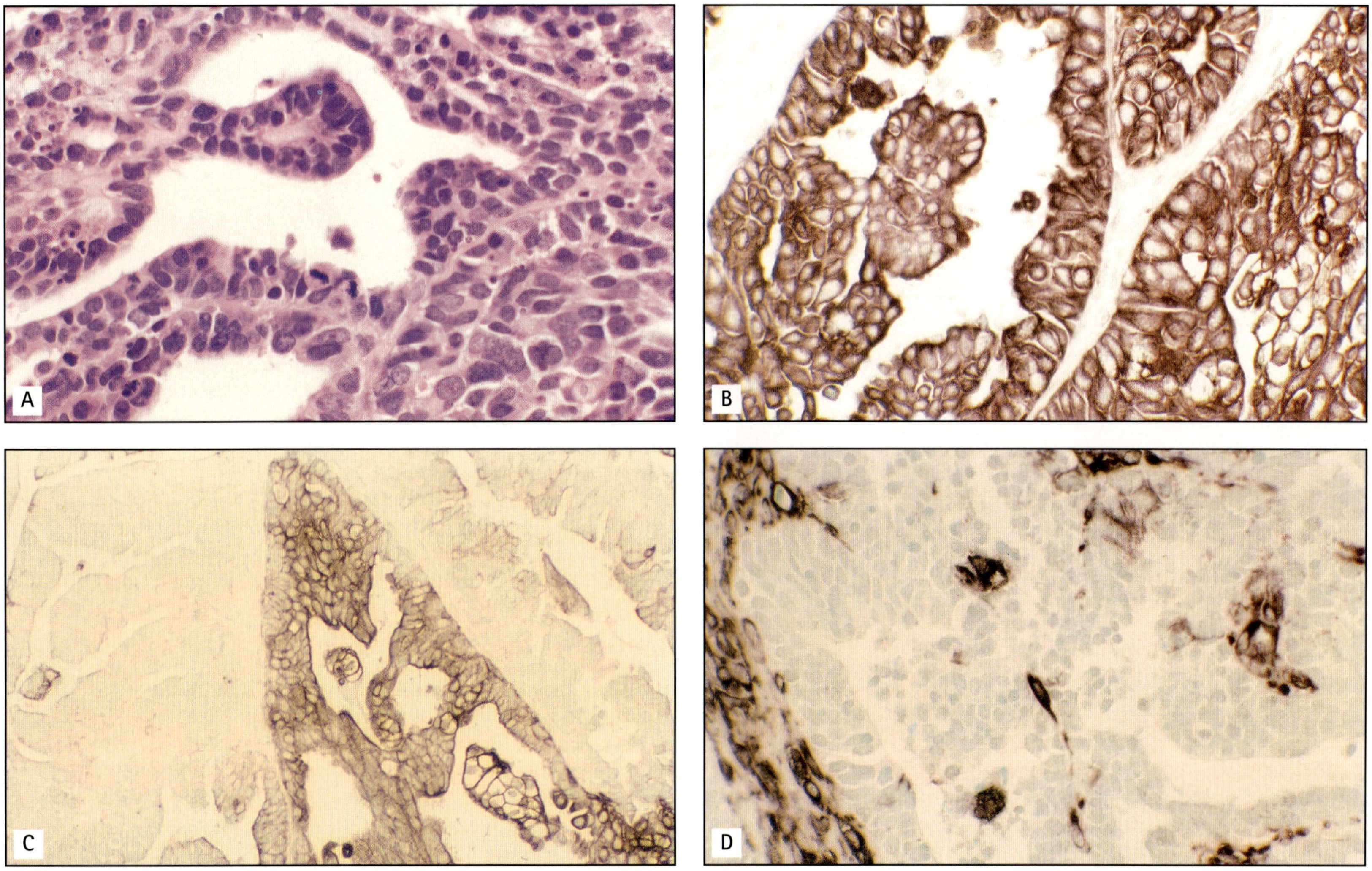

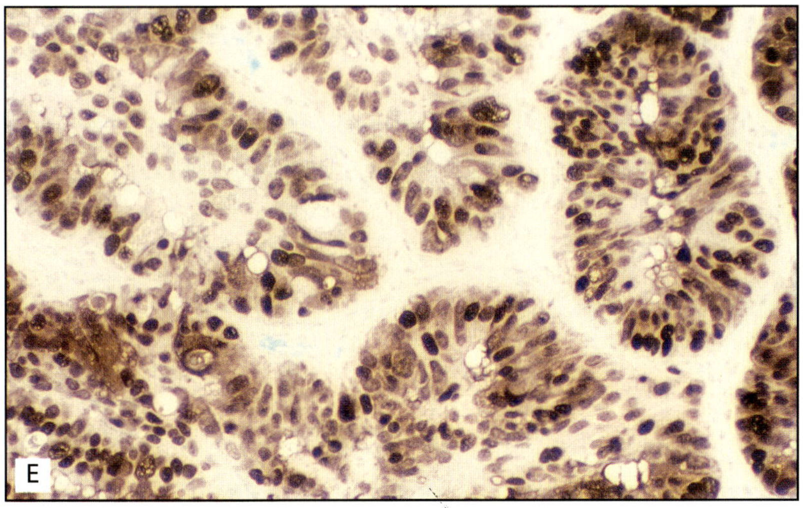

FIGURES 12-8.

Serous papillary carcinoma. **A**, Serous papillary carcinoma (hematoxylin and eosin) is the most common form of ovarian cancer, particularly in the postmenopausal age group. The tumor has a fairly characteristic, albeit not distinctive, immunophenotype. The normal cell counterpart to serous papillary carcinoma is the ovarian surface epithelium, which is a modified type of mesothelium; thus there are similarities but also important differences between the immunophenotype of abdominal mesotheliomas and serous papillary carcinomas of the ovary [26]. **B–E**, The typical immunophenotype of serous papillary carcinoma is featured. **B**, Uniform low molecular weight cytokeratin expression (antibody 35βH11 to cytokeratin 8) is seen. **C**, In contrast, there is only patchy expression of high molecular weight cytokeratin (antibody 34βE12), and an absence of vimentin coexpression (**D**). **D**, Note expression of vimentin only in the stromal vessels and scattered macrophages. **E**, Approximately 70% of ovarian carcinomas possess mutations at the p53 locus [27], with concomitant accumulation of mutant p53 protein in the nucleus.

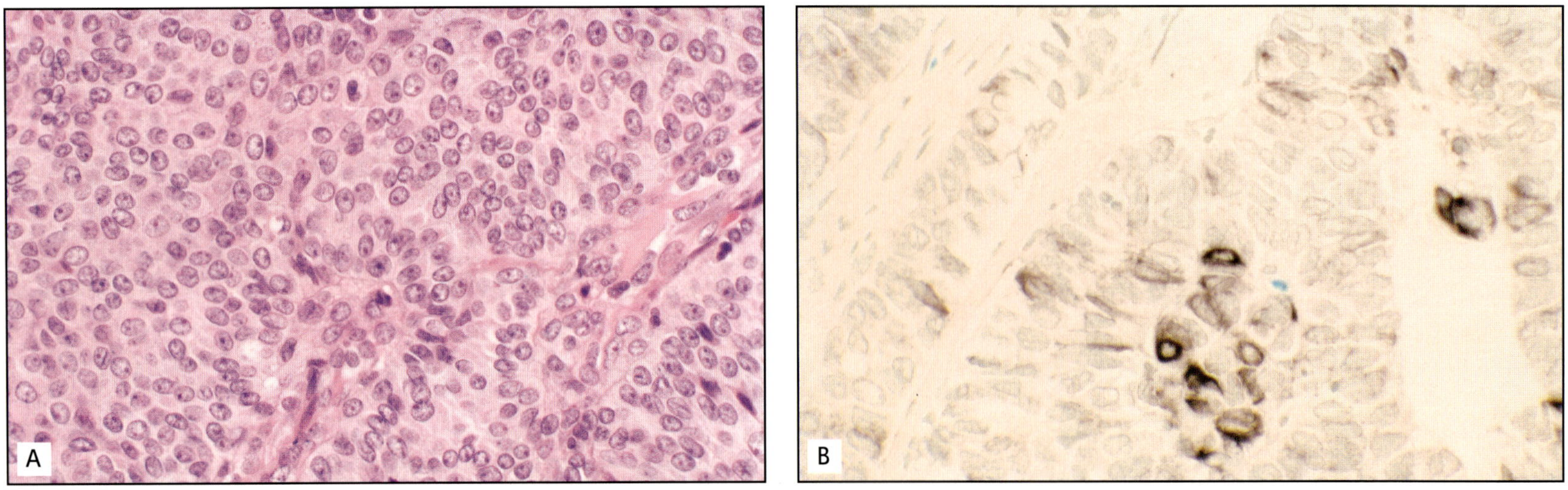

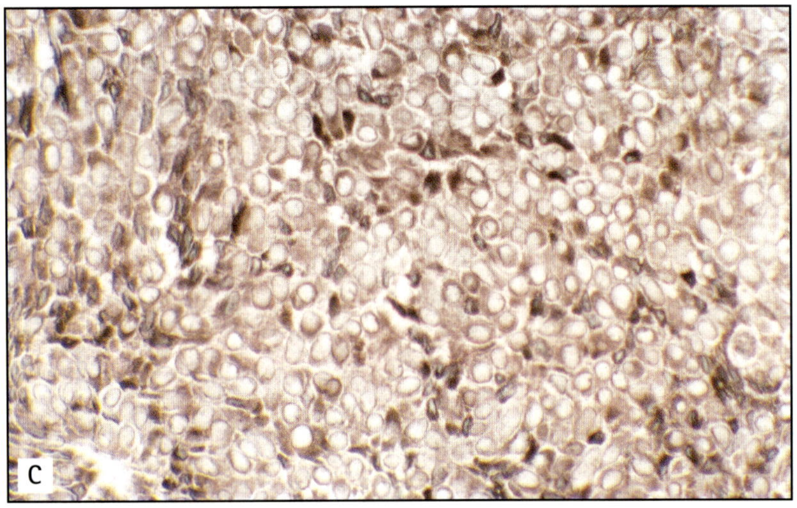

FIGURES 12-9.
Granulosa cell tumor (adult type). Granulosa cell tumor is a type of ovarian sex-cord–stromal tumor that generally occurs in the postmenopausal setting. **A**, The histologic appearance (hematoxylin and eosin) is often distinctive, with the presence of round to ovoid cells with a longitudinal nuclear groove. Occasionally, however, granulosa cell tumors can have a histologic appearance that suggests a carcinoma, with the cells forming follicle-like cysts. Immunocytochemical studies can be very helpful in positively identifying granulosa cell tumors, and distinguishing them from ovarian epithelial tumors [28], despite the ability of granulosa cell tumors to express cytokeratin [29]. **B** However, cytokeratin expression (antibody 35βH11 to cytokeratin 8), in granulosa cell tumors is generally limited to a subset of tumor cells, and often has a punctate or perinuclear distribution in the tumor cell population. Granulosa cell tumors, similar to all ovarian sex cord stromal tumors, frequently show evidence of a partial smooth muscle phenotype, *eg*, expression of smooth muscle actins (not shown) [30]. Recently, however, inhibin alpha has been described as an important marker for granulosa cell tumors [31–33]. **C**, Uniform expression of the alpha subunit of inhibin by the tumor cells is demonstrated. Inhibin alpha, although not expressed by epithelial tumors of the ovary, is also expressed by other sex-cord–stromal tumors [33].

IMMUNOPHENOTYPES OF GERM CELL TUMORS

	Dysgerminoma	Yolk sac tumor	Embryonal carcinoma	Choriocarcinoma
Cytokeratin (low MW)	❍	❑	❑	❑
Vimentin	❑	❍	▼	❍
α-Fetoprotein	❍	❑	▼	❍
Chorionic gonadotropin	❍	❍	❍	❑
CD30	❍	❍	❑	❍

KEY
❑ *Usually positive*
▼ *Sometimes positive*
❍ *Usually negative*

FIGURE 12-10.
Immunophenotypes of germ cell tumors. MW—molecular weight.

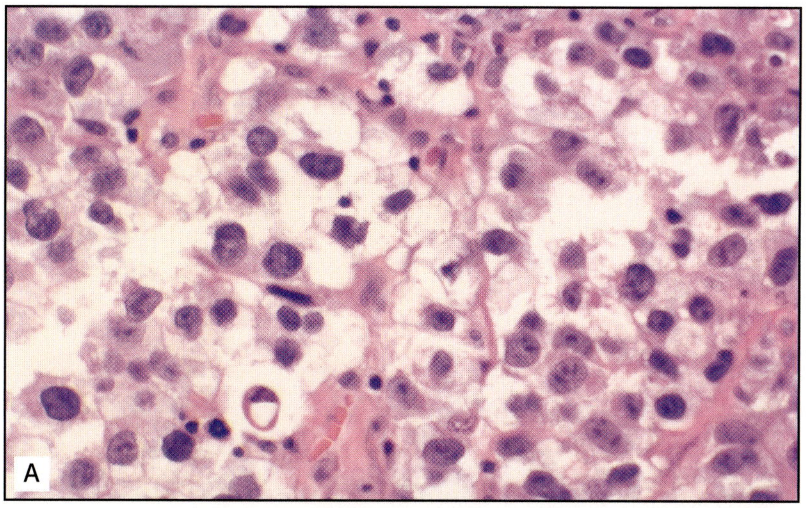

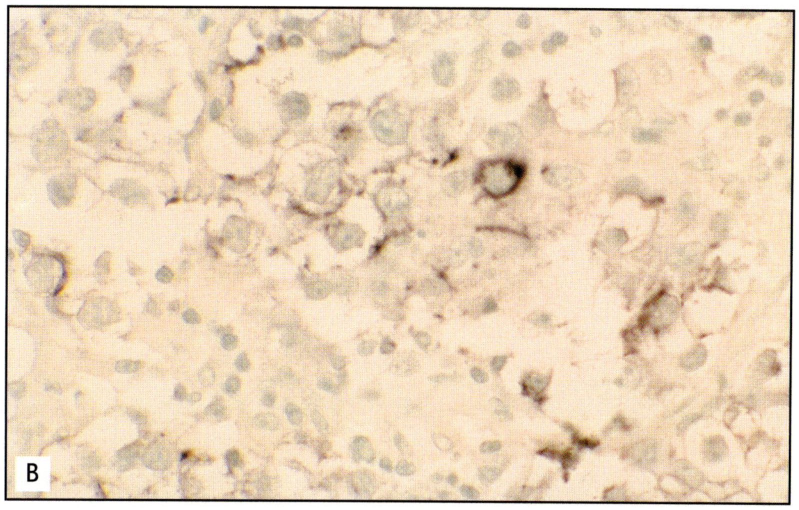

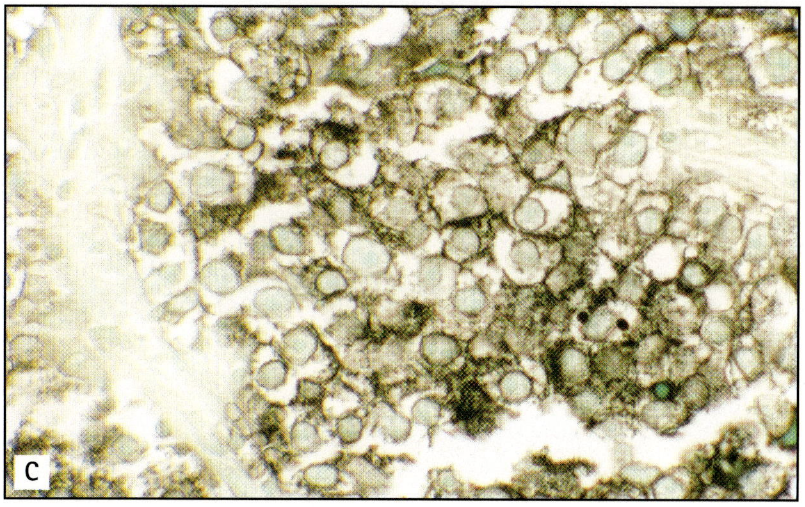

FIGURE 12-11.
Dysgerminoma. Dysgerminoma is a type of ovarian germ cell tumor which characteristically arises in patients between the ages of 10 and 30. **A**, Its histologic appearance is identical to seminoma of the testis: it is characterized by sheets of cells with large nuclei and clear cytoplasm (hematoxylin and eosin). Dysgerminomas also have a characteristic immunophenotype. **B**, Although these tumors, along with their testicular counterparts, seminomas, generally do not express cytokeratin, immunocytochemical studies often reveal the presence of scattered cytokeratin-positive tumor cells (antibody 35bH11 to low molecular weight cytokeratin); these rare cytokeratin-positive cells may represent scattered cells manifesting trophoblastic differentiation. However, a recent report suggests that dysgerminomas may manifest other forms of "further differentiation, albeit at a primitive level," as evidenced by focal desmin and glial fibrillary acidic protein positivity, too [34]. The classic marker for both dysgerminomas and seminomas is uniform expression of placental alkaline phosphatase (PLAP) by the tumor cell population. PLAP expression per se is not specific for dysgerminoma (*ie*, it can be expressed by other germ cell tumors), but in the absence of other germ cell–associated markers (*eg*, α-fetoprotein, CD30) PLAP expression can be considered characteristic of dysgerminoma or seminoma [35,36]. **C**, Characteristic uniform expression of PLAP in dysgerminoma is shown, highlighting its cytoplasmic and membranous immunostaining pattern.

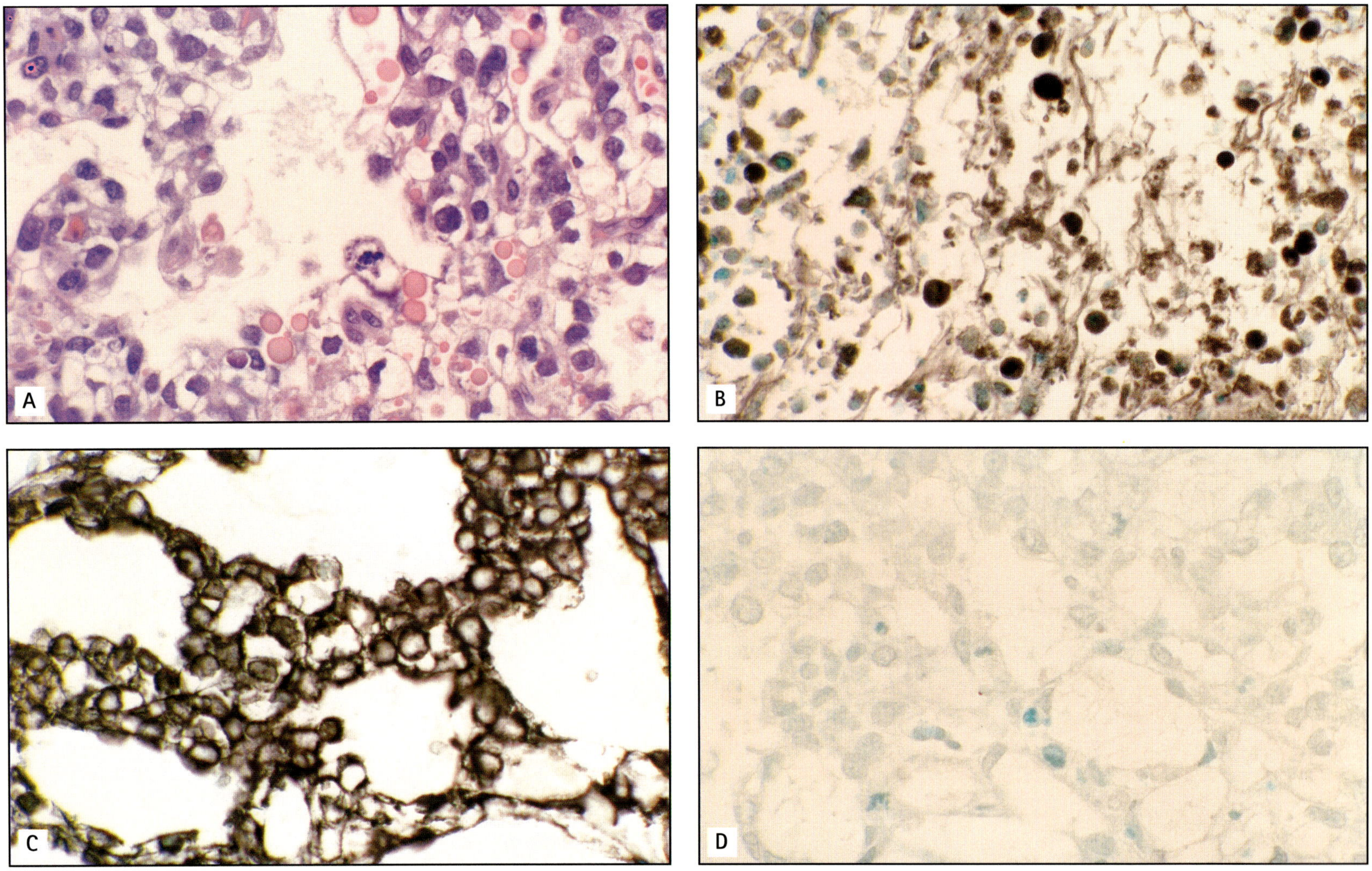

FIGURES 12-12.

Yolk sac tumor. A second form of germ cell tumor, typically occurring in teenage patients, is the yolk sac tumor (or endodermal sinus tumor). This relatively rare tumor is quite protean and can manifest a number of histologic appearances, only some of which are reminiscent of the yolk sac of the developing embryo. Typically, however, yolk sac tumors manifest a loose network of spaces and cystlike structures; there may or may not be glandlike structures present. **A**, Hematoxylin and eosin tissue stain depicts a yolk sac tumor composed of sheetlike arrangements of tumor cells; as in virtually all yolk sac tumors, independent of its morphologic variations, the presence of eosinophilic hyaline droplets (that are periodic acid–Schiff positive) can be documented. **B**, Strong expression of α-fetoprotein (antibodies to α-fetoprotein) is a hallmark of yolk sac tumors; this figure also demonstrates the localization of α fetoprotein to the eosinophilic droplets. **C**, The tumor cells, unlike those of dysgerminoma, are uniformly positive for cytokeratin expression (antibody 35βH11 to low molecular weight cytokeratin), *ie*, the tumor can be considered a subtype of carcinoma. **D**, Unlike true embryonal carcinoma, this tumor is negative for the marker CD30 (antibody BerH2 to CD30) [37].

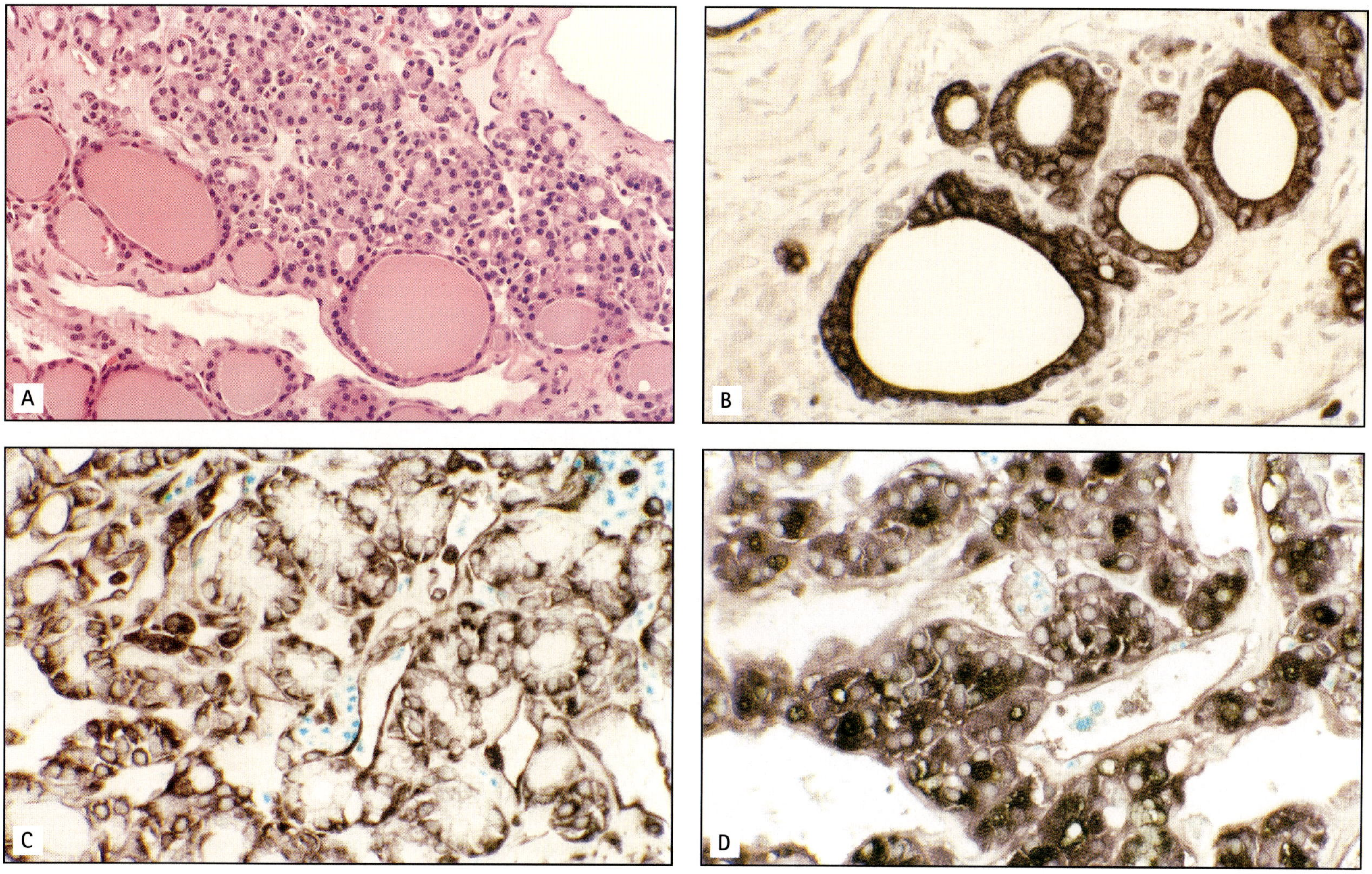

FIGURE 12-13.

Struma ovarii. **A**, Struma ovarii is a form of benign teratoma of the ovary in which thyroid tissue is the only, or at least predominant, component. Occasionally, it can demonstrate many of the same changes that are seen in thyroid tissue, *ie*, thyroiditis, hyperplasia, adenoma, and even carcinoma. When entirely cystic, the attenuated thyroid epithelium lining these cysts can be overlooked. **B**, When necessary, it is possible to definitively identify structures in the ovary as representing thyroid epithelium by demonstrating their expression of cytokeratin (antibody 35βH11 to low molecular weight cytokeratin) and coexpression of vimentin (**C**) (antibody V9 to vimentin), a feature that is characteristic of thyroid epithelium [38,39]. The latter is not a feature unique to thyroid epithelium, however, and for certainty in the diagnosis, the demonstration of the expression of thyroglobulin is essential (**D**) (anti-thyroglobulin antibody) [40]. Struma ovarii may recapitulate other aspects of thyroid tissue, too, including the presence of C cells [41].

REFERENCES

1. Franquemont DW, Ward BE, Andersen WA, Crum CP: Prediction of "high-risk" cervical papillomavirus infection by biopsy morphology [see comments]. *Am J Clin Pathol* 1989, 92:577–582.
2. Payne S, Kernohan NM, Walker F: Proliferation in the normal cervix and in preinvasive cervical lesions. *J Clin Pathol* 1996, 49:667–671.
3. Dunton CJ, van Hoeven KH, Kovatich AJ, *et al.*: Ki-67 antigen staining as an adjunct to identifying cervical intraepithelial neoplasia. *Gynecol Oncol* 1997, 64:451–455.
4. Dabbs DJ, Sturtz K, Zaino RJ:J The immunohistochemical discrimination of endometrioid adenocarcinomas. *Hum Pathol* 1996, 27:172–177.
5. Dallenbach H-G, Lang AE-G, Hahn U. The value of immunohistochemistry in the differential diagnosis of endometrial carcinomas. APMIS Suppl 1991, 23:91–99.
6. Gown AM, Vogel AM: Monoclonal antibodies to human intermediate filament proteins, III. Analysis of tumors. *Am J Clin Pathol* 1985, 84:413–424.
7. Segreti EM, Novotny DB, Soper JT, *et al.*: Endometrial cancer: histologic correlates of immunohistochemical localization of progesterone receptor and estrogen receptor. *Obstet Gynecol* 1989, 73(5 Pt 1):780–785.
8. Ciocca DR, Puy LA, Fasoli LC. Study of estrogen receptor, progesterone receptor, and the estrogen-regulated Mr 24,000 protein in patients with carcinomas of the endometrium and cervix. *Cancer Res* 1989, 49:4298–4304.
9. Palmer DC, Muir IM, Alexander AI, *et al.*: The prognostic importance of steroid receptors in endometrial carcinoma. *Obstet Gynecol* 1988, 72(3 Pt 1):388–393.

10. Pertschuk LP, Masood S, Simone J, *et al.*: Estrogen receptor immunocytochemistry in endometrial carcinoma: a prognostic marker for survival. *Gynecol Oncol* 1996, 63:28–33.
11. Costa MJ, Khan R, Judd R. Carcinoma (malignant mixed mullerian [mesodermal] tumor) of the uterus and ovary: correlation of clinical, pathologic, and immunohistochemical features in 29 cases. *Arch Pathol Lab Med* 1991, 115:583–590.
12. Meis JM, Lawrence WD: The immunohistochemical profile of malignant mixed mullerian tumor: overlap with endometrial adenocarcinoma [see comments]. *Am J Clin Pathol* 1990, 94:1–7.
13. Cattoretti G, Becker MH, Key G, *et al.*: Monoclonal antibodies against recombinant parts of the Ki-67 antigen (MIB 1 and MIB 3) detect proliferating cells in microwave-processed formalin-fixed paraffin sections. *J Pathol* 1992, 168:357–363.
14. Tsukada T, McNutt MA, Ross R, Gown AM. HHF35, a muscle actin-specific monoclonal antibody. II. Reactivity in normal, reactive, and neoplastic human tissues. *Am J Pathol* 1987, 127:389–402.
15. Tsukada T, Tippens D, Gordon D, *et al.*: HHF35, a muscle-actin-specific monoclonal antibody, I: Immunocytochemical and biochemical characterization. *Am J Pathol* 1987, 126:51–60.
16. Traweek ST, Kandalaft PL, Mehta P, Battifora H: The human hematopoietic progenitor cell antigen (CD34) in vascular neoplasia. *Am J Clin Pathol* 1991, 96(1):25–31.
17. Fina L, Molgaard HV, Robertson D, *et al.*: Expression of the CD34 gene in vascular endothelial cells. *Blood* 1990, 75:2417–2426.
18. Gown AM, Boyd HC, Chang Y, *et al.*: Smooth muscle cells can express cytokeratins of "simple" epithelium: immunocytochemical and biochemical studies in vitro and in vivo. *Am J Pathol* 1988, 132:223–232.
19. Norton AJ, Thomas JA, Isaacson PG: Cytokeratin-specific monoclonal antibodies are reactive with tumours of smooth muscle derivation: an immunocytochemical and biochemical study using antibodies to intermediate filament cytoskeletal proteins. *Histopathology* 1987, 11:487–499.
20. Brown DC, Theaker JM, Banks PM, *et al.*: Cytokeratin expression in smooth muscle and smooth muscle tumours. *Histopathology* 1987, 11:477–486.
21. Doglioni C, Tos AP, Laurino L, *et al.*: Calretinin: a novel immunocytochemical marker for mesothelioma. *Am J Surg Pathol* 1996;20:1037–1046.
22. Chang KL, Crabtree GS, Lim T-SK *et al.*: Primary uterine endometrial stromal neoplasms: a clinicopathologic study of 117 cases. *Am J Surg Pathol* 1990, 14:415–438.
23. Farhood AI, Abrams J: Immunohistochemistry of endometrial stromal sarcoma. *Hum Pathol* 1991, 22:224–230.
24. Franquemont DW, Frierson HF Jr, Mills SE: An immunohistochemical study of normal endometrial stroma and endometrial stromal neoplasms: evidence for smooth muscle differentiation. *Am J Surg Pathol* 1991, 15:861–870.
25. Binder SW, Nieberg RK, Cheng L, *et al.*: Histologic and immunohistochemical analysis of nine endometrial stromal tumors: an unexpected high frequency of keratin protein positivity. *Int J Gynecol Pathol* 1991, 10(2):191–197.
26. Khoury N, Raju U, Crissman JD, *et al.*: A comparative immunohistochemical study of peritoneal and ovarian serous tumors, and mesotheliomas. *Hum Pathol* 1990, 21:811–819.
27. Porter PL, Gown AM, Kramp SG, Coltrera MD: Widespread p53 overexpression in human malignant tumors: an immunohistochemical study using methacarn-fixed, embedded tissue. *Am J Pathol* 1992, 140:145–153.
28. Gitsch G, Kohlberger P, Hanzal E, *et al.*: Immunohistochemical differentiation between ovarian granulosa cell tumors and ovarian carcinomas. *Arch Gynecol Obstet* 1991, 249:173–177.
29. Otis CN, Powell JL, Barbuto D, Carcangiu ML: Intermediate filamentous proteins in adult granulosa cell tumors: an immunohistochemical study of 25 cases. *Am J Surg Pathol* 1992, 16:962–968.
30. Santini D, Ceccarelli C, Leone O, *et al.*: Smooth muscle differentiation in normal human ovaries, ovarian stromal hyperplasia and ovarian granulosa–stromal cell tumors. *Mod Pathol* 1995, 8:25–30.
31. Arora DS, Cooke IE, Ganesan TS, *et al.*: Immunohistochemical expression of inhibin/activin subunits in epithelial and granulosa cell tumours of the ovary. *J Pathol* 1997, 181:413–418.
32. McCluggage WG, Maxwell P, Sloan JM: Immunohistochemical staining of ovarian granulosa cell tumors with monoclonal antibody against inhibin. *Hum Pathol* 1997, 28:1034–1038.
33. Rishi M, Howard LN, Bratthauer GL, Tavassoli FA: Use of monoclonal antibody against human inhibin as a marker for sex cord-stromal tumors of the ovary. *Am J Surg Pathol* 1997, 21:583–589.
34. Lifschitz M-B, Walt H, Kushnir I, *et al.*: Differentiation potential of ovarian dysgerminoma: an immunohistochemical study of 15 cases. *Hum Pathol* 1995, 26:62–66.
35. Hustin J, Collette J, Franchimont P: Immunohistochemical demonstration of placental alkaline phosphatase in various states of testicular development and in germ cell tumours. *Int J Androl* 1987, 10:29–35.
36. Hustin J, Gillerot Y, Collette J, Franchimont P: Placental alkaline phosphatase in developing normal and abnormal gonads and in germ-cell tumours. *Virchows Arch A Pathol Anat Histopathol* 1990,, 417:67–72.
37. Ferreiro JA: Ber-H2 expression in testicular germ cell tumors. *Hum Pathol* 1994, 25:522–524.
38. Azumi N, Battifora H. The distribution of vimentin and keratin in epithelial and nonepithelial neoplasms: a comprehensive immunohistochemical study on formalin- and alcohol-fixed tumors. *Am J Clin Pathol* 1987, 88:286–296.
39. McNutt MA, Bolen JW, Gown AM, *et al.*: Coexpression of intermediate filaments in human epithelial neoplasms. *Ultrastruct Pathol* 1985, 9:31–43.
40. Young RH: New and unusual aspects of ovarian germ cell tumors. *Am J Surg Pathol* 1993, 17:1210–1224.
41. Stagno PA, Petras RE, Hart WR: Strumal carcinoids of the ovary: an immunohistologic and ultrastructural study. *Arch Pathol Lab Med* 1987, 111:440–446.

Index

(*Continued on next page*)

D

E

(*Continued on next page*)

F

G

H

I

P

R

S

(*Continued on next page*)

T

U

V

W

Y